Stories of Children's Pain

Linking Evidence to Practice

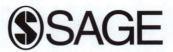

Stories of Children's Pain

Linking Evidence to Practice

Bernie Carter
and Joan Simons

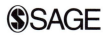

Los Angeles | London | New Delhi
Singapore | Washington DC

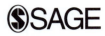

Los Angeles | London | New Delhi
Singapore | Washington DC

SAGE Publications Ltd
1 Oliver's Yard
55 City Road
London EC1Y 1SP

SAGE Publications Inc.
2455 Teller Road
Thousand Oaks, California 91320

SAGE Publications India Pvt Ltd
B 1/I 1 Mohan Cooperative Industrial Area
Mathura Road
New Delhi 110 044

SAGE Publications Asia-Pacific Pte Ltd
3 Church Street
#10-04 Samsung Hub
Singapore 049483

Editor: Becky Taylor
Associate editor: Emma Milman
Production editor: Katie Forsythe
Copyeditor: Rose James
Proofreader: Audrey Scriven
Indexer: Silvia Benvenuto
Marketing manager: Tamara Navaratnam
Cover design: Naomi Robinson
Typeset by: C&M Digitals (P) Ltd, Chennai, India
Printed and bound by CPI Group (UK) Ltd,
Croydon, CR0 4YY

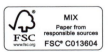

MIX
Paper from
responsible sources
FSC® C013604

First published 2014

Library of Congress Control Number: 2014931025

British Library Cataloguing in Publication data

A catalogue record for this book is available from
the British Library

ISBN 978-1-4462-0760-4
ISBN 978-1-4462-0761-1 (pbk)

Contents

List of Figures and Tables

About the Authors

Bernie Carter is Professor of Children's Nursing at the University of Central Lancashire and Alder Hey Children's NHS Foundation Trust in the United Kingdom. She is a Clinical Professor at the University of Tasmania and Editor-in-Chief for the *Journal of Child Health Care*. She was made a Fellow of the Royal College of Nursing in recognition of her contributions to the field of children's pain.

Bernie's research and writing focuses on children's pain experiences and the assessment of children's pain. She is particularly interested in improving the lives of children with complex health care needs and life limiting/threatening illness. Bernie's research work draws particularly on narrative and appreciative inquiry and on arts-based methods as a means of engaging with children and eliciting stories of their experiences, hopes, beliefs and concerns. Bernie believes that stories are at the heart of the connections we make with children, families and their experiences of pain.

Joan Simons is Assistant Head of Department in the faculty of Health and Social Care at The Open University. She has worked in the field of children's pain for over 20 years and has observed significant developments which have come about through the passion and dedication of practitioners. However, as the content of this demonstrates, there is still some way to go to consistently deliver effective pain management to children and their families.

Acknowledgements

When we set out to write this book we knew that the success of our endeavour would hinge on the support of many people. We requested stories from across the world, and were humbled by the time and effort put in by all those who wrote down their stories and shared their experiences. We have not been able to use every story we were sent and we had to make some difficult choices about which ones we included in the book.

The stories we received have come from Australia, Bahrain, Ireland, Kenya, New Zealand, South Africa, Sweden, the United Kingdom and the United States of America. There are stories from each of these countries in the book.

We would like to say a very big thank you to the people who provided stories but wished to remain anonymous and to the following people who gave permission for us to acknowledge their contributions:

Dave Barton, Nikki Brown, Ruth and Adrian Davies, Annette Dickinson, Maria Forsner, Jayne Francis Sharma, Karen Harrison Janet Mattsson, Julie Mullett, James Mwaura, Stefan and Katerina Nilsson, Judy Rollins, Carole Shaw, Sharon Skowronski, Anne Smith, Sekayi Tangayi and Amanda Williamson.

We are especially thankful to the children and young people who contributed their stories and drawings. Some of you chose to remain anonymous and some of you were happy for your names to appear in the book. We wish that you did not have stories of pain to tell us. We hope that you have a pain-free future or if this is not possible that your pain is always managed well by health care professionals. Thank you to:

Justice Addo, Hattie, Sandra Jonsson, Kamau, Tanya Tia Kerr, Samantha Llannwarne, Luci McDougall, Fauzana Nakaigozi, Nabila Nakigou, Nazra Sesay, 'Noah', Shantell.

Bernie Carter: To my sisters, Bridget and Claire, for all the stories we have shared and we will share together. To Art Frank 'narrative guru' and friend. And, as always and forever, for Jon.

Joan Simons: To my father, Paddy Keely, a renowned storyteller; to Clodagh and Sorcha whose stories are still unfolding; and to Tom for his unwavering belief and support no matter what the story.

Publisher's Acknowledgements

All of the stories in this book are reproduced with permission, and with ethics approval. Ethics approval was granted by The University of Central Lancashire.

Introduction

In the beginning ...

Stories are fundamentally about life and the lives we lead, the experiences we have and our determination to share, connect and make sense of the things that happen to us and other people. Pain stories are ways of reaching out, asking for help, explaining actions and inactions and positioning pain within the world. In health care settings which are often dominated by measurable organisational storylines of efficiency, throughput, outcomes, and performance indicators, stories are often overlooked. Yet it is through attending to stories that we have a chance to start to understand what is important to the children, young people and families for whom we care. If we ignore their stories, we are ignoring who they are as well as what we can do for and with them.

Pain stories are important stories to attend to because they have the capacity to shape our thinking and our professional practice. Stories create connections between people and experiences. When we hear a child's or a parent's pain story, it connects us to the other children and parents we have heard tell stories about their pain. When we hear a professional's pain story we connect to it through our own experiences of caring for children and families in similar situations. Pain stories make us think. They are affective, not just shaping and changing our thinking but also creating emotional ties and new empathic understanding of how we can better engage with and manage people's pain.

The stories in this book represent just the tiniest fraction of the pain stories that are told. If, as a practitioner, you take time to stop and listen you will find yourself surrounded by stories that resonate with the ones that children, parents and professionals shared with us. Inherent in all of the stories we share are 'moral moments' – moments that demand of us a response and where that response 'declares our moral self'. We defy anyone to read the stories we share without experiencing moral moments. In fact, if all that readers did was to read the stories and gain a stronger sense of how they wish to be present in the lives of children and their families, then this book will have achieved a great deal.

Throughout the creation of the book, we have lived with the stories. They have accompanied us, guided us, and challenged us. They have wrapped themselves around our thinking and our emotions. We felt and still feel that the stories were entrusted to us. We actively sought stories from children, parents and professionals as these are the people most caught up in pain stories. Rather than focusing just on stories from our own back yard, we sought stories from further afield. Although the geography and context are different, the stories resonate regardless of the setting. Pain is a human experience and pain stories tell us of that experience. When we first thought of the book we asked ourselves two key questions: first, 'should we do it?' and second, 'could we do it'? Each was important – the 'should we?' question required us to think through the ethics of collecting pain stories and then publishing them. A considerable amount of paperwork resulted in us gaining ethics clearance to send out a request for stories. In thinking through 'should we?' we knew that once we publicly shared the stories, they would have a public life of their own. Although this is what we wanted, we were aware that they would be out of our control. We would not be able to predict or define how other people connected with the stories, what they would do with them. However, the nature of stories is that they are never really under our control. All of the stories in this book represent stories that the storytellers wanted to share: they knew that by telling us their stories for a book, they would be setting these free to roam and change people's hearts and minds. When we have been given permission to use the storyteller's name we have done so, where pseudonyms were supplied we have used these. Where names were withheld, we have taken the liberty of choosing names for the children as we felt that a story had more life when the person in it was named. We have done almost no editing of the stories; instead we have – for the most part – let them stand as they were told. Tiny changes to punctuation or micro-editing have been done to assist the narrative flow or to remove identifiers such as names or settings where the storyteller requested this.

The stories came to us by email, post and face-to-face. Some stories were handwritten, others were word processed. Some – we were told – were written in a passionate outpouring, others were crafted over time. Some stories were written specifically for the purpose of the book, others were built from diary extracts. Some built over time with episodes of the story being shared with us gradually. Each story in its own way disrupted and distracted our thinking as we read it. Amongst much of the mundanity of everyday emails and post, these stories demanded attention and many shook us to our core. When you read these, give yourself time to absorb them and prepare to be affected.

The second question we asked was 'could we do it?' and we didn't really know the answer to that until very near to the point we were due to submit the manuscript to Sage. For much of the time we were not sure we could do it. Both of us have said that putting together the chapters for this book has been the hardest thing we have ever written. Both of us have experienced the sense of trepidation of starting with a child's, parent's or professional's story and trying to both honour and respect and interpret it but also to *use* it (and we use the word use deliberately here) as a starting point for a chapter. Both of us have felt somewhat trapped by the stories at times – this is perhaps a natural consequence of spending so much time with them. In many ways our experience of being haunted by some of the stories reflects the experiences of the children, parents and professionals. They told stories that deeply affected them, so it is hardly surprising that they affected us as we strove to write with and about them and link them to evidence, theory, science and practice. In many cases we have shared the chapters with the storytellers, partly perhaps reflecting a nervousness on our part that we had done justice to the stories, got things right. In each case, the storytellers have come back to us with more stories and reflections: stories do beget stories. We have also shared the chapters with professionals and experts, in this case perhaps reflecting a nervousness about whether or not we have got the 'facts right', and again we have been overwhelmed not just by the confirmation that things are correct but also by stories of their own. As we have been trying to tie the book down, we have been collecting new stories, new ideas and some new beginnings.

We chose a story-based approach because we know stories are powerful in being able to shape thinking *and* feeling. There is a wealth of excellent research evidence and literature that guides what we should be doing but it does not always change practice. We hope that in a small way, this book will help shape the way that professionals approach the care of children and young people who are in pain. The stories in this book should act as guides – not guidelines – to practice; we hope these will affect and effect pain practice. We also hope that the stories that the children, young people and professionals have shared with us will become stories that you share with other people and that you start to tell and learn from your own stories. Amongst many of the eloquent things that Frank (2010: 60) says about letting stories breathe, is that 'stories will not leave people alone'. This is how it should be with stories of pain: we should not simply hear a pain story, shrug our shoulders and say 'nothing to do with me'. Children's pain and their stories about their pain are intimately and absolutely to do with each of us. As we have come to know the children in the stories, we have tried to care for the stories as we would hope we would care for them in real life. In some ways, we have nursed these children and their parents and we have come to know the professionals as colleagues.

This book is about the stories that people tell about children's pain and how these touch and affect the lives of the children, their parents and the professionals involved in them. The notion of learning through stories is not new. To a greater or lesser extent all of our lives have been shaped by the stories we have been told or read. The stories we read or that we were read as children often have a strong sense of explaining the rules of the society in which we are growing up – "do this ... " or "don't do this because ... ". Fables, folk tales, and many other story forms often give guidance about or insights into living a good life.

Before turning to the stories of real experiences and trying to shed light on children's pain, we turn to a children's story called 'Crow and Weasel' (Lopez 1993). It is a mythical story about a journey taken by Crow and Weasel as they learn about themselves, respect for other people and their traditions, and their obligations to other people. It is a story about 'how things should be' and how to live a life worth living. They learn from the animals, like Mouse and Grizzly Bear and the Inuit people they meet. Towards the end of their journey, Crow and Weasel meet Badger. The lesson that Badger teaches is about the importance of caring for stories and her words are as apposite to us as professionals caring for children in pain as they were to Crow and Weasel:

'I would ask you to remember only this one thing,' said Badger. 'The stories people tell have a way of taking care of them. If stories come to you, care for them. And learn to give them away where they are needed. Sometimes a person needs a story more than food to stay alive. That is why we put these stories in each other's memory. This is how people care for themselves. One day you will be good story-tellers. Never forget these obligations.' (Lopez 1992)

Badger says that the stories people tell 'have a way of taking care of them'. You can see this in the stories we share in the rest of the book. We want you to care for the pain stories that come to you – to attend to the stories in this book and to the stories that you are told in practice. Listen to them, think with the stories and understand why these are being told. Grow with the stories – use them as food to sustain and enhance your practice. The people who have told their stories have 'given them away'. The people who shared these stories with us 'put these stories' into our memories. In turn, we want these stories to become both part of your memory and part of your future. Practise with these and your own stories in your mind and in your heart. If you do this then you will be shaping a more connected, child-centred and human approach to managing children's pain. Badger warns that we should 'never forget [our] obligations'; pain stories illuminate the path to help shape better pain stories for children and their families.

References

Frank, A. W. (2010) *Letting Stories Breathe: A Socio-narratology*. Chicago, IL: University of Chicago Press.
Lopez, B. (1992) *Crow and Weasel*. New York: Harper Perennial.

Chapter 1

Managing Neonatal Pain

Lucas's and Lily's Stories

Lucas's story

I think one of the most difficult aspects of being a neonatal nurse is anticipating the behavioural cues of neonates to ensure that their needs are met. When babies are very immature it is difficult to interpret their cues and easy to forget that although the baby may not cry or show obvious signs of pain that they are still feeling pain from procedures we undertake. At our NHS Trust we have a Guideline for the Assessment and Management of Pain and Sedation in Neonates which acts as a clear reminder to us all about the importance of ensuring good pain relief prior to undertaking invasive procedures. For a baby requiring intensive care, assessment of pain should be undertaken hourly, however in critical situations I'm not always sure we remember as well as we should.

The little boy I was caring for, called Lucas, was ventilated on synchronised intermittent mandatory ventilation with pressures of 18/4 and a rate of 60bpm. He had a morphine infusion running at 20mcgs/kg/hour. Lucas started becoming agitated and there had been a slight drop in his oxygen saturations. I could also see some secretions in his ET tube so decided to undertake ET suction to clear the tube. This can be an uncomfortable procedure. As Lucas was already on a morphine infusion I asked his mother to utilise the 'containment technique' while I undertook the suction. His mum placed her hands gently but continuously over Lucas's head and legs to comfort him while I undertook the procedure. Containment has been shown to speed recovery from procedures with babies demonstrating less oxygen desaturations, lower heart rates and less behavioural cues demonstrating pain. I quickly undertook the suction and he recovered quickly. By undertaking containment his mum was able to undertake a vital care role for him and his stress and pain levels during the procedure were reduced.

Lily's story

This story involves the management of neonatal pain during the insertion of a chest drain by an Advanced Neonatal Nurse Practitioner (ANNP). The little girl called Lily was born at 24 weeks gestation and was 48 hours old when she developed a pneumothorax and required insertion of a chest drain. This is a very invasive procedure and is known to be very painful. I needed to ensure that Lily was kept as pain-free as possible during the procedure, and I didn't want to cause any undue stress that could impact on her condition further.

The Trust Guideline for the Assessment and Management of Pain and Sedation in Neonates asks us to consider if the procedure definitely needs to happen, could the procedure wait until later, or could a less painful procedure be used. Due to the emergency nature of her condition the answer to all of these (except the first one) was no and it was essential that the chest drain was inserted straight away. The little girl was already receiving a morphine infusion as she was being ventilated. I discussed with the consultant neonatologist if Lily also required some local lignocaine around the insertion site or if a bolus of morphine to sedate Lily further would be more appropriate. We decided not to use the local lignocaine as the type of chest drains we use involve the insertion of a single needle as would an injection of lignocaine. So as she was ventilated I prescribed and gave a bolus of 100mcgs/kgs of morphine in addition to her maintenance morphine to increase her pain relief. I asked the staff nurse caring for her to perform containment to try to reduce her stress further using non-pharmacological methods. The insertion was undertaken as quickly as possible. As she was so premature it was very difficult to interpret her stress cues but I hope that Lily had adequate relief by using both pharmacological and non-pharmacological methods.

Introduction

Both Lucas's and Lily's pain stories clearly demonstrate the daily challenge of meeting the needs of premature babies requiring intensive care. The nurses telling these stories demonstrated concern in minimising the level of pain experienced by the babies while they carried out essential procedures, not knowing if these vulnerable infants were actually experiencing pain or not. These stories articulate some of the complexities involved in managing neonatal pain.

This chapter will first explore the historical perspective that still influences the management of neonatal pain. This will be followed by an exploration of the amount of pain typically encountered by babies in neonatal intensive care units (NICUs) and the need for proactive pain management by nurses. A number of pain tools which have been designed for assessment of neonatal pain will be considered while acknowledging the challenges in identifying or recognising pain in very premature babies. Many essential painful procedures are undertaken with neonates, and require nurses to act to minimise their negative impact. Non-pharmacological methods of pain relief as outlined in the two stories will be explored as well as the part parents can play in helping to manage their babies' pain, followed by a focus on what pain management guidelines are available to assist nurses and parents in this particularly challenging area of pain management.

Neonatal pain in context

Babies often experience high levels of pain in NICU. One study suggests that premature babies experience 100–150 painful procedures in the first week of life (Herrington 2007). Most of these procedures are considered to be minor, such as a heel prick, the insertion of an intravenous cannula or suctioning. However, cumulatively

these minor painful procedures make up the largest part of painful exposure for premature babies. Stevens et al. (2003) reported that neonates underwent more than 10
painful procedures a day, with those at highest risk receiving more painful procedures and being administered the least amount of analgesia during the first days of
life. This is exemplified in Lily's story, where a very premature baby, two days old,
required a painful life-saving procedure.

Every year in England and Wales one in eight babies is born prematurely. In the
United States the incidence is also one in eight or 540,000 babies annually (March
of Dimes 2011). It is known that the rate of premature births is rising (WHO 2012)
and with improved technology and advances in neonatology very premature babies
are surviving. These very premature babies require intensive care involving both very
close monitoring and repeated procedural interventions which are essential for their
survival. However, these repeated unavoidable painful procedures produce significant painful cortical responses (Slater et al. 2006), and pose a real challenge for
neonatal nurses to recognise and respond to effectively. At the end of Lily's story the
nurse expresses her concern for Lily and hopes she had adequate pain relief, suggesting that managing pain well in neonates is a real challenge for nurses, and may cause
them anxiety and stress. However, the nature of their treatment means painful procedures are unavoidable.

Anand (2001), recognised as a pioneer in the research of infant pain, suggests that
premature infants have the necessary neurotransmitters to transmit pain, but are
poorly equipped physiologically to inhibit pain, leaving them hypersensitive to acute
pain. This hypersensitivity to pain can lead, over time, to a lowering of their pain
threshold and result in preterm babies interpreting ordinary non-painful stimulus,
such as holding, as painful. The consequences also endure over time as demonstrated
by a classic study conducted by Grunau et al. (1994) who compared the pain perceptions of two groups of toddlers: one group had extremely low birthweights and had
experienced repeated painful procedures as neonates; the second group had received
minimal painful procedures. At three years and four-and-a-half years the children in
the extremely low birthweight group had significantly higher scores for pain hypersensitivity than the children in the full-term group.

The effect of the cumulative pain experience in NICU

There is something quite unique in relation to the topic of pain in neonates. This
group of babies are incredibly vulnerable to the experience of pain due to their
immaturity and yet it is their very immaturity that demands the need for intensive
care for their survival. However, intensive care of this nature includes life-saving
procedures that are often very painful, a good example of which is Lily's story of
needing a chest drain. It is necessary to consider the consequences of this high incidence of pain on this vulnerable group.

The newborn period is a time of rapid brain development and therefore makes
premature babies very vulnerable (Kostovic and Judas 2010). Despite this recognition
however, it is not yet fully understood what effect early pain-related stress has on the

newborn neurologically. Brummelte et al. (2012), in the only study of its kind to date, conducted brain scans on 86 babies born very prematurely (24–32 weeks), collecting detailed information on the number of painful procedures between scans. The results demonstrated effects on subcortical structures in the brain, suggesting that repeated early procedural pain may be linked with impaired brain development.

The time a premature baby spends in a Neonatal Intensive Care Unit (NICU) is critical for their overall growth and neurodevelopment. Therefore procedures carried out during this period may effect the neurological development of their early life (Fabrizi and Slater 2012).

Bouza (2009) suggests that preterm neonates are more vulnerable to stress and painful procedures and have heightened responses to successive stimuli. There is a need therefore for therapeutic interventions to provide comfort and analgesia for preterm babies. Bauer et al. (2004) studied the stress demonstrated by neonates in response to the experience of pain. They found an increase in oxygen consumption, energy expenditure and heart rate. Slater et al. (2012) found a significant relationship between procedural pain and oxidative stress in preterm neonates. It is clear that stress and increased energy expenditure are likely to have a negative impact on the babies' resources for cognitive and physiological development and maturity, with the result that the length of time in hospital in likely to be increased.

Longer-term consequences of pain have also been explored: Walker et al. (2009) performed quantitative sensory testing in 43 babies born extremely prematurely (recruited from the EPICure study, babies born at less than 26 weeks gestation in 1995) and found a generalised decreased sensitivity to all thermal modalities. They concluded that changes in neurological functioning can be detected many years after an extreme preterm birth. In Lucas's story the nurse described containment for a heel prick procedure. This is an example of a pain-minimising intervention for one of the most common painful procedures carried out in NICU.

Having considered the amount of pain neonates experience in NICU and the likely impact of that pain, there is a real need for pain to be effectively managed. This will be explored in the next section.

Management of neonatal pain

Neonatal pain is often poorly managed and many painful procedures are carried out without any effort to relieve pain. A survey of neonatal pain management across the UK (Robins 2007) found varying standards of pain management of neonates. More than half of neonatal units did not have a protocol for pain relief, less than half administered analgesia before chest drain insertion and 75–80 per cent did not give analgesia before cannulation, heel pricks or venepuncture, despite evidence of simple effective measures such as the use of sucrose for pain relief for simple procedures (Kassab et al. 2012). The picture is one of a lack of priority given to dealing with or anticipating pain in many NICUs across the UK. A previous study by Rennix et al. (2004) found a similar picture with only 10 per cent of units giving analgesia prior to heel sticks. In Lily's story the nurse recognises the potential for Lily to experience considerable pain. In response to this she considers a local anaesthetic but realises that providing this would mean two painful procedures for the baby rather than one. She therefore opts for a bolus dose of morphine to provide sedation during the painful procedure. This story demonstrates the sort of dilemma neonatal nurses are often faced with, and the need to be well informed in making strategic decisions about what route to take in dealing with neonatal pain.

A study in Norway (Andersen et al. 2007) involving 90 clinical staff in two NICUs found that although the majority rated most of the listed procedures as moderately painful for neonates, analgesics were rarely used. This finding led the authors to conclude that neonatal pain is not sufficiently managed and analgesics as well as comfort measures are under-utilised.

It is worth considering here what the literature has to offer in relation to what influences nurses' pain management which may provide insight into why neonatal pain appears to be poorly managed. Nimbalkar et al. (2012), who surveyed nurses in relation to their knowledge of neonatal pain across a paediatric department, found that nurses' lack of knowledge and their attitudes were hindering pain management. Nurses identified doctors not prescribing analgesics as a barrier to managing neonatal pain. These findings are supported by a study by Latimer et al. (2009) who found that the management of procedural pain for neonates was more likely to be evidence-based when there was higher nurse–doctor collaboration. Other positive influences were identified as caring for higher-intensity infants and where nurses had unexpected increases in work assignments. These findings could suggest that nurses who care for high-intensity infants were more likely to have a neonatal nursing qualification which gave them more confidence and therefore the ability to develop good working relationships with doctors as well as cope with the unpredictability in their role, such as unexpected increases in work assignments.

Despite the wider picture from the literature being quite negative both Lucas's and Lily's stories demonstrate how nurses in NICU can, with some forethought, anticipate a baby's pain and plan to prevent or at least minimise it.

Pain assessment

So far it is clear that painful procedures in NICU are mostly unavoidable and occur in significant numbers with potentially quite detrimental effects for a baby. Nurses and other health care professionals need support to be able to recognise and respond to infant pain. A number of pain assessment tools have been developed to help nurses address the specific needs of neonates on pain. However, due to a baby's inability to self-report there is no recognised gold standard for infant pain assessment, unlike that which exists for older children (Warnock and Lander 2004). The alternative therefore involves physiological and behavioural indicators of pain, making assessing pain in newborns very challenging for nurses. In

Lily's story the nurse articulates her hope that the baby's pain was managed, indicating the difficulty in actually identifying pain cues in premature neonates. When using behavioural indicators, it is not always clear how to distinguish behaviours that indicate hunger, distress or actual pain. Stevens et al. (2007) suggest that although all infants demonstrate withdrawal behaviour in response to pain, the relative intensity and duration of responses are linked to the baby's gestational age and also how ill they are. Assessing pain in infants is challenging as many behavioural cues may indicate distress, but without self-report it is difficult to distinguish pain. Nurses are expected to be able to make the judgement as to whether the infant is in pain. Balda et al. (2000) suggest there is speculation that health professionals under-assess infant pain as a coping strategy when put in a position where the care they deliver necessitates inflicting pain. Such a strategy may be understandable, but inevitably leads to pain being ignored or overlooked.

A systematic review by Duhn and Medves (2004) on infant pain assessment tools found dozens of unidimensional, multidimensional and composite measures for assessing pain in infants. These various tools have a range of feasibility and clinical usefulness, however the number of tools available is also indicative of the lack of an available gold standard for infant pain measurement in response to hospitalisation.

Although infant pain tools are readily available, the uptake of any tool will depend on its acceptability to nurses and its usefulness in determining pain. In a study by Schiller (1999) the clinical utility of PIPP (Stevens et al. 1996) and CRIES (Krechel and Bildner 1995) was evaluated; both tools were deemed clinically useful although CRIES took longer to complete, and PIPP was more acceptable to nurses.

Stevens et al. (2008), who developed PIPP, studied 149 neonates at risk of neurological impairment as a result of painful procedures carried out in neonatal intensive care units. They found that facial actions were rated by clinicians as the most important indicators of neonatal pain. Pain researchers, however, demonstrated a better understanding of the importance of pain indicators than nurses. The indicators identified with the highest accuracy for discriminating pain were brow bulge, eye squeeze, nasolabial furrow and total facial expression. These findings could suggest that nurses recognise the facial features indicating pain but do not necessarily act on them, or it could be that contextual factors in the NICU influence the decisions made by nurses in response to the recognition of pain cues. Perhaps nurses are sensitised to pain or influenced by competing demands such as speed or urgency for a medical painful procedure to be undertaken.

Hutchinson and Hall (2005) suggest that although there are validated pain tools for use with premature neonates, there are various challenges inherent in assessing neonatal pain: in NICU some babies receive paralysing medication while being ventilated. Such babies also undergo various painful procedures, however it is very challenging for nurses to assess their level of pain due to the paralysing agents. Experience of staff can have a dual effect in that experienced staff are likely to have more finely tuned observational skills than less experienced staff, but they are also more likely to be able to carry out painful procedures such as venepuncture with more skill and in a shorter period of time, thereby diminishing the amount of pain experienced by the baby.

The lack of a gold standard for pain assessment has meant ongoing studies for indicators of neonatal pain. A new area under development is the study of biomarkers in relation to pain response in infants (Anand et al. 2007). Relevant biomarkers should be a meaningful signal that reflects the babies' pain system and their response to pain. An example of a readily available biomarker is salivary cortisol. The limitation of biomarkers, however, is their ability to be interpreted meaningfully in relation to infant pain, such as indicating the intensity of a pain sensation. While many biomarkers are available for use in neonatal pain responses, no single biomarker reflects all aspects of a baby's response to pain.

Pain assessment tools

A range of validated pain assessment tools is now available, some of which will be explored here. Three categories of behaviours have been consistently identified in the evaluation of pain for all infants: facial expression, vocalisations and motor activity (Stevens et al. 1998).

The Premature Infant Pain Profile (PIPP) was developed by Stevens et al. (1996) and contains seven indicators. Stevens et al. (2007) studied the pain responses of 149 neonates and categorised the responses. The pain indicators identified were then classified into two main categories: physiological (e.g. gestational age, behavioural state, oxygen saturation, and heart rate) and behavioural (e.g. eye squeeze, nasolabial fold, brow bulge). The findings of the study support the use of PIPP in measuring pain in vulnerable infants. Another study using PIPP was carried out by Badr et al. (2010) on the pain responses of 72 preterm babies to a heel stick procedure, scoring their pain on the Preterm Infant Pain Profile (PIPP) scale. Pain scores were highest for the lowest gestational age group. They concluded that sick premature babies and those who have been exposed to many painful procedures may not demonstrate behavioural or physiological signs of pain, but may be the most likely to benefit from precise pain assessment and careful management. In Lily's story her nurse articulates that the baby's prematurity makes it difficult to interpret her pain cues.

The COMFORT scale has also been adapted for the measurement of pain in premature infants with a gestational age of between 28 and 37 weeks (Caljouw et al. 2007) in the Netherlands. It was found that a combination of the Visual Analogue Scale (VAS) and the adapted COMFORT scale allowed nurses to judge the clinical presence of pain in premature infants.

With such an array of tools, nurses need to be able to discriminate between them as to their usefulness. Spasojevic and Breugun-Doronjski (2011) evaluated the usefulness of four neonatal tools in describing an infant's pain in a clinical setting. The four tools were the Neonatal Infant Pain Scale (NIPS), the Douleur Aigue du Nouvou-ne (DAN), the Neonatal Pain Assessment Scale (NPAS) and the Premature Infant Pain Profile (PIPP). Although PIPP was found to be the most precise pain scale, one shortcoming of PIPP was the need to make a judgement on facial expression, which cannot be easily achieved in ventilated babies or where there is not a clear view of the baby's face.

In response to the need to have a neonatal tool that did not require an assessment of facial expression, Milesi et al. (2010) devised the Faceless Acute Neonatal Pain Scale (FANS), which does not depend on facial expression. FANS relies on an assessment of limb movement, cry and autonomic reaction. A validation study has found this tool to be reliable for use in preterm newborns when facial expression is not accessible (Milesi et al. 2010).

Pain tools are variously designed to determine if a baby has pain and, in some tools, the amount of pain. However, none of the tools differentiate between different causes of pain or actually identify where in the body the pain is located. Due to these and many other limitations of pain assessment tools, nurses need to be holistic in their approach to managing premature babies' pain.

Halimaa (2003) suggests that procedural pain management in preterm babies is a process involving four stages (see Figure 1.1).

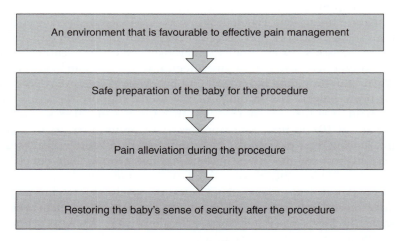

Figure 1.1   Four stages of procedural pain management
Source: Halimaa 2003

Systematic pain management also requires documentation of the whole pain management process.

Having considered tools that may be used to assess a baby's pain, the next section will consider pain-relieving interventions to use with neonates and the involvement of parents.

Pain-relieving interventions and the role of parents

In both Lucas's and Lily's stories the nurses utilised non-pharmacological methods of pain relief which have been found to have a positive impact on infant pain. Nurses are ideally placed not only to utilise such methods but also to promote the use of them to parents to enable them to contribute to the management of their baby's pain.

In the stories of Lucas and Lily, nurses used containment as a pain-relieving intervention. Containment involves restricting premature babies' reflex movements by holding them so that their arms and legs are near their trunk and maintain a flexed *in-utero* position. Containment can increase a neonate's feeling of security and calm agitated babies (Velasco-Whetsell et al. 1992). It has been found in the past to effectively reduce premature babies' pain responses and is adopted as a nursing standard of care in pain management (Corff et al. 1995; Liang et al. 2000). Of other effective non-pharmacological methods used in pain management, swaddling has been found to have a similar effect to containment (Neu and Browne 1997). Leslie and Marlow (2006) suggest that simple non-pharmacological methods such as the use of pacifiers, facilitated tucking and skin-to-skin contact can be effective in relieving neonatal pain. It is clear that parents can and should be encouraged to become involved in recognising, responding to and using non-pharmacological methods of pain relief to help manage their babies' pain.

In a study by Franck et al. (2004) involving 61 parents across nine neonatal units in the UK and US, it was found that parents reported that their infants had experienced moderate to severe pain, which was more than they had expected. Parents received information about pain and how to comfort their baby, but most of this information was verbal. Only 18 per cent of parents were shown signs of infant pain. The authors suggested that parents have unmet needs in relation to information regarding infant pain. It is clear that parents should be supported to become more involved in their babies' pain management. Parents have been found to be more accurate in their assessment of their infant's pain than health professionals (Pillai Riddell and Chambers 2007). However, parents in NICU require help in responding to their babies to help reduce or alleviate their pain. The difficulty in dealing with preterm babies is that their ability to communicate their pain or distress can be extremely limited due to their immaturity. Parents can be effective in helping health professionals recognise their babies' pain. By so doing they enhance the ability of the nurse to respond more readily and ultimately to reduce the long-term consequences of infant pain. Gale et al. (2004) interviewed parents and found that they wanted more information regarding their babies' pain and to be consulted on how they wanted to be involved in helping to manage pain. A developmentally sensitive approach to understanding the needs of both infants and parents is necessary (Pillai Riddell and Chambers 2007).

Parents have a key role to play when their infant undergoes a painful procedure (Curry et al. 2010), but parents need support themselves to be able to provide comfort for their baby. Parents should have the painful procedure and their role in providing comfort explained. The nurse should assess the parents' level of anxiety as an overly anxious parent can inadvertently convey that anxiety to that baby. Axelin et al. (2010) found that mothers are willing to actively participate in their preterm babies' pain care. The involvement in care was found to be influenced by the mothers' experience prior to and during an NICU stay, suggesting that nurses need to assess mothers' preferences to be able to facilitate their involvement effectively. Parents have much to offer in helping to relieve their babies' pain: Johnston et al. (2003) suggest that the presence of parents and the use of touch promote physiological stability and a quiet state in infants. In both Lucas's and Lily's stories parents were included in managing their babies' pain, promoting evidence-based care. Including parents in managing their babies' pain also helps parents: Skene et al. (2011) conducted a study with 11 families that focused on the parents' involvement in their premature babies' pain management. Parents were observed and interviewed over ten months. It was found that including parents in comforting their babies when they undergo painful procedures helps them learn to parent.

Parents can also provide pain relief for babies in other ways. A study by Phillips et al. (2005) demonstrated that breastfeeding and maternal holding were effective pain-relieving strategies for babies undergoing heel prick procedures. An earlier study by Carbajal et al. (2003), of 180 newborn babies, found that breastfeeding during a procedure significantly reduced pain. Clifford et al. (2004) suggest that breastfeeding-induced analgesia appears to use a pain blockade composed of the components of taste, suckle and contact. Other strategies parents can use are consoling measures to manage injection pain and nurses should help parents to provide that support to their babies (Curry et al. 2010).

It would appear that there are many pain-relieving interventions that parents can utilise with the guidance and support of nurses. Being a parent of a premature baby in a NICU who is experiencing repeated painful procedures presents a number of potential obstacles to normal parenting. These include learning to parent their newborn baby, the transfer of responsibility for the baby from the nurse to the parent, and the establishment of attachment behaviour between the newborn baby and parent. A number of guidelines have been produced to guide nurses in dealing with the challenges of neonatal pain. These will be discussed in the next section.

Guidelines on the management of neonatal pain

Anand (2001), who drew up a consensus statement for the prevention and management of pain in the newborn, suggests that practice should be geared to minimise or mitigate against pain. Pain should be anticipated because pain can occur every day and sometimes every hour. Physical aspects of the environment in which the premature baby is cared for, such as light and noise, can have an impact on pain perception and tolerance. Reduced light and noise can enhance physiological stability and therefore have the potential to reduce the babies' pain response.

Urso (2007) suggests that for the past two decades neonatal pain care has been an issue for health care. Now that protocols are being developed they need to be established in NICUs, because they promote assessment of pain, treatment, family involvement and education for caregivers. Guidelines for preventing or treating neonatal pain and its negative consequences include recognition of the sources of pain, routine assessment of pain, avoidance of recurrent painful stimuli, and the use of specific non-pharmacological and pharmacological interventions (Bouza 2009). In both Lucas's and Lily's stories the nurses demonstrated how they pre-empted their pain and consciously planned to reduce or alleviate the babies' pain in advance of the procedure.

A good source of guidance for pain management is provided by the APA (2012). In relation to neonatal pain it is recommended that sucrose or other sweet solutions can be used for procedural pain and non-pharmacological measures including tactile stimulation, breastfeeding, non-nutritive sucking, 'kangaroo care', and massage of the heel can be used for heel prick blood sampling. In Lucas's and Lily's stories, sucrose was not used but touch was in the form of containment.

Conclusion

Lily's and Lucas's stories highlight the degree of pain that some neonates experience in NICU, as well as the regular challenge that nurses face in dealing with such pain. The cumulative effect of painful procedures can have a detrimental effect on neonates, in the short term by using up vital resources needed for growth, and in the longer term by sensitising them to painful procedures and distorting their perception of pain. The acceptance of the need for an accurate assessment of pain has led to a number of studies to develop validated pain assessment tools. Nurses now have a range of tools to use, but there is still a real challenge in reading the pain cues of very premature babies. The role parents play in dealing with their baby's pain has considerable potential but needs to be supported and guided by nurses. Nurses also need support to provide evidence-based care for premature babies whose survival involves regular, often life-saving, painful procedures.

Key Points

- The rate of premature births is rising, meaning more very premature babies are requiring intensive care involving unavoidable painful procedures.
- Cumulative pain in the neonatal period can have long-lasting consequences.
- Analgesics and comfort measures have been found to be under-used with neonates experiencing painful procedures.
- There are a number of challenges for nurses in the use of validated neonatal pain assessment tools.
- Parents have a key role to play in the management of neonatal pain.
- Pain guidelines suggest that pain in neonates should be anticipated and comfort measures should be used to help relieve pain.

Additional Resources and Reading

- You may want to learn more about neonates and neonatal care. Three resources are outlined here.
  - o The EPICure study was the largest of its kind focusing on the long term consequences of being born premature. Costeloe K., Hennessy E., Gibson A.T., Marlow N. and Wilkinson A.R. (2000) 'The EPICure Study: outcomes to discharge from hospital for infants born at the threshold of viability', *Pediatrics*, 106 (4): 659–71.
  - o The National Neonatal Audit Programme (NNAP) has been established with the aim of informing good clinical practice in aspects of neonatal care by auditing national standards: www.rcpch.ac.uk/child-health/standards-care/clinical-audits/national-neonatal-audit-programme-nnap/national-neonatal
  - o Bliss is the UK charity working to provide the best possible care and support for all premature and sick babies and their families: www.bliss.org.uk/

References

Anand, K.J.S. and the International Evidence-Based Group for Neonatal Pain (2001) 'Consensus Statement for the Prevention and Management of Pain in the Newborn', *Archives of Pediatric & Adolescent Medicine*, 155: 173–80.

Anand, .K.J.S., Stevens, B.J. and McGrath, B.J. (eds) (2007) *Pain in Neonates and Infants*, 3rd edition. Amsterdam: Elsevier.

Andersen, R.D., Greve-Isdahl, M. and Jylli, L. (2007) 'The opinions of clinical staff regarding neonatal procedural pain in two Norwegian neonatal intensive care units', *Acta Paeditrica*, 96 (7): 1000–03.

Association of Paediatric Anaesthetists (APA) (2012) *Good Practice in Postoperative and Procedural Pain*, 2nd edition. London: APA.

Axelin, A., Lehtonen, L., Pelander, T. and Salenterä, S. (2010) 'Mothers' different styles of involvement in preterm infant pain care', *Journal of Obstetric Gynecology and Neonatal Nursing*, 39: 415–24.

Badr, L.K., Abdallah, B., Hawari, M., Sidani, S., Kassar, M., Nakad, P. and Breidi J. (2010) 'Determinants of premature infant pain responses to heel sticks', *Pediatric Nursing*, 36 (3): 129–36.

Balda, R.C.X., Guinsburg, R., de Almeida, M.F.B., de Araújo Peres, C., Miyoshi, M.H., and Kopelman, B.I. (2000) 'The recognition of facial expression of pain in full-term newborns by parents and health professionals', *Archives of Pediatric & Adolescent Medicine*, 54(10): 1009–16.

Bauer, K., Ketteler, J., Hellwig, M., Laurenz, M. and Versmold, H. (2004) 'Oral glucose before venepuncture relieves neonates of pain, but stress is still evidenced by increase in oxygen consumption, energy expenditure and heart rate', *Pediatric Research*, 55: 695–700.

Bouza, H. (2009) 'The impact of pain in the immature brain', *Journal of Maternal-Fetal and Neonatal Medicine*, 22 (9): 722–32.

Brummelte, S., Grunau, R.E., Chau, V., Poskitt, K.J., Brant R., Vinall, J., Gover, A., Synnes, A.R. and Miller, S.P. (2012) 'Procedural pain and brain development in premature newborns', *American Neurological Association*, 71: 385–96.

Caljouw, M.A.A., Kloos, M.A.C., Olivier, M.Y., Heemskerk, I.W., Pison, W.C.R., Stigter, G.D. and Verhoef, A.M.J.H. (2007) 'Measurement of pain in premature infants with a gestational age between 28 to 37 weeks: validation of the adapted COMFORT scale', *Journal of Neonatal Nursing*, 13: 13–18.

Carbajal, R., Paupe, A., Hoenn, E., Lenclen, R. and Olivier-Martin, M. (1997) 'DAN a compartmentalised scale of assessment of acute pain in neonates", *Archives of Pediatrics*, 4: 623–8.

Carbajal, R., Veerapen, S., Couderc, S., Jugie, M. and Ville, Y. (2003) 'Analagesic effect of breast feeding in term neonates: randomised controlled trial', *British Medical Journal*, 326(7379): 13.

Clifford, P.A., Stringer, M., Christensen, H. and Mountain, D. (2004) 'Pain assessment and intervention for term neonates', *Journal of Midwifery and Women's Health*, 49 (6): 514–19.

Corff, K.E., Seideman, R., Venkataraman, P.S., Lutes, L. and Yates, B. (1995) 'Facilitated tucking: a non pharmacologic comfort measure for pain in preterm neonates', *Journal of Obstetric Gynecologic and Neonatal Nursing*, 24 (2): 143–7.

Costeloe, K., Hennessy, E., Gibson, A.T., Marlow, N. and Wilkinson, A.R. (2000) 'The EPICure study: outcomes to discharge from hospital for infants born at the threshold of viability ', *Pediatrics*, 106 (4): 659–71.

Curry, D., Brown, C. and Wrona, S. (2010) 'Effectiveness of oral sucrose for pain management in infants during immunizations', *Pain Management Nursing*, 13 (3): 139–49.

Duhn, L.J. and Medves, J.M. (2004) 'A systematic integrative review of infant pain assessment tools', *Advances in Neonatal Care*, 4: 126–40.

Fabrizi, L. and Slater, R. (2012) 'Exploring the relationship of pain and development in the neonatal intensive care unit', Editorial. *Pain*, 153: 1340–1.

Franck, L.S., Cox, S., Allen, A. and Winter, I. (2004) 'Parental concern and distress about infant pain', *Archives of Diseases in Childhood – Fetal and Neonatal Edition*, 89: F71–F75.

Gale, G., Franck, L.S., Kools, S. and Lynch, M.(2004) 'Parents' perceptions of their infant's pain experience in the NICU', *International Journal of Nursing Studies*, 41(1): 51–8.

Grunau, R.V., Whitfield, M.F., Petrie, J.H. and Fryer, E.L. (1994) 'Early pain experience, child and family factors, as precursors of somatization: a prospective study of extremely premature and fullterm children', *Pain*, 56 (3): 353–9.

Halimaa, S.L. (2003) 'Pain management in nursing procedures on premature babies', *Journal of Advanced Nursing*, 42 (6): 587–97.

Herrington, C.J. (2007) 'Reducing pain of heelstick in premature infants with Gentle Human Touch'. PhD Dissertation. Wayne State University, Detroit, Michigan.

Hutchinson, F. and Hall, C. (2005) 'Managing neonatal pain', *Journal of Neonatal Nursing*, 11: 28–32.

Johnston, C.C., Stevens, B., Pinelli, J., Gibbins, S., Filion, F., Jack A., Steele, S., Boyer, K. and Veilleux, A. (2003) 'Kangaroo care is effective in diminishing pain response in preterm neonates', *Archives of Pediatric & Adolescent Medicine*, 157(11): 1084–88.

Kassab, M.I., Roydhouse, J.K., Fowler, C. and Foureur, M. (2012) 'The effectiveness of glucose in reducing needle-related procedural pain in infants', *Journal of Pediatric Nursing*, 27(1): 3–17.

Kostovic, I. and Judas, M. (2010) 'The development of the subplate and thalamocortical connections in the human foetal brain', *Acta Pediatrica*, 99: 1119–27.

Krechel, S.W. and Bildner, J. (1995) 'CRIES: a new neonatal postoperative pain measurement score: initial testing of validity and reliability', *Pediatric Anesthesia*, 5(1): 53–61.

Latimer, M.A., Johnston, C.C, Ritchie, J.A., Clarke, S.P. and Gilin, D. (2009) 'Factors affecting delivery of evidence-based procedural pain care in hospitalized neonates', *Journal of Obstetrics Gynecologic and Neonatal Nursing*, 38 (2): 182–94.

Leslie, A. and Marlow, N. (2006) 'Non-pharmacological pain relief', *Seminars in Neonatal Medicine*, 11: 246–50.

Liang, S.R., Wang, Rh., Chang, Y.K. and Wang, M.S. (2000) 'Study of containment for premature infants in alleviating pain from heelstick', *Medical Research (Chinese)*, 20 (7): 368–76.

March of Dimes (2011) *Prematurity Campaign. The Serious Problem of Premature Birth.* Available at www.marchofdimes.com/mission/prematurity/html (accessed 8 December 2012).

Milesi, C., Cambonie, G., Jacquot, A., Barbotte, E., Mesnege, R., Masson, F., Pidoux, O., Ferragu, F., Thevenot, P., Mariette, J.B. and Picaud, J.C. (2010) 'Validation of a neonatal pain scale adapted to the new practices in caring for preterm newborns', *Archives of Diseases in Childhood – Fetal and Neonatal Edition*, 95: F263–F266.

Neu, M. and Browne, J.V. (1997) 'Infant physiologic and behavioural organization during swaddled versus unsaddled weighing', *Journal of Perinatology*, 17 (3): 193–8.

Nimbalkar, A., Dongara, A.R., Phatak, A.G. and Nimbalkar, S.M. (2012) 'Knowledge and attitudes regarding neonatal pain among nursing staff of pediatric department: an Indian experience', *Pain Management Nursing*. Available at www.sciencedirect.com/science/article/pii/S1524904212000847 (accessed 17 June 2013).

Pillai Riddell, R.R. and Chambers, C.T. (2007) 'Parenting and pain during infancy', in K.J. Anand, B.J. Stevens and B.J. McGrath (eds), *Pain in Neonates and Infants*, 3rd edition. Amsterdam: Elsevier.

Phillips, R.M., Chantry, C.J. and Gallagher, M.P. (2005) 'Analgesic effects of breast-feeding or pacifier use with maternal holding in term infants', *Ambulatory Pediatrics,* 5: 359–64.

Rennix, C., Manjunatha, C.M. and Ibhanesebhor, S.E. (2004) 'Pain relief during common neonatal procedures: a survey', *Archives of Diseases in Childhood – Fetal Neonatal Edition*, 89: F563.

Robins, J. (2007) '"Post code ouch": a survey of neonatal pain management prior to painful procedures within the United Kingdom', *Journal of Neonatal Nursing*, 13: 113–17.

Schiller, C.J. (1999) 'Clinical utility of two neonatal pain assessment measures', Master's Thesis, University of Toronto.

Skene, C., Curtis, P., Gerrish, K. and Franck, L. (2011) 'Parental involvement in neonatal pain management', *Archives of Diseases in Childhood – Fetal and Neonatal Edition*, 96: Fa7–Fa8.

Slater, L., Asmerom, Y., Boskovic, D.S., Bahjri, K., Plank, M.S., Angeles, K.R., Philips, R., Deming, D., Ashwal, S., Hougland, K., Fayard, E. and Angeles, D.M. (2012) 'Procedural pain and oxidative stress in premature neonates', *Journal of Pain*, 13 (6): 590–7.

Slater, R., Cantarella, A., Gallella, S., Worley, A., Boyd, S., Meek, J. and Fitzgerald, M. (2006) 'Cortical pain responses in human infants', *Journal of Neuroscience*, 26: 3662–6.

Spasojevic, S. and Breugun-Doronjski, A. (2011) 'A simultaneous comparison of four neonatal pain scales in clinical settings', *Journal of Maternal-Fetal and Neonatal Medicine*, 24 (4): 590–4.

Stevens, B., Franck, L.S., Gibbins, S., McGrath, P., Dupuis, A. and Yamada, J. (2007) 'Determining the structure of acute pain responses in vulnerable neonates', *Clinical Journal of Neonatal Nursing*, 39 (2): 32–47.

Stevens, B., Johnston, C. and Gibbons, S. (1998) 'Assessment of pain in the neonate', in K.J.S. Anand, B.J. Stevens and P.J. McGrath (eds), *Pain in Neonates and Infants*, 2nd edn. New York: Elsevier.

Stevens, B., Johnston, C., Petryshen, P. and Taddio, A. (1996) 'Infant Pain Profile: development and initial validation', *Clinical Journal of Pain*, 12: 13–22.

Stevens, B., McGrath, P., Dupuis A., Gibbins, S., Beyene, J., Breau, L., Camfield, C., Finley, A., Franck, L., Hewlett, A., Johnston, C., McKeever, P., O'Brien, K., Ohlsson, A. and Yamada J. (2008) 'Indicators of pain in neonates at risk for neurological impairment', *Journal of Advanced Nursing*, 65 (2): 285–96.

Stevens, B., McGrath, P., Gibbins,S., Beyene, J., Breau, L., Camfield, C., Finley, A., Franck, L., Hewlett, A., McKeever, P., O'Brien, K., Ohlsson, A. and Yamada J. (2003) 'Procedural pain in newborns at risk for neurologic impairment', *Pain*, 105 (1–2): 27–35.

Urso, A.M. (2007) 'The reality of neonatal pain and the resulting effects', *Journal of Neonatal Nursing*, 13: 236–8.

Velasco-Whetsell, M., Even, J.C. and Wang, M.S. (1992) 'Do postsuctioning transcutaneous PO_2 values change when a neonate's movements are restrained?', *Journal of Perinatology*, 12: 333–7.

Walker, S.M., Franck, L.S., Fitzgerald, M., Myles, J., Stocks, J. and Marlow, N. (2009) 'Long-term impact of neonatal intensive care and surgery on somatosensory perception in children born extremely preterm', *Pain*, 141: 79–87.

Warnock, F. and Lander J. (2004) 'Foundations of knowledge about neonatal pain', *Journal of Pain and Symptom Management*, 27(2): 170–79.

WHO (2012) *Preterm Birth Factsheet No. 363*. Available at www.who.int/mediacentre/factsheets/fs363/en/index.html (accessed 17 June 2013).

Chapter 2

Pain Management: Advice on Discharge

Holly's story

Jill's and Holly's story

A young girl (16 months old) with complex health problems including cognitive impairment, called Holly, on my caseload underwent abdominal surgery for insertion of a gastrostomy tube. As she was discharged just before a long bank holiday weekend, this child was at home for four days before I was able to make a post-operative home visit. On arrival, I found her parents to be anxious and angry that their daughter had been crying and unsettled for much of the time since her discharge. The parents reported the nurse discharging the child from the regional specialist unit had instructed them 'not to give analgesia regularly but just paracetamol when she cries!'

Holly was discharged home earlier than had been expected and at the time the community children's nursing team was not notified. If they had known, the on-call nurse could have contacted the family over the weekend.

Having spent lots of time preparing this family pre-operatively for their daughter's surgery, I was extremely frustrated at this inappropriate pain management advice, which resulted in such a painful and distressing post-operative experience for the whole family. As a Community Children's Nurse, I regularly visit families who are given little or incorrect information to manage their child's pain on discharge from hospital. This leads to children experiencing unrelieved pain unnecessarily and can impact significantly on the family by increasing the distress caused by the whole illness and hospitalisation experience.

Following an assessment of this child's pain, a management plan was then easily negotiated with her parents, agreeing on an analgesic regime of paracetamol and addition of a non-steroidal anti-inflammatory drug (NSAID). On re-evaluation the following day, effective pain relief had been achieved simply by the regular administration of analgesics. Since completing a module in the management of pain in children, I feel much more confident in my knowledge and ability to deliver evidence-based practice in pain management to the children and families in my care. Training in pain management needs to become an integral and essential part of nurse education, to prevent any child experiencing unnecessary pain and ensure all children and families can benefit from evidenced-based best practice in any setting.

From the above story it is evident that there are two extremes of practice taking place. On the one hand there is Jill, the community children's nurse, who engaged with the child and family to prepare them for the operation, and post-discharge picked up the pieces of a distressing and frustrating situation and within 24 hours had managed to provide pain relief for Holly. On the other hand there is the apparently casual attitude of the discharging nurse providing advice that runs contrary to current guidelines, which resulted in causing Holly considerable distress and left her parents feeling angry and upset.

In order to explore this situation, this chapter will first focus on the current advice on children's pain management in order to establish what advice should have been given on discharge that could have prevented Holly and her family experiencing a distressing weekend before being seen by their community nurse.

From Jennie's story, it is clear that Holly and her mother did not receive evidence-based care in relation to the management of her pain. To explore this it is necessary to focus on what it is that is recommended in such a situation. There is no shortage of current information or guidance on how pain should be managed. In fact it is true to say that, since the beginning of the twenty-first century, there has been a revolution in the knowledge of children's pain management, with guidance being developed by a wide range of international groups. The Royal College of Nursing published its first guideline on children's pain in 1999, followed by the Joint Commission on Accreditation of Healthcare Organisations (JCAHO) in America bringing out standards that called for effective assessment, management and evaluation of pain in health care settings (Berry and Dahl 2000). In 2008 the Association of Paediatric Anaesthetists published a *Good Practice Guide on Postoperative and Procedural Pain in Children* (APA 2008), updated in 2012, and in 2009 the Royal College of Nursing published its updated version of *The Recognition and Assessment of Acute Pain in Children*. The Australian and New Zealand College of Anaesthetists have published their third edition of Scientific Evidence on acute pain management (ANZCA 2010). These guidelines provide ample accessible and current information on how to effectively manage children's pain. However, despite the availability of such evidence, hospitalised children still report high levels of pain (Van Hulle 2007).

In the UK, the Children's National Service Framework (DH, 2004) stated that children had a right to effective pain management, followed by the IASP Special Interest Group bringing out a position statement in 2005 entitled *Children's Pain Matters!*, asking why children's pain is dealt with inadequately around the world (IASP 2005). In Jennie's story it is clear that the advice Holly's mother was given on discharge was not based on current guidelines and the lack of appropriate discharge advice and support led to Holly experiencing unnecessary pain over a long bank holiday weekend without support.

Current recommendations for the management of pain in children

Two recent guides which will be looked at are those from the Association of Paediatric Anaesthetists (APA 2012) and the Royal College of Nursing (2009).

The Association of Paediatric Anaesthetists (APA 2012) has updated *Good Practice Guidelines for Procedural and Postoperative Pain*. These guidelines are designed to provide evidence-based information on the assessment of pain and the efficacy of pain management strategies, such that an informed plan of effective analgesia can be formulated that is appropriate for the patient and clinical setting. Two general principles of pain assessment suggested are that children's self-report of their pain is the preferred approach, and that health care professionals and parents/carers should receive information, education and training in pain assessment. The APA (2012: 33) note that:

- Prior to discharge from the hospital, patients and their families should be given clearly presented information and advice regarding the assessment of pain and the administration of analgesia at home.
- Post-operative analgesia should be appropriate to developmental age, surgical procedure and clinical setting.
- Providers of post-operative care should understand the general principles of good pain management in children and the use of analgesics at different developmental ages.

It is clear that Holly's care did not meet this level of good practice, however it also suggests that the nurse providing the discharge advice did not have the appropriate knowledge in pain management.

The Royal College of Nursing (RCN 2009) guidelines state that pain in neonates and children should be anticipated at all times. This recommendation would suggest that nurses need to be proactive in their pain management practices and should ask children about their pain when it can be anticipated that specific procedures or surgery make it likely that they will experience pain. The recommendations also suggest nurses should use a validated pain assessment tool and for children unable to self-report to use a behavioural or composite tool and not rely on isolated indicators to assess pain. The final recommendation is that nurses should assess, record and re-evaluate pain at regular intervals, with the frequency of assessment determined by the individual child's needs.

It is interesting to note that not only was the discharging nurse's advice unhelpful, it was also in fact the opposite to what should have been advised. Holly's mother was told not to give any medicine unless Holly cried, whereas the guidelines clearly promote pre-empting children's pain. The notion of attempting to prevent pain is not new: as far back as 1988 Patrick Wall proposed the concept of pre-emptive treatment because pain relief was more effective if given before pain was experienced. This has been reinforced by Lloyd-Thomas (1998) and Taddio et al. (1997) who demonstrated that pre-emptive analgesia resulted in long-term behavioural benefits. However, in the second decade of the twenty-first century pain is still not being consistently pre-empted.

So why is available knowledge not being utilised?

Breivik and Stubhaug (2008) suggest that guidelines and directives, even from the Department of Health, are not enough to change practice. There is also recognition of the challenges nurses face in attempting to manage children's pain, and the cost to them emotionally. Nurses have the responsibility and accountability for pain management, but are sometimes unable to give the amount of analgesic they would like to (Blondal and Halldorsdottir 2009). On the other hand, studies suggest that nurses under-medicate children in pain due to a lack of knowledge and inadequate assessment skills (Mackintosh and Bowles 2000; Simons and Moseley 2009).

One reason could be that there is a need for a better provision of nurse education on pain. A number of studies have found that nurses lack knowledge of pain management (Czarnecki et al. 2010;Vincent 2005) while other studies found that some nurses recognise their lack of knowledge on pain management (Simons 2002) and express a desire to rectify that lack of knowledge (Simons and Macdonald 2004). However, it is recognised that the provision of education on pain in children is not available or easily accessible to many nurses caring for children in pain. Where provision is available, there is the added complication of the current economic constraints of getting support to attend a course on pain management. Nurses' knowledge will be further explored later in this chapter.

One of the good practice points suggested by the APA (2012) is that providers of post-operative care should understand the general principles of good pain management in children. These include knowledge of assessment techniques and the use of analgesics at different developmental ages. Walker (2004) on the other hand suggests that the emphasis on tools and drugs is partly to blame for the poor care some patients receive. Poor care could also be a consequence of patient expectations being low, as found by Twycross and Collins (2011), resulting in nurses having little demanded of them (Picker 2009).The low expectation on the part of children and parents is likely to be contributing to the status quo of poor pain management, as nurses may take parents' lack of demands in relation to pain management as a sign of satisfaction with how pain is managed or a sign of lack of pain being experienced by children. If parents were encouraged to be more active in the management of their children's pain, it is likely that Holly's mother would have felt able to challenge the nurse who provided the poor advice to not give analgesia unless Holly cried. However, it has been found that many parents are not actively involved in managing their children's pain (Simons and Roberson 2002) and do not feel comfortable asking nurses for help when their child is in pain.

Parents and pain

Holly's mother needed to understand Holly's pain and have the confidence to deal with it over the long weekend following Holly's discharge home. Instead the misguided information left her unable to manage Holly's pain effectively. A significant amount of literature focuses on parents and their children's pain, and can provide insight into the role of parents in managing their children's pain.

Knowledge of pain management could contribute greatly to families' confidence in their children's treatment, but parents tend to under-medicate because of the difficulty of estimating the degree of their child's pain, the absence of instruction in how to assess pain and a lack of knowledge of appropriate actions to take. Parents tend to only use methods to relieve their child's pain that are familiar to them. When parents are involved in pain management they help to reduce their child's pain and feel that they have contributed to their child's care. Parents need more information to feel confident to manage pain (Gorodzinsky et al. 2013; Kankkunen et al. 2003).

Although some nurses appear to recognise that parents need information regarding their child's pain, the nature of the information appears to be problematic for parents. Kankkunen et al. (2005) carried out a literature review of families and their children's post-operative pain. They found that parents criticised pain-related instructions provided by hospital staff, and they described difficulties in managing pain at home. In an attempt to ascertain the availability of advice for parents to help them support their child experiencing procedural pain, Power et al. (2007) found that there was little published information to guide parents on how to deal with their children's pain. Information provision is an overlooked aspect of the care of children.

Although nurses recognise the need for parents to have information there is a lack of supporting mechanisms to ensure that parents receive information that is accurate and supports them in managing their child's pain. Simons and Roberson (2002) conducted a study on parents' support and satisfaction with their child's post-operative care, and carried out interviews and a survey with 20 parents. It was found that there was a discrepancy in the perceptions of parents and nurses in relation to the support parents received. Nurses felt that parents were receiving more support from them than that which parents felt they were receiving. There seemed to be a gap in communication between parents and nurses, with nurses tending to keep their distance from parents. Without communicating effectively with parents as to how much support a parent needs or receives, nurses are at risk of basing nursing care on assumptions.

Parents can find their child's hospitalisation a stressful and bewildering experiennence, as found in Darbyshire's (1994) seminal work where resident parents felt they were sleeping in someone else's workplace, i.e. that of nurses. Parents are likely to be stressed and anxious if their child is undergoing surgery and are unlikely to initiate a conversation with nurses who appear busy and unapproachable.

Holly's pain

Holly had undergone abdominal surgery for the insertion of a gastrostomy tube, but her mother was advised not to give her anything for pain unless she cried. Such advice suggests that the nurse did not consider that the surgery involved was likely to cause Holly pain. However, there is reliable evidence that surgery causes pain. A seminal study by Asprey (1994) explored what it is about surgery that is painful and found that pain is caused by multiple factors. These factors include the incision itself, severing nerve fibres in the skin, cutting and stretching muscle fibres, chemical irritation from cell breakage, discomfort and stiffness from lying on the operating table for a period of time in one position and endotracheal intubation (Eland 1988). It is clear therefore that pain after surgery can be assumed, regardless of the child's behaviour.

Day case surgery

Holly's surgery was performed as a short-stay admission. Day case surgery is common in paediatric practice (Blacoe et al. 2008), however, the provision of effective analgesia after ambulatory surgery remains poor. In a Swedish nationwide survey of day case surgery, pain was the most common problem at follow-up after discharge in a paediatric population (Segerdahl et al. 2008). Although it is clear that Holly's nurse did not provide appropriate or helpful advice regarding the administration of adequate analgesia, similar poor practice has been found elsewhere. Wilson and Helgadottir (2006) studied the patterns of pain and use of analgesia in 68 Icelandic children aged 3–7 years during the first three days post-tonsillectomy. It was found that only 40 per cent of children received therapeutic analgesic doses in the first 24 hours post-operatively, while still in hospital. However, that figure dropped to only 10 per cent in the subsequent 24 hours when the children were at home being cared for by parents. This study demonstrates the real need for a change in practice in relation to how young children are discharged home, when it is clear that analgesics will be required while being cared for at home by parents.

Other researchers have focused on addressing the issue of poor post-operative pain management. Lonnqvist and Morton (2005) conducted a review of post-operative analgesia in children and outlined a pragmatic approach to children's pain management that has been developed and used in many paediatric centres. The aims are to recognise pain in children, to minimise moderate and severe pain safely in all children, to prevent pain where it is predictable, to bring pain rapidly under control and to continue pain control after discharge from hospital.

In Holly's story her post-operative pain and the challenge for her mother to deal with it was compounded by her inability to tell her mother how she felt about her pain due to her age and cognitive impairment. This will be explored next.

Pain in a non-verbal child

Dubois et al. (2008) carried out a study on the vocal and verbal expression of pain in preschoolers in America: 47 children aged 1–6 years were observed post-operatively as to their vocalisation of pain. Young pre-verbal children were unable to express their pain accurately due to immaturity of speech and cognitive skills, which are necessary to be able to report how they are feeling and how much pain they are experiencing. The majority of children under two years of age use cry vocalisation to express their pain, and during the post-operative period the frequency of the vocalisation increased (von Baeyer and Spagrud 2007). It is clear from Holly's story that she was vocalising her distress to her parents during the weekend following her surgery. Assessing pain in children can be difficult, and in non-verbal children it is even more challenging. In response to such challenges Herr et al. (2006) developed recommendations approved by the American Pain Society which states that pain is a subjective experience, and no objective tests exist to measure it as illustrated in Box 2.1.

> ## Box 2.1   Recommendation for dealing with pain in non-verbal patients (Herr et al. 2006)
>
> 1. A hierarchy of pain assessment techniques:
>   - Self-report: attempts should be made to obtain self-report from all patients.
>   - Search for potential causes of pain:
>   - o Observe patient behaviour.
>   - o Surrogate reporting of pain and behaviour/activity changes.
>   - o Attempt an analgesic trial.
> 2. Establish a procedure for pain assessment.
> 3. Use behavioural pain assessment tools as appropriate.
> 4. Minimise emphasis on physiologic indicators – they are not sensitive in discriminating pain from other sources of distress.
> 5. Reassess and document – after intervention and regularly over time the patient should be reassessed.

In infants and toddlers, although no single behavioural scale has been shown to be superior to others, a scale should be selected that is appropriate to the patient and the types of pain on which is has been tested. Behavioural pain tools should be used for initial and ongoing pain assessment. In Holly's case she is particularly susceptible to poor pain management due to her age, stage of development and cognitive impairment. It is likely that the discharging nurse's inappropriate advice was a result of her lack of knowledge of effective pain management and lack of insight into the needs of children with cognitive impairment.

Nurses' knowledge

As far back as 1996 it was accepted that the responsibility for alleviating post-operative pain rests with the nurse (Romsing 1996). Nurses play a crucial role in the assessment and management of a child's pain, because they are the only health professional that provides 24-hour bedside care, spending the most direct time with the child and family (Zhang et al. 2008). This unique position in relation to children's pain places considerable responsibility on nurses to manage pain effectively and to have the relevant knowledge to do so.

There is considerable literature exploring nurses' knowledge in relation to pain management. Twycross (2010) conducted a review of research published in the past 15 years, exploring factors that impact on the management of pain in children, and found that possible explanations included knowledge deficits, incorrect or outdated beliefs about pain and pain management, the decision-making strategies used and organisational strategies. These findings suggest that there are many complex influences that determine how children's pain is managed, and it is not down to one single nurse to get it right. In Holly's story organisational strategies could have been put in place to ensure a smoother discharge procedure, in the shape of written advice for the management of pain on discharge. Such a strategy would ensure that there was a standardised approach to discharge advice and avoid the poor advice given to Holly's mother.

Nurses' knowledge and attitudes have been found to affect nursing decisions about patient care (Rieman and Gordon 2007), which indicates that nurses need to understand pain in order to be able to recognise, assess and manage pain to improve the quality of children's pain management. Gimbler-Berglund et al. (2008) found that the way nurses manage pain in children is influenced by cooperation between nurses and physicians and nurses and parents, children's behaviour, routines in the organisation, and the experience and knowledge of nurses. Holly's admission to hospital was brief and it is unlikely that she or her mother developed a relationship with the nurses in that time.

In an attempt to understand nurses' perspectives on the barriers to pain management Twycross and Collins (2011) observed pain management practice on two children's wards in an English hospital. They found that more than half of the children observed complained of severe pain with a quarter experiencing moderate pain. However, both parents and children felt their pain was of an acceptable level or good, demonstrating the low expectations of parents and children. This low expectation could be seen as an obstacle to the effective management of pain as a lack of reporting pain by the child and family is likely to be interpreted as no pain by nurses, and therefore no intervention is required. The study also found that when parents were involved in their child's pain management it was usually initiated by them, suggesting that nurses did not encourage parents to help manage their child's pain. It would appear that the relationship between nurses and parents needs attention to redress the balance of power in relation to how pain is managed.

Wong (2003) suggests feminist theorisations are helpful by understanding power as a relational, multidimensional web, with four key types of power emerging:

Box 2.2   Wong's (2003) web of power

Power-from-within	Personal power, the psychological power derived from self-confidence, self-esteem and self-respect.
Power-to	The ability to take action, the power to participate and mobilise change.
Power-with	Collective force as people come together and cooperate to solve problems and achieve goals which they would be unable to realise alone.
Power-over	A resisting force which can be negative when used to force someone to do something against their will, but also positive when used to overrule dominance and inequality.

It could be suggested that nurses have 'power-from-within' in relation to pain management because they are more experienced than parents. Nurses also have 'power-to' in that they are in a position to engage with the management or not of a child's pain. What appears to be missing is 'power-with', where nurses could work as a collective with parents to solve pain management issues. There is real potential for nurses working with parents to achieve the desired goal of alleviating children's post-operative pain. However, by not communicating with parents, nurses leave parents powerless and disadvantaged in relation to how they can comfort the child in pain and influence the pain management process.

Having considered some of the influencing factors in the management of children's pain, it is necessary to consider what barriers there are that both parents and nurses encounter.

Barriers to pain management

The management of children's pain is complicated by how pain is identified or recognised. Children need to alert their parents to their pain. Parents in turn need to notify nurses, and nurses need the cooperation of doctors in order to have the correct prescription to administer a therapeutic dose of analgesia. This fourfold interconnected chain of events makes the likelihood of the delivery of effective pain management precarious: this process can be undermined by any one of the four stakeholders not communicating effectively with another. Several studies have explored barriers to effective pain management of children's pain. Czarnecki et al. (2010) explored nurses' (n = 272) perceptions of barriers to pain management. The four most significant barriers were insufficient analgesic prescriptions, insufficient time to medicate children prior to painful procedures, the perception of a low priority given to pain management by medical staff and parents' reluctance to have children receive analgesics. Twycross and Collins (2011) explored the views of nurses (n = 30) in a UK hospital, and identified a number of barriers to effective pain management, including a lack of knowledge about pain management on the part of nurses and doctors, staff shortages and a heavy workload and sometimes insufficient prescriptions for analgesics. The authors concluded that nurses appeared not to take as active a role as they could do in managing children's pain, preferring to view it as the parents' and child's responsibility to let them know when they are experiencing pain. Nurses also felt that parents exaggerated their child's pain and asked for analgesic drugs before their child needed them. This finding would suggest that parents are pre-empting their child's pain but that their nurses are not recognising this.

Nurses' lack of involvement of parents in the management of children's pain may contribute to poor or ineffective pain management. The issue of parents' involvement in their child's pain was explored by Simons and Roberson (2002) who interviewed 20 nurses and 20 parents in a UK children's hospital. Nurses had deficits in their pain management knowledge, yet they had unrealistic expectations of the level of knowledge parents had of pain management. They found that nurses' poor communication with parents (i.e. expecting them to notify nurses when their child had pain, yet not communicating that expectation to parents) created obstacles to effective pain management. However, it is necessary to acknowledge that dealing with children in pain can be distressing and emotionally challenging for nurses. Byrne et al. (2001) focused on emotional influences on communication by exploring how nurses construed patients who were in pain, and how these constructions were related to the emotional challenge of children's pain and to deficits in communication. The study found that nurses viewed and managed children according to a schedule of objective behavioural milestones that denied the reality or urgency of their pain and distress. These findings appear to be highly critical of nurses, however, such attitudes could be as a result of a lack of institutional support for nurses managing pain.

One of the RCN (2009) pain management guidelines states that acknowledging pain makes pain visible. It could be suggested that a number of the studies that have highlighted the barriers that prevent effective pain management have one thing in common: the barriers appear to work against the acknowledgement of the existence of pain. If pain is acknowledged, and therefore made visible, it is difficult to deny it or not to attend to the child in pain. The barriers that were identified, in relation to communication between nurses and parents, could be in place in order for nurses to avoid being confronted with pain which they either do not feel confident in dealing with, or do not place a high enough priority on to fit it into their already busy schedule.

In Holly's story the solution to the problem of controlling her pain appeared to be achieved with ease by the community children's nurse. However, it is important to acknowledge that the community nurses' confident approach was related to having studied how to effectively manage children's pain. The nurse recognised Holly's pain and confidently set about administering not only paracetamol but also an NSAID (BNFC 2012–2013) to achieve sufficient pain relief to make Holly comfortable. Many nurses do not possess this same level of confidence in administration of analgesics to children. The confidence felt by Holly's community children's nurse meant that it is likely that Holly was administered therapeutic doses of two complementary analgesics which had very good effect.

Pharmacological management of Holly's pain

Although Holly did not have effective analgesia for the first few days postoperatively, when she was reviewed by her community children's nurse she was commenced on paracetamol and ibuprofen which were effective in reducing her pain. Paracetamol (acetaminophen) is effective for mild pain in children (Anderson 2008), it has similar efficacy to non-selective NSAIDs, and may be a useful adjunct to other treatments for more severe pain.

NSAIDs are effective analgesic agents for mild to moderate pain. Although the product information states that safety in children less than 2 years old is not established, NSAIDs have been studied and used in all age groups including infants (Eustace and O'Hare 2007).

Clinical studies suggest a similar efficacy of NSAIDs and paracetamol (Hiller et al. 2006; Riad and Moussa 2007), as long as equi-effective doses are being given. Combining NSAIDs and paracetamol has been shown to improve analgesia and/or decrease the need for additional analgesia after adenoidectomy in a number of minor operative procedures (Viitanen et al. 2003; Hiller et al. 2006; Gazal and Mackie 2007; Riad and Moussa 2007).

Jennie recognised the need to give regular analgesia for a number of days so as to alleviate Holly's pain and provide reassurance to Holly's mother. By ensuring steady plasma concentrations of the analgesics, Holly's pain was well controlled. Jennie re-evaluated the effectiveness of the doses the next day. By adhering to the current guidelines, effective pain management was achieved in a short period of time. However, it is not known what the long-term consequences are of having been left in pain for several days due to misguided and inaccurate advice from the discharging nurse.

Conclusion

In the story of Holly's experience of pain, two sorts of pain management are described: the nurse who discharged Holly and her mother from hospital with inaccurate advice, and Jennie who had spent time preparing Holly and her mother for hospital, and who picked up the pieces and managed Holly's pain effectively while she was at home. The end result is that Holly's pain was eventually managed well, which demonstrates that evidence-based practice was being carried out. What is needed is that all practice becomes evidence-based and is a part of everyday norms rather than a pocket of isolated good practice. To achieve such a shift there is a need for nurses to have the educational support to be confident in their ability to intervene effectively to relieve pain, and through that confidence involve parents to continue to participate in effective pain management at home.

Key Points

- Nurses need to be proactive in their pain management practice and should ask children about their pain when it is anticipated that a procedure is likely to cause pain.
- Parents tend to under-medicate their child at home because of the difficulty of estimating the degree of their child's pain.
- Prior to discharge from hospital, children and their families should be given clearly presented information and advice regarding managing pain at home.

- Assessing pain in a non-verbal child is challenging.
- A behavioural assessment tool should be used to assess pain in young children.
- There is a need to redress the balance of power between parents and nurses in relation to pain management.

Additional Resources and Reading

- An online resource developed for parents whose children have had surgery can be found at http://mychildisinpain.org.uk/
  - o This website has been developed by researchers working with parents of children who have had day case surgery and with health care professionals who are experts in pain management. The information is especially useful for parents whose children are 2–6 years old.
- You may wish to further explore the issue of managing pain in the non-verbal patient.
  - o Herr, K., Coyne, P.J., Key, T., Manworren, R., McCaffery, M., Merken, S., Pelosi-Kelly, J. and Wild, L. (2006) 'Pain assessment in the nonverbal patient: position statement with clinical practice recommendations', *Pain Management Nursing*, 7 (2): 44–52.
- If you are interested in exploring feminist issues of power, you could read the article by Wong. Although this paper does not focus on health care it does make many pertinent points about power that can be related to how nurses work with parents, and the influence power can have in a working relationship.
  - o Wong, K.F. (2003) 'Empowerment as a panacea for poverty – old wine in new bottles? Reflections on the World Bank's conception of power', *Progress in Development Studies*, 3 (4): 307–22.

References

Anderson B.J. (2008) 'What we don't know about paracetamol in children', *Paediatric Anaesthesia*, 8(6): 451–60.

Association of Paediatric Anaesthetists (APA) (2008) *Good Practice in Postoperative and Procedural Pain*. London: APA.

Asprey, J.R. (1994) 'Postoperative analgesic prescription and administration in a pediatric population', *Journal of Pediatric Nursing*, 9 (3): 150–7.

ANZCA (Australian and New Zealand College of Anaesthetists) (2010) *Acute Pain Management: Scientific Evidence*, 3rd edn. Melbourne: Australian and New Zealand College of Anaesthetists and Faculty of Pain Medicine.

Berry. P.H. and Dahl, J.L. (2000) 'The new JCAHO pain standards: implications for pain management nurses', *Pain Management Nursing*, 1(1): 3–12.

Blacoe, D.A., Cunning, E. and Bell, G. (2008) 'Paediatric day-case surgery: an audit of unplanned hospital admission Royal Hospital for Sick Children, Glasgow', *Anaesthesia*, 63: 610–15.

Blondal, K. and Halldorsdottir, S. (2009) 'The challenge of caring for patients in pain: the nurse's perspective', *Journal of Clinical Nursing*, 18: 2897–906.

BNFC (2012–2013) *British National Formulary for Children*. Paediatric Formulary Committee. London: Pharmaceutical Press.

Breivik, H. and Stubhaug, A. (2008) 'Management of acute postoperative pain: still a long way to go!', *Pain*, 137 (2): 233–4.

Byrne, A., Morton, J. and Salmon, P. (2001) 'Defending against patients' pain: a qualitative analysis of nurses' responses to children's postoperative pain', *Journal of Psychosomatic Research*, 50: 69–76.

Czarnecki, M.L., Simon, K., Thompson, J.J., Armus, C.L., Hanson, T.C., Berg, K.A., Petrie, J.L., Xiang, Q. and Malin, S. (2010) 'Barriers to pediatric pain management: a nursing perspective', *Pain Management Nursing*, 11 (1): 15–25.

Darbyshire, P. (1994) 'Hoping for the best: live-in parents' experiences', in D.A. Gaut and A. Boykin (eds), *Caring as Healing, Renewal through Hope*. New York: National League for Nursing, pp. 183–95.

Department of Health UK (2004) *Getting the Right Start: National Service Framework for Children: Standard for Hospital Services*. London: Department of Health.

Dubois, A., Bringuier, S., Capdevilla, X. and Pry, R. (2008) 'Vocal and verbal expression of postoperative pain in preschoolers', *Pain Management Nursing*, 9 (4): 160–5.

Eland, J.M. (1988) 'Pharmacologic management of acute and chronic pediatric pain', *Issues in Comprehensive Pediatric Nursing*, 11: 93–111.

Eustace, N. and O'Hare, B. (2007) 'Use of nonsteroidal anti-inflammatory drugs in infants: a survey of members of the Association of Paediatric Anaesthetists of Great Britain and Ireland', 17 (5): 464–69.

Gazal, G. and Mackie, I.C. (2007) 'A comparison of paracetamol, ibuprofen or their combination for pain relief following extractions in children under general anaesthesia: a randomized controlled trial', *International Journal of Paediatric Dentistry*, 17 (3): 169–77.

Gimbler-Berglund, I., Ljusegren, G. and Enskar, K. (2008) 'Factors influencing pain management in children', *Paediatric Nursing*, 20 (10): 21–4.

Gorodzinsky, A.Y., Davies, W.H. and Drendel, A.L. (2013) 'Parents treatment of their children's pain at home: pharmacological and nonpharmacological approaches', *Journal of Pediatric Health Care*. Electronic Linking Issn 08915245. In press, corrected proof available at www.sciencedirect.com/science/article/pii/S0891524512003021.

Herr, K., Coyne, P.J., Key, T., Manworren, R., McCaffery, M., Merken, S., Pelosi-Kelly, J. and Wild, L. (2006) 'Pain assessment in the nonverbal patient: position statement with clinical practice recommendations', *Pain Management Nursing*, 7 (2): 44–52.

Hiller, A., Meretoja, O.A., Korpela, R. et al. (2006) 'The analgesic efficacy of acetaminophen, ketoprofen, or their combination for pediatric surgical patients having soft tissue or orthopedic procedures', *Anesthesia and Analgesia*, 102 (5): 1365–71.

IASP (International Association for the Study of Pain Special Interest Group on Pain in Childhood) (2005) *Children's Pain Matters! Priority on Pain in Infants, Children and Adolescents. A Position Statement from the Special Interest Group*. Available at www.childpain.org (accessed 12 January 2013).

Kankkunen, P., Pietila, A.M. and Vehvilainen-Julkunen. K. (2005) 'Families' and children's postoperative pain – literature review', *Journal of Pediatric Nursing*, 19 (2): 133–9.

Kankkunen, P., Vehviläinen-Julkunen, K., Pietilä, A.M., Kokki, H. and Halonen, P. (2003) 'Parents' perceptions and use of analgesics at home after children's day surgery', *Pediatric Anesthesia*, 13 (2): 132–40.

Lloyd-Thomas, A. (1998) 'Pre-emptive analgesia – relevant to children?', *Acute Pain*, 1 (2): 20–6.

Lonnqvist, P.A. and Morton, N.S. (2005) 'Postoperative analgesia in infants and children', *British Journal of Anaesthesia*, 95 (1): 59–68.

McCaffery, M. and Pasero, C. (1999) *Pain: Clinical Manual*, 2nd edn. St. Louis, MO: Mosby Inc.

Mackintosh, C. and Bowles, S. (2000) 'The effect of an acute pain service on nurses knowledge and beliefs about post-operative pain', *Journal of Clinical Nursing*, 9: 119–26.

Picker (2009) *Key Findings Report: Inpatients Survey Results*. Oxford: Picker Institute Europe.

Power, N., Liossi, C. and Franck, L. (2007) 'Helping parents to help their child with procedural and everyday pain: practical, evidence-based advice', *Journal of Specialists in Pediatric Nursing*, 12 (3): 203–9.

Riad, W. and Moussa, A. (2007) 'Pre-operative analgesia with rectal diclofenac and/or paracetamol in children undergoing inguinal hernia repair', *Anaesthesia*, 62 (12): 1241–5.

Rieman, M.T. and Gordon, M. (2007) 'Pain management competency evidenced by a survey of pediatric nurses' knowledge and attitude', *Pediatric Nursing*, 33 (4): 307–12.

Romsing, J. (1996) 'Assessment of nurses' judgement for analgesic requirements of postoperative children', *Journal of Clinical Pharmacy and Therapeutics*, 21: 159–63.

Royal College of Nursing (2009) *The Recognition and Assessment of Acute Pain in Children*. Update of full guideline. London: Royal College of Nursing.

Segerdahl, M., Warren-Stomberg, M., Rawal, N. et al. (2008) 'Clinical practice and routines for day surgery in Sweden: results from a nation-wide survey', *Acta Anaesthesiologica Scandinavica*, 52 (1): 117–24.

Simons, J. (2002) 'Parents' support and satisfaction with their child's postoperative care', *British Journal of Nursing*, 11 (22): 1442–9.

Simons, J. and Macdonald, L.M. (2004) 'Pain assessment tools: children's nurses' views', *Journal of Child Health Care*, 8 (4): 264–78.

Simons, J. and Moseley, L. (2009) 'Influences on nurses' scoring of children's post-operative pain', *Journal of Child Health Care*, 13 (2): 101–15.

Simons, J. and Roberson, E. (2002) 'Poor communication and knowledge deficits: obstacles to effective management of children's postoperative pain', *Journal of Advanced Nursing*, 40 (1): 78–86.

Taddio, A., Katz, J., Ilersich, A.L. and Koren, G. (1997)'Effect of neonatal circumcision on pain response during subsequent routine vaccination', *Lancet*, 349: 599–603.

Twycross, A. (2010) 'Managing pain in children: where to from here?', *Journal of Clinical Nursing*, 19: 2090–9.

Twycross, A. and Collins, S. (2011) 'Nurses' views about the barriers and facilitators to effective management of pediatric pain', *Pain Management Nursing*, pp. 1–9. In press, corrected proof available at www.sciencedirect.com/science/article/pii/S1524904211001937 (accessed 12 January 2013).

van Hulle, V. (2007) 'Nurses' perceptions of children's pain: a pilot study of cognitive representations', *Journal of Pain and Symptom Management*, 33 (3): 290–301.

Viitanen, H., Tuominen, N., Vaaraniemi, H. et al. (2003)'Analgesic efficacy of rectal acetaminophen and ibuprofen alone or in combination for paediatric day-case adenoidectomy', *British Journal of Anaesthesia*, 91 (3): 363–7.

Vincent, C.V. (2005) 'Nurses knowledge, attitudes and practices regarding children's pain', *American Journal of Maternal and Child Nursing*, 30 (3): 177–183.

von Baeyer, C.L. and Spagrud, L.J. (2007) 'Systematic review of observational (behavioral) measures of pain for children and adolescents aged 3 to 18 years', *Pain*, 127 (1–2): 140–50.

Walker, J. (2004) 'The nature and purpose of pain management', Editorial. *Journal of Nursing Management*, 12 (3): 147–51.

Wall, P.D. (1988) 'The prevention of postoperative pain', *Pain*, 33 (3): 289–90.

Wilson, M.E. and Helgadottir, H.L. (2006) 'Patterns of pain and analgesic use in 3 to 7 year old children after tonsillectomy', *Pain Management Nursing*, 7 (4): 159–66.

Wong, K.F. (2003) 'Empowerment as a panacea for poverty – old wine in new bottles? Reflections on the World Bank's conception of power', *Progress in Development Studies*, 3 (4): 307–22.

Zhang, C.H., Hsu, L., Bi-Rong, Z., Jian-Fang, L., Hong-Ying, W. and Huang, J. (2008) 'Effects of a pain education program on nurses' pain knowledge, attitudes and pain assessment practices in China', *Journal of Pain and Symptom Management*, 36 (6): 616–26.

Chapter 3

Managing Procedural Pain

Tilli's, Alice's and Toby's Stories

Georgina's and Tilli's story

Our little girl was taken into hospital for five days with an acute infection of the kidneys and secondary sepsis. At no time did anyone assess her pain regarding the infection despite her rubbing her tummy. Paracetamol was prescribed for pyrexia: as a nurse I knew this may help with the pain but if I hadn't been then how would I know this? Although the tummy pain was present the most painful episodes were the cannulations. We accept that while we were being transferred by ambulance and within resus at A&E, pain control was not a priority (BM 0.8, O$_2$ sats 85 per cent, tachycardia, hypertension) and that it was important that IV access was gained. However, later when she was transferred to the wards, this should have been managed.

When I asked for 'Emla cream' (a vague memory from my A&E days some years ago) I was treated like I was asking for something very much out of the ordinary and was told that the ice spray would be better. I agreed, I'm not a children's nurse and I believed them. The spray was useless and the next time I did insist on the cream, much to the nurse's disgust, what an effort to have to get that out of the cupboard!! Many, many attempts were made; each time, cannulas tissued. This involved us pinning her down while she screamed and cried. Only one doctor showed any kindness to her, the rest treated her like a piece of meat. To my absolute disgust, when I went down to the café to get food (I'm pregnant and felt faint) a trainee doctor was allowed to practise on her: my husband's not medical, he did not know he was a trainee. As I came back and 'caught' him I finally lost my temper. No one had asked us if this was okay, and as a Senior Lecturer in Health I know that our student nurses would have to ask for consent, why are doctors above this? He spoiled the last of her little veins and did not even seem to care as long as he had got his practice in.

My last bit of faith in the NHS has gone now. I know technological and medical advances are important and save lives, I know that without the IVI [intra venous infusion] she may have died, but what about compassion, empathy and basic human kindness – has this been lost amongst all our 'advances'? At a recent trip to the GP, Tilli had a panic attack when she saw a nurse in a blue tunic: she screamed and tried to get out of the doors, she was terrified.

Nikki's and Alice's story

I was looking after Alice, an 8-year-old girl who was scheduled to have a liver biopsy that morning. She had been prescribed an intramuscular premedication. I explained to her mother that she would need an injection. I also explained that I thought it might help to gain Alice's cooperation if she was allowed to choose where the injection would be administered. Alice started to cry when told she was to have an injection, then she agreed to cooperate. However, she kept changing her mind about where to have the injection – first one leg, then 'No, the other leg' and then 'Not in the treatment room, I want to be in my room'. This went on for some time. Finally her mother turned to me and said: 'Just get on with it!', so I did.

On reflection, I realised that my attempts to offer an 8-year-old child some choice in the decision were well meaning, but perhaps did not take into account that when confronted by such a stressful situation, children sometimes regress. Furthermore, it did not even occur to me to question why the premedication had to be an injection. I can see I tried to do the right thing, but I really think that I could have done a better job of thinking through the whole situation.

Sharon and Toby's story

Many years ago, when I was an RSCN student, I was asked to assist a doctor who was going to insert a cannula and take blood from Toby, who was about 5 years old. I went into the treatment room where the child was sitting on his mother's knee with the doctor poised to insert a cannula. As I was taking over from the senior nurse I assumed that Toby had been fully prepared for the procedure. The doctor who was new to the paediatric ward attempted to insert the cannula and this was unsuccessful. Toby then became distressed as a second and third attempt failed. At this point Toby and his mother were distressed. So the mum left the room and the father came in to hold the child and the fourth attempt was made. At this point the doctor was beginning to show signs of lacking confidence as she attempted to once again insert the cannula unsuccessfully. With all the distress and anxiety that was in the room, I decided to ask the doctor if she would like somebody else to have a try or could we give Toby a break to settle him down. Initially the doctor disagreed, but after I mentioned that I would need to speak with my senior nurse the doctor agreed. Toby was given time to settle by being allowed into the playroom and the parents given support and reassurance. In the end a paediatric anaesthetist inserted the cannula even though the child was distressed.

After the experience I discussed the situation with the senior nurse as I felt that the situation could have been handled in a different way, and I found that the child or parents had not been adequately prepared for the procedure by either the play specialist or nurse. On reflection I learnt a lot from this experience and this has helped me to further develop my practice. It made me aware of the importance of advance preparation of the child and family and to check that this has been carried out rather than to assume. It has also taught me that I can and should act as an advocate for the child and if a situation is spiralling out of control it is better to take control of the situation so as not to cause further distress. I have also learnt that there is no shame in saying that we have to get assistance and that we cannot do the procedure without help. The importance of preparation has also been highlighted.

Introduction

Georgina's story reflects the anguish of a mother who witnessed her child suffering pain from repeated cannulation. Georgina clearly articulates the ways in which she feels that her daughter was failed by the people caring for her. Her daughter presented at A&E with abdominal pain, pyrexia and in need of fluid resuscitation. She was diagnosed with an acute urinary tract infection and secondary sepsis, but despite being life-threatening these issues almost fade into insignificance: as Georgina said 'The most painful episodes were the cannulations'. While this story is central to the chapter, we have woven in two stories shared by nurses about their own experiences of procedural pain. These also illuminate the vital role that the nurse has as an advocate for the child and their family.

Procedures and interventions are an inevitable part of health care. What may seem to be a routine and vital intervention to a health professional will be perceived differently by the child and their parents. Many procedures are invasive; they are often painful and can be frightening. How we manage medical procedures and the potential pain associated with them is a benchmark for our commitment to caring for children in a way that predicts their needs, promotes their rights and protects them from harm. Effective management of iatrogenic pain is an ethical and moral imperative; we dare not get it wrong.

In this chapter we will explore some of the issues related to preventing and managing pain associated with procedures and interventions. We will examine what is meant by procedural pain and the incidence, extent, nature and impact of pain associated with procedures. We will also explore the importance of preparing the child and their family, and approaches which can be used to mitigate the experience. We will then consider the issues of clinical holding and advocacy as these are central to good management of procedural pain.

Procedure-related pain: definition, incidence and cause

Many of the procedures commonly used in health care to diagnose, treat or palliate can also produce acute pain (Czarnecki et al. 2011; Luthy et al. 2012). This creates an awkward paradox: while the procedures are almost always necessary, the pain and the accompanying distress are unwelcome for the child, their family and for health care professionals.

Medical procedures which can evoke pain are commonplace in health care settings. These loci are as diverse as ambulances, emergency departments, wards, clinics, dental practices, and general practitioners' surgeries, as well as in schools and, for some children, their own homes (Czarnecki et al. 2011; Curtis et al. 2012). While the procedures themselves are usually of short duration, the impact and outcomes can be long-lasting. Like other pain experiences, procedural pain results from a 'complex interplay of genetic, experiential, and developmental factors' (Walco 2008: S125).

The term procedural pain covers a wide range of procedures, the most common being immunisation. Estimates vary between studies as to how many skin-puncturing injections the average child will have experienced by the time they have completed the recommended schedule of vaccination. These estimates vary from a minimum of 18 (Curtis et al. 2012) to more than 20 (McMurtry et al. 2007; Noel et al. 2012) or 35 (Luthy et al. 2012) needles. So, although the immunisation schedule aims to protect children and keep them healthy, it also sets the context for many children's early experiences of procedural pain. Many children experience other potentially pain-evoking procedures such as intravenous cannulation, injections, heel stick and capillary blood sampling (Stinson et al. 2008; Bice et al. 2013). More substantial procedures include lumbar puncture, central venous port access, wound dressings (Nilsson et al. 2008), incision and drainage (Uspal et al. 2013), insertion of a nasogastric tube, urinary catherisation (APA 2012), nasal aspiration, joint aspiration, biopsies (Curtis et al. 2012) and endotracheal suctioning (Pillai Riddell et al. 2012). What can be described as a pain-evoking procedure is also dependent, to a degree, on developmental factors. So, for example, nappy change and weighing procedures can be deemed to be painful procedures for preterm infants (Pillai Riddell et al. 2012).

Considering the range of procedures which can cause pain, it becomes clear that hospitalised children are likely to experience at least one painful procedure during any one admission. Stevens et al. (2012) retrospectively studied children (n = 3822) in eight Canadian paediatric hospitals and found that in the 24-hour study period, a total of 18,929 procedures were recorded, and 87 per cent of the children had one or more painful procedures (mean, 6.3 painful procedures per child).

Procedures can and do cause pain and both professionals and the literature talk of 'painful procedures'. However, it is within the gift of health care professionals to ensure that these procedures are not painful. As such it would perhaps be better to talk of potentially painful procedures.

How well are we doing in managing procedural pain?

The picture is mixed in terms of how well procedural pain is being managed and this, perhaps, is reflective of the broader state of play in terms of the assessment and management of children's pain. There are reports of excellent practice, quality improvement and a real commitment to ensuring that children feel safe and comfortable during potentially painful procedures (Carrier and Walden 2001; Kolcaba and DiMarco 2005). However, despite the ubiquity of procedural pain, it is not always well-managed, even though both non-pharmacological and pharmacological interventions are available to mitigate the nociceptive effects of the procedures (APA 2012; Curtis et al. 2012). Bice et al.'s (2013) review concludes that prophylactic measures for managing procedural pain are under-utilised. Oligoanalgesia or the under-treatment of procedural pain may occur for a number of different reasons such as poor knowledge, skill, communication and attitudes, a lack of resources including time, and non-use of protocols.

In each of the stories with which we started the chapter, there are indications of the factors which result in under-treatment. In Georgina's story a mix of poor attitudes, lack of knowledge and compassion, and a lack of commitment to protecting Tilli and managing her pain results in Tilli's situation spiralling from bad to worse. In Nikki's story we see a nurse trying to do the right things for 8-year-old Alice but – despite her best efforts – getting things wrong. Nikki's story reflects the need to be careful in the promises that we make to children and the challenge inherent in getting things right for every child.

Evidence from a Cochrane review identifies two major issues which can inhibit practice enhancement: (1) an inconclusive or absent evidence base, and (2) robust evidence but problems associated with knowledge translation (Curtis et al. 2012). Quality improvement can increase the utilisation of procedural pain interventions (Bice et al. 2013) and protocols can improve pain management (Cregin et al. 2008).

However, even where protocols are used to guide practice, Kolcaba and DiMarco (2005: 187) argue that they are 'directed more to pain relief than to the comfort of each child'. This is almost certainly the case as the success of pain management is often measured through the single metric of pain intensity. This means that while comfort is important, it is frequently an overlooked outcome.

Impact and outcomes of procedural pain

Much of the work focusing on the impact of pain on children and the longer term sequelae primarily comes from evidence of infants who have been exposed to early and repeated painful experiences (Lidow 2002). As part of the life-saving treatments and monitoring of their health status in NICU, neonates often require repeated tissue-damaging procedures over a period of weeks or months; these are often painful. An increasing body of evidence suggests that early exposure to painful experiences has a wide range of consequences including increasing the gain in pain pathways (Hohmeister et al. 2009), acute and long-term effects on nociception (Knaepen et al. 2013) and 'increased anxiety, altered pain sensitivity, stress disorders, hyperactivity/attention deficit disorder, leading to impaired social skills and patterns of self-destructive behaviour' (Anand and Scalzo 2000: 69). While there is clear evidence of the noxious effects of procedural and other pain on neonates and infants, there is also evidence of the adverse effects on older children. For some children the experience of painful or distressing procedures can result in short-term and longer-term trauma which can have a major impact on their lives and well-being (Forgey and Bursch 2013). Rennick et al. (2002: 133) studied children who were hospitalised on a general ward and those on PICU and found that irrespective of the setting, it was the younger, more severely ill children who had experienced the most invasive procedures who had more medical fears six months post-discharge.

Procedural pain is a multidimensional experience for the child, inducing physical and emotional suffering, anxiety and distress. The child not only has to deal with the pain itself but also with other elements of the procedure such as being positioned in a particular way, the intrusion of catheters and needles into their body, the close proximity of the health care professionals undertaking the procedure, and strange sights, sounds and smells as well as uncertainty about what is going to happen. Kortesluoma et al.'s (2004, 2006, 2008,) work shows how children have particular and personal ways of framing pain that are based on their past experience. Such experiences will shape the way they are able to cope with future medical procedures. Walco (2008: S129) notes two major types of harm to children – the suffering during the procedure and the long-term consequences.

Increasing evidence shows that children's pain memories are powerful (Liossi and Fitzgerald 2012) and play an important role in their experience of distress during repeated stressful medical procedures (Noel et al. 2012). Children will not necessarily differentiate between the experience of pain and the distress, anxiety or fear that accompanies it. The painful procedure is experienced as a whole: this is why management is so important. Chen et al.'s (2000) study of children undergoing lumbar puncture, found they remembered both negative (length of needle) and positive (parental support) factual details.

It is fundamental to take a long view when managing children's procedural pain. Tilli's panic attack when she saw the nurse in a blue tunic at the GP's is linked to her memories of the painful procedures she endured; these memories are so vivid that they create high levels of distress and anxiety long after the event. McMurtry et al. (2011) noted that children who had a negative reaction to the blood tests had higher fear ratings than those who did not have negative reactions. Like other researchers, they also noted poor levels of agreement between the parents' and children's report of fear. While poorly managed pain associated with medical procedures can result in children being fearful of future procedures during childhood, it can also result in long-term consequences into adulthood (Pate et al. 1996).

Some research considers health care professionals' perceptions of procedures and how painful and/or distressing they are for children. Babl et al. (2008) surveyed medical and nursing staff working in an emergency department and found that the procedures perceived by staff as being the most painful were supra-pubic aspiration, intramuscular injection and lumbar puncture, and the most distressing were nasogastric tube insertion, intravenous insertion and lumbar puncture. These findings were consistent regardless of the experience level of the staff.

Health care professionals may also be affected by being part of a painful and distressing medical procedure (McCarthy and Kleiber 2006) and also being part of improved pain management can enhance their job satisfaction and their relationship with children (Papa and Zempsky 2010). This is borne out by Nikki's and Sharon's stories. Both of them have very clear memories of these particular 'stand out' moments of practice: they have taken these memories of practice to heart, reflected on them, learnt and chosen to reveal and share them with other people. At the heart of their stories are moral moments that have acted as crucibles for their subsequent nursing practice, forging a new commitment to advocacy and better pain practice.

Advocacy and comfort, rights and responsibilities

While it may be, and often is, necessary for children to undergo medical and nursing procedures, it is ethically unacceptable for a child to be exposed to pain that could have been prevented or treated. Procedures which may seem to be routine, minor and fairly inconsequential to health professionals can be perceived very differently by children. Some of the worst pains that children experience in hospital are related to procedures (Cummings et al. 1996). Needle-related pain is rated by children as one of the worst pains (Goodenough et al. 2000; Spagrud et al. 2008). Preventing or relieving suffering and advocacy is fundamental to good nursing practice and effective pain care (Vaartio et al. 2008). Advocacy requires us to analyse, counsel and respond to situations (Vaartio et al. 2009) and to do this we need to feel empowered and be courageous.

Sharon's story of acting as an advocate for the child shows how there are times when we need to intervene and ensure that the child is not lost within the drive to complete the procedure. Acting as an advocate can mean taking control of the situation and ensuring that the child's rights are protected. As a student nurse, Sharon acted courageously in urging the doctor to desist; by so doing she created a space for Toby to recover and ensured that no further attempts were made by the inexperienced doctor.

One of our responsibilities as health care professionals is to carefully consider the child's comfort (Stephens et al. 1999; Kolcaba and DiMarco 2005) before, during and after the procedure. Regardless of the urgency of the procedure, we should act with kindness and compassion and provide affirmative support to the child and family. If the health care professionals had acted with greater compassion towards Tilli and her parents, her mother may not have felt so betrayed by the 'lack of basic human kindness' when she saw her daughter being 'treated like a piece of meat'. It is unlikely that the doctor set out to be unkind and heartless, but Georgina clearly perceived and will remember the experience as being devastating.

Planning a potentially painful procedure

Good preparation does not increase the overall time required to undertake the procedure (Benore and Enlow 2013), and good planning involves understanding the factors that influence a child's response (McCarthy and Kleiber 2006).

Factors that can influence a child's response to a painful procedure

A child's response to a potentially painful procedure is a complex, multidimensional and subjective experience that is composed of physiological, emotional, sensory, developmental, social, cognitive and behavioural elements. These all need to be considered when trying to understand how and why children respond as they do to procedures. Understanding the responses that a child may have also helps us understand why non-pharmacological and pharmacological measures can contribute so effectively to pain prevention and management.

McCarthy and Kleiber (2006) present a model of the factors influencing children's responses to a painful procedure when their parents are acting as distraction coaches. Elements from this model and work by other authors can be translated into a visual depiction of the core child-parent-procedural factors which influence a child's response to a painful procedure (see Figure 3.1). A complex mix of child-related factors works alongside an equally complex set of parent-related factors. Both of these

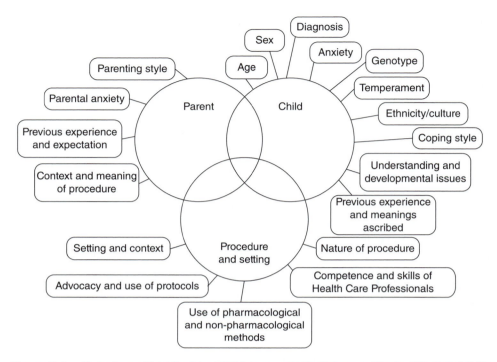

Figure 3.1   Overview of key factors which can negatively or positively affect a child's distress and coping

Developed from Frank et al. (1995); Blount et al. (1989), McMurtry et al. (2007) and Nilsson et al. (2011)

sets of factors are linked to procedural and setting factors. Attending to all three major elements (child, parent and procedure/setting) is likely to result in the best care and support of the child.

Factors which influence a child's distress and coping associated with a procedure

While good pain management is fundamental in any procedure, it is also important to manage the child's distress and support their coping strategies, as fear and anxiety can 'wind up' the pain experience. Factors can either heighten (e.g. criticism, apologies, poor planning) or mitigate (e.g. humour, commands to cope, non-procedural talk, engaging the child and using non-pharmacological techniques) the amount of distress that the child experiences. It is important for health care professionals to ensure that the child feels secure, prepared, able to participate in the procedure if they so wish and can draw on their own coping strategies. Kortesluoma et al. (2008) found that children used different coping strategies including thought-stopping, positive self-talk and positive actions.

Planning for good practice

While health care professionals should attend to the actual physical task they are performing (e.g., lumbar puncture, cannulation) this should not be at the cost of the wider elements of their performance. A narrow preoccupation with the actual task has been suggested as a contributing factor to poor pain management (Curtis and Morrell 2006) whereas psycho-educational preparation can have beneficial effects on parental anxiety and reduced children's behavioural distress (Benore and Enlow 2013).

Children are often held during the procedure to ensure that they do not move. Clinical holding can take many forms, from gentle, supportive cradling to a form of restraint. Jacobsen et al. (1990) noted that 39 per cent of children required to be physically restrained during venepuncture. Bray et al.'s (2013) study of clinical holding during medical procedures also noted that parents and professionals tended to perceive that a child's short-term distress was acceptable if the procedure could be completed quickly and that parents and professionals persevered to complete procedures in spite of the difficulties they experienced. However, they also noted that preparation and support and praise could result in children having fairly positive outcomes. Figure 3.2 provides a visual 'map' of the child's response to the experience; the faces reflect the child's emotion and the height of the 'lollipop' stick shows the intensity of the expressed emotion.

Ensuring good practice occurs requires paying careful attention to the following stages: (1) before the procedure when a plan needs to be established and the team, child and family prepared; (2) during the procedure; and (3) after the procedure (see Table 3.1); evaluation should be ongoing. The children in Nilsson et al.'s (2011) study expressed the importance of their nurses noticing their total pain experience and making them feel safe.

Saying the right thing to a child

How we talk to children before, during and after a procedure is important, but despite our best efforts we can get this wrong. Much of the work looking at language and communication has focused on child distress during procedures rather than looking specifically at pain. Parental reassurance is conveyed through a combination of the language used, the intonation of the words (e.g. a soothing tone) and the facial expression of the parent (McMurtry et al. 2006). Although the evidence is reasonably strong in relation to parental reassurance and immunisation and injections, there is little evidence about reassurance in older children and/or children experiencing other medical procedures.

McMurtry et al. (2006, 2007) conclude that parental 'reassurance can hurt' rather than support their child. McMurtry et al.'s (2011, 2010) work and that of others (Manimala et al. 2000; Chambers et al. 2002) suggests that what parents should be saying to young children is in fact the opposite of what they tend instinctively to say. Most studies, apart from Gonzalez et al.'s (1993), have found that parental reassurance

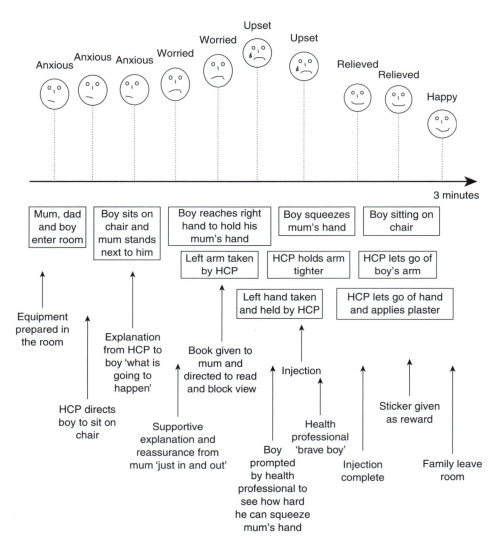

Figure 3.2 'Lollipop' map showing child's responses, actions taken by parents and HCP and key events during venipuncture

Table 3.1 Good practice for the management of potentially painful procedures

Before the procedure: establishing a plan and preparing the team

- Protect the child from unnecessary procedures.
- Avoid multiple procedures, wherever possible, plan the timing of procedures to minimise frequency.
- Consider whether modification of the procedure could reduce the child's experience of pain.
- Consider the developmental differences in the response to pain and analgesic efficacy when planning analgesia.
- Identify pharmacological and non-pharmacological interventions that are appropriate to the child, taking into account their individual needs, their previous pain history and response to procedural pain.
- Work with the child (and their family as appropriate) to develop a mutually agreed plan using appropriate methods such as distraction to help the child to cope before, during and after the procedure.
- Consider whether the child's particular circumstances (e.g. previous exposure, distressed response to painful procedures, need to remain still for a long time, level of pain and/or invasiveness) mean that sedation or general anaesthesia may be required for a safe and satisfactory outcome.
- Identify whether the planned environment is suitable. Ideally, this should be a quiet, calm place with suitable distractions such as toys, games, music, and preferably not the child's hospital room.
- Ensure that health care staff who possess the necessary technical, support and communication skills and competence are available.
- Allow sufficient time for analgesic drugs and other analgesic measures to be effective.
- Ensure there is a clear action plan of what will happen if initial pain measure(s) do not work or if the procedure fails, including the option that the procedure will be stopped.
- Ensure that the health care staff are prepared and establish the specific roles (e.g., undertaking procedure, assessing child's pain, holding, coaching) that each will take during the procedure (if more than one person involved).
- Ensure that there are sufficient staff to undertake the procedure safely.

Before the procedure: preparing the child and family

- Determine any concerns or anxieties that the child and family have in relation to the procedure and take these into account.
- Ensure that appropriate information and education are provided that meet the child's (and family's) particular needs.
- Determine whether the child's mother/father/caregiver is planning to stay with the child and help them to understand the procedure, their role as a support to their child and/or how to hold their child, if needed.
- Ensure that the child and family are clear about the technique they will be using within the procedure to help them cope.
- Determine with the child how they will communicate during the procedure any unrelieved pain or anxiety.

(Continued)

Table 3.1   (Continued)

During the procedure

- Ensure that the agreed support techniques, such as distraction, are used during the procedure.
- Ensure that the coach/health care staff use appropriate tone and language to communicate with and reassure the child.
- Ensure that assessment of the child's pain and/or anxiety is ongoing throughout the procedure and that the planned measures are taken if the child's pain and/or anxiety are not effectively managed. Add in extra pharmacological and/or non-pharmacological support as needed, and/or halt the procedure if necessary.
- Maintain a safe, relaxed, supportive atmosphere and environment, and identify and act on any issues of concern.

After the procedure

- Ensure that the child and/or their family have an opportunity to provide feedback about their experience of the procedure.
- Ensure that the procedure, the measures taken and the child's/family's responses to it are documented.
- Refine the plan used for this procedure based on the knowledge gained from how this procedure went.
- Ensure that assessment of the child's comfort is undertaken after completion of the procedure to ensure any further pain interventions are provided as necessary.

Developed from APA (2012) and Czarnecki et al. (2011)

is linked to child distress. Research undertaken with 4–6-year-olds being immunised strongly suggests that parental reassurance can actually result in greater amounts of distress, a greater likelihood of the need for restraint and more verbal fear than is the case with children using attention control or distraction (Manimala et al. 2000).

Parental reassurance such as 'don't worry, it's going to be alright' or 'this won't hurt much' is likely to trigger a young child's concerns about what is going to happen, what they should be worrying about and that it will hurt. Three mechanisms potentially explain the link between children's distress and parental reassurance are (1) reassurance may warn the child of their parents' anxiety about what is about to happen; (2) reassurance may reinforce the child's distress behaviour in a cyclical manner with the child expressing more distress and gaining more reassurance; and (3) parental reassurance may create the opportunity for the child to express their negative emotions (McMurtry et al. 2006).

Parents should be encouraged to use affirmative language that positively reinforces the child's sense of control such as 'You're doing really well' and 'You're holding your arm beautifully still'. There is not much evidence about the language that should be used by health care professionals, although it is likely we should also be talking affirmatively, clearly and directly to the children and avoiding negative language that can trigger worries.

Pharmacological and non-pharmacological interventions for managing pain associated with procedures

Since medical procedures can be accompanied by pain, distress and anxiety it is important for health care professionals to have access to a broad repertoire of interventions. The APA (2012) recommend that, whenever possible, both pharmacological and non-pharmacological strategies should be employed. Although medical procedures which evoke pain are commonplace, surprisingly little robust evidence exists to underpin practice in all but the most frequently performed procedures (see Table 3.2 and APA 2012).

Pharmacological interventions for managing procedural pain

The ideal pharmacological agent would be easy to administer, quick-acting, have no adverse effects, not add to the distress and anxiety associated with a procedure, be acceptable to the child, family and health care professionals, and not delay or decrease the success rate of the procedure. One of the reasons why pharmacological

Table 3.2 Overview of specific recommendations for procedural pain in older children

Procedure	Recommendations	Grading		
		A	B	C
Blood sampling and intravenous cannulation	Topical local anaesthetic (LA) should be used for intravenous cannulation.			
	Psychological strategies, e.g., distraction or hypnosis, to reduce pain and anxiety should be used.	✓		
Lumbar puncture (LP)	Behavioural techniques of pain management should be used to reduce LP pain.	✓		
	Topical LA and LA infiltration are effective for LP pain and do not decrease success rates.		✓	
	50% nitrous oxide in oxygen should be offered to children willing and able to cooperate.			✓
Bladder catheterisation and related urine sampling procedures	Psychological preparation and psychological and behavioural interventions should be used during bladder catheterisation and invasive investigations of the renal tract.		✓	
	Infants: consider procedure modification as urethral catheterisation is less painful than supra pubic aspiration (SPA) for urine sampling.		✓	

(Continued)

Table 3.2   (Continued)

Procedure	Recommendations	Grading		
		A	B	C
Immunisation and intramuscular injection	Psychological strategies such as distraction should be used for infants and children undergoing vaccination.	✓		
	Consider additional procedure modifications such as vaccine formulation, order of vaccines (least painful first) needle size, depth of injection (25mm, 25-gauge needle) or the use of a vapocoolant spray.	✓		
	Swaddling, breastfeeding or a pacifier, and sucrose should be considered in infants undergoing vaccination.	✓		
Laceration repair	For repair of simple low-tension lacerations, tissue adhesives should be considered as they are less painful, quick to use, and have a similar cosmetic outcome to sutures or adhesive skin closures (steri-strips).	✓		
	Topical anaesthetic preparations, for example, LAT (lidocaine-adrenaline-tetracaine) if available, can be used in preference to injected LA, as they are less painful to apply; it is not necessary to use a preparation containing cocaine.	✓		
	Buffering injected lidocaine with sodium bicarbonate should be considered.	✓		
	Hair apposition technique (HAT) should be considered for scalp lacerations. It is less painful than suturing, does not require shaving, and produces a similar outcome.		✓	
	If injected lidocaine is used, pre-treatment of the wound with a topical anaesthetic preparation, for example, lidocaine-adrenaline-tetracaine (LAT) gel, reduces the pain of subsequent injection.		✓	
	50% nitrous oxide reduces pain and anxiety during laceration repair.		✓	
Dressing change in children with burns	Potent opioid analgesia given by oral, transmucosal, or nasal routes according to patient preference and availability of suitable preparations should be considered for dressing changes in burned children.	✓		
	Non-pharmacological therapies such as distraction and relaxation should be considered as part of pain management for dressing changes in burned children.		✓	

Developed from APA (2012)

agents are not used or used ineffectively is because they do not necessarily meet these criteria for clinical utility. For example, EMLA® works well but only if it has been applied properly and left on the skin for long enough. Conversely, a vapocoolant spray wears off very quickly, so cannulation must take place within seconds of its application. As with any medication prescribed for a child, the health care professional should be clear about how to administer it and how it works, as inappropriate usage impacts on its potential therapeutic impact.

Georgina's story is distressing because, until she asked for EMLA cream, no attempt was made to pharmacologically intervene with the pain of gaining IV access. Georgina talks of being treated as if she was 'asking for something very much out of the ordinary', yet in reality a topical anaesthetic should routinely be available for use as part of procedural management. Georgina's recollection of the apparent 'effort to have to get [the EMLA] out of the cupboard' reflects really badly on the health care professionals providing care. Nothing we do should ever look like it is an effort, and while pain management might be challenging it should never be too much trouble.

A wide range of different pharmacological agents is proposed for procedural pain. The choice of pharmacological agent will be dependent, to a degree, on factors related to the child, parent and procedure and setting (see Figure 3.1) and choices must be made based on a clear assessment and pain management plan. Within this chapter attention is paid to three common procedures.

Blood sampling and intravenous cannulation

High quality evidence exists for the use of topical local anaesthetics such as EMLA®, amethocaine (AMETOP®) and buffered lidocaine in the management of venous cannulation (Koh et al. 2004). When compared with EMLA®, amethocaine is often seen to be superior (Stinson et al. 2008; Curtis et al. 2012), as it has a faster onset of action (30 minutes compared to at least 60 minutes), which is particularly useful in settings where it is necessary to undertake the procedure without delay. Amethocaine also has a duration of 4–6 hours compared to 1–2 hours for EMLA® after application (O'Brien et al. 2005).

The stories that both Georgina and Sharon told could have been vastly different if a topical agent such as amethocaine had been used. Most failures to manage cannulation/blood sampling pain result from 'operator failure'; for example, insufficient time from application of the product to the procedure taking place or the product 'not working' because of delays to the procedure. If cannulation is expected to be tricky then an experienced person should undertake the procedure and it can also be helpful to apply the agent in several places so that if cannulation fails at site A, then the opportunity is there for a pain-free attempt at site B. Although there are no specific guidelines on how many attempts it is acceptable to make, individual professionals should not have multiple attempts to cannulate. Adopting this approach could certainly have helped to protect Toby from an inexperienced doctor's attempts to cannulate him. As a student nurse, Sharon acted well – although maybe a little late – in standing up for Toby. Giving a child a chance to recover between attempts and reconsidering the pain management plan are important. If the health care professionals caring for Tilli had taken this stance then much of the distress she experienced could have been avoided.

Vapocoolant spray has a less robust evidence base than either EMLA® or ame-thocaine with mixed evidence supporting its use. Farion et al. (2008) showed good pain reduction results and no delay in cannulation, whereas Costello et al. (2006) showed no difference between children treated with vapocoolant spray and the controls and Moore et al.'s (2009) review of eight randomised trials of coolant sprays concluded the results were ambiguous and difficult to explain. Georgina's experience of the ice spray used on Tilli was that it was 'useless'. However, it could have been that it was not applied correctly or that the attempted insertion of the cannula was undertaken when the very short-term effect of the coolant had worn off.

Nasogastric tube insertion

Nasogastric tube insertion is invasive, distressing and painful and there is little direct evidence to support best practice in children (APA 2012). Evidence from adult studies suggests that the use of a lubricant and topical local anaesthesia can reduce pain. Nebulised lidocaine has also been shown to be effective in adults, although Kuo et al. (2010) note that there is 'insufficient evidence to recommend the dosage, concentration, or delivery method'. Babl et al.'s (2009) study of the use of nebulised lidocaine during nasogastric insertion showed no benefit to children aged between 1–5 years.

Immunisation and intramuscular injection

Injections and immunisations are recognised as being painful and they can be distressing for children. The APA (2012) recommend that wherever possible intra-muscular injections should not be given as part of a child's routine care.

Not only can children be highly distressed but parents can also be distressed by vaccine-associated pain; this may result in them avoiding taking their child for vac-cination (Luthy et al. 2012). Immunisation pain can be managed with vapocoolant spray (Cohen Reis and Holubkov 1997) and EMLA®. The APA further note that where possible the vaccination procedure should be modified; for example, where more than one vaccine is being given, the least painful vaccine should be given first (Taddio et al. 2009) and the size of the needle and depth of injection should be carefully considered (Diggle et al. 2006).

Nikki's story of Alice and the intramuscular premedication is a story of a nurse who honours the child's agency. Nikki tries hard to gain Alice's cooperation but fails to set boundaries and 8–year-old Alice is astute enough to use some excellent delaying tactics. Having relinquished control to the child, Nikki finds it difficult to regain it and eventually Alice's mother takes partial control of the situation by demanding that Nikki 'just gets on with it'. The situation however remains muddled; neither Nikki nor Alice/her mother gain effective control again. Nikki admits she could have done a 'better job of thinking through the whole situation'. Advanced planning could have resulted in everyone being better prepared and Nikki might have been able to ques-tion the appropriateness of premedication being given by the intramuscular route.

Non-pharmacological interventions for managing procedural pain

Although there is little systematic research (Polkki et al. 2003) there is increasingly sound evidence for a core number of non-pharmacological interventions. This evidence demonstrates that when used appropriately, they can effectively contribute to mitigating a child's experience of pain during a medical procedure (American Academy of Pediatrics et al. 2001), as well as having the effect of reducing anticipatory and procedural anxiety. Yet despite this, they are not routinely or consistently used in practice. The child's own preferences for which intervention to use should be taken into account (Koller and Goldman 2012). A wide range of non-pharmacological methods can be used both in terms of preparing the child for and supporting them throughout the procedure.

Non-pharmacological interventions work by modifying cognitive and affective pathways, thus reducing the child's fear and anxiety and increasing their sense of control. Non-pharmacological methods include making changes to the physical techniques used in a procedure, such as modifying the way an injection is given (Taddio et al. 2009), use of cold therapy (Ebner 1996) and the use of TENS (Lander and Fowler-Kerry 1993); however, the evidence is often contradictory and inconclusive. Modifications to the child's environment and surroundings, such as the use of calming language (McMurtry 2010) and the creation of a secure (Nilsson et al. 2011) calm atmosphere, have also been shown to be helpful. Cognitive-behavioural techniques such as hypnosis (Richardson et al. 2006), guided imagery (Mosiman and Pile 2013), procedural preparation (Cohen and MacLaren 2007; Jaaniste et al. 2007) and distraction (Miller et al. 2011; Schmitt et al. 2011) have been found to be helpful. Stinson et al.'s (2008) review of systematic reviews showed that hypnosis and distraction had the best evidence base for their effectiveness, although Curtis et al. (2012) note that distraction is not always successful.

Distraction

Distraction is by far the most commonly used method in practice and it encompasses a wide range of approaches. Distraction is a means by which a child becomes engaged in an activity or behaviour that shifts their attention from the pain (Koller and Goldman 2012) and the child's role can be active or passive (Kleiber and Harper 1999) (see Figure 3.3). Generally, active distraction methods are perceived as better than passive methods, as they more fully demand the child's attention and engagement, although the findings are not really conclusive (Koller and Goldman 2012). Some children, due to illness, cognitive impairment or disability, may prefer or only be able to engage in passive approaches such as watching television during a venepuncture; these can be successful (Bellieni et al. 2006).

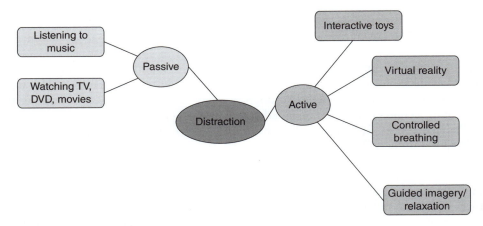

Figure 3.3   Active and passive distraction techniques

New technologies create possibilities for new forms of distraction, such as interactive toys (Jameson et al. 2011) and immersive and non-immersive virtual reality (Windich-Biermeier et al. 2007; Malloy and Milling 2010; Schmitt et al. 2011). These create absorbing environments for children and engage many of their senses: as one child explained 'I was relaxed, I did not notice that she removed the stitches' (Nilsson et al. 2011: 1453). However, techniques such as virtual reality are quite complex and costly and seem to work best when the game is tailored to the child and the situation.

Audio-visual distraction techniques, which engage the children in different activities such as playing games on an iPad, watching cartoons, DVDs, the TV or using distraction cards, have all had some success (Bagnasco et al. 2012; Downey and Zun 2012; Inal and Kelleci 2012; Luthy et al. 2012; McQueen et al. 2012).

Measures such as controlled breathing in bubble blowing (Sparks 2001), guided imagery and relaxation (Huth et al. 2004; Cregin et al. 2008) and asking a child to squeeze a soft ball during a procedure (Sadeghi et al. 2013) are simple, less costly and less reliant on technology. They are also simple to learn and use, can be undertaken in nearly any setting and are measures that the child can use for themselves.

Health care professionals need to have a basic understanding of these approaches and then implement them as appropriate with the children they care for.

Conclusion

Despite knowing that many procedures are inherently painful and that children often become distressed before, during and after procedures, there is still a high level of inconsistency in how health care professionals manage procedure-related pain. The stories that triggered this chapter on procedural pain all reflect different facets of procedural pain management. Georgina clearly understood that 'without the IV [Tilly] may have died'. Within Georgina's story there are two plotlines; the first is about technical and medical competence. The second and much more impassioned storyline is about the lack of 'compassion, empathy and basic human kindness'. While Sharon's story is also about technical competence, she reflects on the tensions she experienced in acting as Toby's advocate. Nikki's story is of a nurse who 'tried to do the right thing … but could have done a better job of thinking through the whole situation'. We can learn from these stories about the technical skills we need to care for children and their parents. We can also learn about the need to underpin our relationships with children undergoing procedures with compassion or 'intelligent kindness' (Commissioning Board Chief Nursing Officer and DH Chief Nursing Adviser 2012: 13).

Poor management of pain associated with medical procedures is not only an issue for individual health care professionals, it is also an organisational and health policy issue (Latimer et al. 2010). Stevens et al. (2011) call for clinicians and researchers to become engaged in developing strategies to improve caregiving.

This does not seem to be too much to ask of health care professionals. Optimal prevention and/or management of the pain that we are directly responsible for inflicting should be the very least that children and families can expect of us.

Key Points

- Managing medical procedures and the associated potential pain should reflect a commitment to caring for children in a way that predicts their needs, promotes their rights and protects them from harm.
- Procedural pain is a multi-dimensional experience for the child that can, unless managed well, induce physical and emotional suffering, anxiety and distress.
- Health care professionals should attend to the actual physical task they are performing but this should not be at the cost of the wider elements of their perfomance.
- Parents should be encouraged to use affirmative language that positively reinforces the child's sense of control.
- Since medical procedures can be accompanied by pain, distress and anxiety, health care professionals should have access to a broad repertoire of pharmacological and non-pharmacological interventions.
- Our relationships with children undergoing procedures should be underpinned by with compassion and 'intelligent kindness'.

Additional Resources and Reading

- For more information on managing pain arising from procedures and operations see APA 2012; Curtis et al. 2012; Pillai Riddell et al. 2012.
- For detailed information on different analgesics and local anaesthetic agents (e.g., doses, routes, adverse effects), go to the *British National Formulary for Children* (BNFC), available at www.bnf.org/bnf/org_450055.htm
- The Medicines for Children website (www.medicinesforchildren.org.uk/) gives parents practical and reliable advice about giving medicine to their child.

References

American Academy of Pediatrics, Committee on Psychosocial Aspects of Child and Family Health and American Pain Society, Task Force on Pain in Infants, Children, and Adolescents (2001) 'The assessment and management of acute pain in infants, children, and adolescents', *Pediatrics*, 108 (3): 793–7.

Anand, K.J.S. and Scalzo, F.M. (2000) 'Can adverse neonatal experiences alter brain development and subsequent behavior?', *Biology of the Neonate*, 77 (2): 69–82.

Association of Paediatric Anaesthetists (APA) (2012) '*Good Practice in Postoperative and Procedural Pain Management*, 2nd edn', *Pediatric Anesthesia*, 22 (Supplement 1): 1–79.

Babl, F.E., Goldfinch, C., Mandrawa, C., Crellin, D., O'Sullivan, R. and Donath, S. (2009) 'Does nebulized lidocaine reduce the pain and distress of nasogastric tube insertion in young children? A randomized, double-blind, placebo-controlled trial', *Pediatrics*, 123 (6): 1548–55.

Babl, F.E., Mandrawa, C., O'Sullivan, R. and Crellin, D. (2008) 'Procedural pain and distress in young children as perceived by medical and nursing staff', *Pediatric Anesthesia*, 18 (5): 412–19.

Bagnasco, A., Pezzi, E., Rosa, F., Fornonil, L. and Sasso, L. (2012) 'Distraction techniques in children during venipuncture: an Italian experience', *Journal of Preventive Medicine and Hygiene*, 53 (1): 44–8.

Bellieni, C.V., Cordelli, D.M., Raffaelli, M., Ricci, B., Morgese, G. and Buonocore, G. (2006) 'Analgesic effect of watching TV during venipuncture', *Archives of Disease in Childhood*, 91 (12): 1015–17.

Benore, E. and Enlow, T. (2013) 'Improving pediatric compliance with EEG: decreasing procedural anxiety and behavioral distress', *Epilepsy & Behavior*, 27 (1): 169–73.

Bice, A.A., Gunther, M. and Wyatt, T. (2013) 'Increasing nursing treatment for pediatric procedural pain', *Pain Management Nursing*, in press corrected proof, doi: 10.1016/j. pmn.2012.004.

Bray, L., Snodin, J., McArthur, E., Traynor, H., Carter, B. and Twigg, E. (2013) 'Clinically holding children and young people for procedures or interventions within a children's hospital'. Unpublished Report.

Carrier, C.T. and Walden, M. (2001) 'Integrating research and standards to improve pain management practices for newborns and infants', *Newborn and Infant Nursing Reviews*, 1 (2): 122–31.

Chambers, C.T., Craig, K.D. and Bennett, S.M. (2002) 'The impact of maternal behavior on children's pain experiences: an experimental analysis', *Journal of Pediatric Psychology*, (27): 293–302.

Chen, E., Zeltzer, L.K., Craske, M.G. and Katz, E.R. (2000) 'Children's memories for painful cancer treatment procedures: implications for distress', *Child Development*, 71 (4): 933–47.

Cohen, L.L. and MacLaren, J.E. (2007) 'Breaking down the barriers to pediatric procedural preparation', *Clinical Psychology: Science and Practice*, 14 (2): 14428.

Cohen Reis, E. and Holubkov, R. (1997) 'Vapocoolant spray is equally effective as EMLA cream in reducing immunization pain in school-aged children', *Pediatrics*, 100 (6): E5–E5.

Commissioning Board Chief Nursing Officer and DH Chief Nursing Adviser (2012) *Compassion in Practice*. Department of Health, NHS Commissioning Board. Available at www.commissioningboard.nhs.uk (accessed 8 August 2013).

Costello, M., Ramundo, M., Christopher, N.C. and Powell, K.R. (2006) 'Ethyl vinyl chloride vapocoolant spray fails to decrease pain associated with intravenous cannulation in children', *Clinical Pediatrics*, 45 (7): 628–32.

Cregin, R., Rappaport, A.S., Montagnino, G., Sabogal, G., Moreau, H. and Abularrage, J.J. (2008) 'Improving pain management for pediatric patients undergoing nonurgent painful procedures', *AJHP: Official Journal of the American Society of Health-System Pharmacists*, 65 (8): 723–7.

Cummings, E.A., Reid, G.J., Finley, G.A., McGrath, P.J. and Ritchie, J.A. (1996) 'Prevalence and source of pain in pediatric inpatients', *Pain*, 68: 25–31.

Curtis, L.A. and Morrell, T.D. (2006) 'Pain management in the emergency department', *Emergency Medicine Practice*, 8 (7): 1–28.

Curtis, S., Wingert, A. and Ali, S. (2012) 'The Cochrane Library and procedural pain in children: an overview of reviews', *Evidence-Based Child Health*, 7 (5): 1363.

Czarnecki, M.L., Turner, H.N., Collins, P.M., Doellman, D., Wrona, S. and Reynolds, J. (2011) 'Procedural pain management: a position statement with clinical practice recommendations', *Pain Management Nursing*, 12 (2): 95–111.

Diggle, L., Deeks, J.J. and Pollard, A.J. (2006) 'Effect of needle size on immunogenicity and reactogenicity of vaccines in infants: randomised controlled trial', *British Medical Journal (International Edition)*, 333 (7568): 571–4.

Downey, L.V.A. and Zun, L.S. (2012) 'The impact of watching cartoons for distraction during painful procedures in the emergency department', *Pediatric Emergency Care*, 28 (10): 1033–5.

Ebner, C.A. (1996) 'Cold therapy and its effect on procedural pain in children', *Issues in Comprehensive Pediatric Nursing*, 19 (3): 197–208.

Farion, K.J., Splinter, K.L., Newhook, K., Gaboury, I. and Splinter, W.M. (2008) 'The effect of vapocoolant spray on pain due to intravenous cannulation in children: a randomized controlled trial', *CMAJ*, 179 (1): 31–6.

Forgey, M. and Bursch, B. (2013) 'Assessment and management of pediatric iatrogenic medical trauma', *Current Psychiatry Reports*, 15 (2): 340.

Gonzalez, J.C., Routh, D.K. and Armstrong, F.D. (1993) 'Effects of maternal distraction versus reassurance on children's reactions to injections', *Journal of Pediatric Psychology*, 18 (5): 593–604.

Goodenough, B., Perrott, D.A., Champion, G.D. and Thomas, W. (2000) 'Painful pricks and prickle pains: is there a relation between children's ratings of venipuncture pain and parental assessments of usual reaction to other pains?', *Clinical Journal of Pain*, 16 (2): 135–43.

Hohmeister, J., Demirakça, S., Zohsel, K., Flor, H. and Hermann, C. (2009) 'Responses to pain in school-aged children with experience in a neonatal intensive care unit: cognitive aspects and maternal influences', *European Journal of Pain*, 13 (1): 94–102.

Huth, M.M., Broome, M.E. and Good, M. (2004) 'Imagery reduces children's post-operative pain', *Pain*, 110 (1–2): 439–48.

Inal, S. and Kelleci, M. (2012) 'Distracting children during blood draw: looking through distraction cards is effective in pain relief of children during blood draw', *International Journal of Nursing Practice*, 18 (2): 210–19.

Jaaniste, T., Hayes, B. and von Baeyer, C.L. (2007) 'Providing children with information about forthcoming medical procedures: a review and synthesis', *Clinical Psychology: Science and Practice*, 14 (2): 124–43.

Jacobsen, P.B., Manne, S.L., Gorfinkle, K., Schorr, O., Rapkin, B. and Redd, W.H. (1990) 'Analysis of child and parent behavior during painful medical procedures', *Health Psychology*, 9 (5): 559–76.

Jameson, E., Trevena, J. and Swain, N. (2011) 'Electronic gaming as pain distraction', *Pain Research & Management*, 16 (1): 27–32.

Kleiber, C. and Harper, D.C. (1999) 'Effects of distraction on children's pain and distress during medical procedures: a meta-analysis', *Nursing Research*, 48 (1): 44–9.

Knaepen, L., Patijn, J., van Kleef, M., Mulder, M., Tibboel, D. and Joosten, E.A. (2013) 'Neonatal repetitive needle pricking: plasticity of the spinal nociceptive circuit and extended postoperative pain in later life', *Developmental Neurobiology*, 73 (1): 85–97.

Koh, J.L., Harrison, D., Myers, R., Dembinski, R., Turner, H. and McGraw, T. (2004) 'A randomized, double-blind comparison study of EMLA and ELA-Max for topical anesthesia in children undergoing intravenous insertion', *Paediatric Anaesthesia*, 14 (12): 977–82.

Kolcaba, K. and DiMarco, M.A. (2005) 'Comfort theory and its application to pediatric nursing', *Pediatric Nursing*, 31 (3): 187–94.

Koller, D. and Goldman, R.D. (2012) 'Distraction techniques for children undergoing procedures: a critical review of pediatric research', *Journal of Pediatric Nursing*, 27 (6): 652–81.

Kortesluoma, R. and Nikkonen, M. (2004) '"I had this horrible pain": the sources and causes of pain experiences in 4- to 11-year-old hospitalized children', *Journal of Child Health Care*, 8 (3): 210–31.

Kortesluoma, R. and Nikkonen, M. (2006) '"The most disgusting ever": children's pain descriptions and views of the purpose of pain', *Journal of Child Health Care*, 10 (3): 213–27.

Kortesluoma, R., Nikkonen, M. and Serlo, W. (2008) '"You just have to make the pain go away" – children's experiences of pain management', *Pain Management Nursing*, 9 (4): 143–9.

Kuo, Y., Yen, M., Fetzer, S. and Lee, J. (2010) 'Reducing the pain of nasogastric tube intubation with nebulized and atomized lidocaine: a systematic review and meta-analysis', *Journal of Pain and Symptom Management*, 40 (4): 613–20.

Lander, J. and Fowler-Kerry, S. (1993) 'TENS for children's procedural pain', *Pain*, 52 (2): 209–16.

Latimer, M.A., Ritchie, J.A. and Johnston, C.C. (2010) 'Individual nurse and organizational context considerations for better knowledge use in pain care', *Journal of Pediatric Nursing*, 25 (4): 274–81.

Lidow, M.S. (2002) 'Long-term effects of neonatal pain on nociceptive systems', *Pain*, 99 (3): 377–83.

Liossi, C. and Fitzgerald, M. (2012) 'Remember, remember, a child's pain experience', *Pain*, 153 (8): 1543–4.

Luthy, K.E., Beckstrand, R.L. and Pulsipher, A. (2012) 'Evaluation of methods to relieve parental perceptions of vaccine-associated pain and anxiety in children: a pilot study (in press)', *Journal of Pediatric Health Care*, 27 (5): 351–8.

Malloy, K.M. and Milling, L.S. (2010) 'The effectiveness of virtual reality distraction for pain reduction: a systematic review', *Clinical Psychology Review*, 30 (8): 1011–18.

Manimala, M.R., Blount, R.L. and Cohen, L.L. (2000) 'The effects of parental reassurance versus distraction on child distress and coping during immunizations', *Children's Health Care*, 29 (3): 161–77.

McCarthy, A.M. and Kleiber, C. (2006) 'A conceptual model of factors influencing children's responses to a painful procedure when parents are distraction coaches', *Journal of Pediatric Nursing*, 21 (2): 88–98.

McMurtry, C.M. (2010) *A Multi-method Examination of Adult Reassurance During Children's Painful Medical Procedures*. Unpublished doctoral dissertation. Halifax, Nova Scotia: Dalhousie University.

McMurtry, C.M., McGrath, P.J., Asp, E. and Chambers, C.T. (2007) 'Parental reassurance and pediatric procedural pain: a linguistic description', *The Journal of Pain*, 8 (2): 95–101.

McMurtry, C.M., McGrath, P.J. and Chambers, C.T. (2006) 'Reassurance can hurt: parental behavior and painful medical procedures', *Journal of Pediatrics*, 148 (4): 560–1.

McMurtry, C.M., Noel, M., Chambers, C.T. and McGrath, P.J. (2011) 'Children's fear during procedural pain: preliminary investigation of the Children's Fear Scale', *Health Psychology*, 30 (6): 780–8.

McQueen, A., Cress, C. and Tothy, A. (2012) 'Using a tablet computer during pediatric procedures a case series and review of the "apps"', *Pediatric Emergency Care*, 28 (7): 712–14.

Miller, K., Rodger, S., Kipping, B. and Kimble, R.M. (2011) 'A novel technology approach to pain management in children with burns: a prospective randomized controlled trial', *Burns*, 37 (3): 395–405.

Moore, A., Straube, S. and McQuay, H. (2009) 'Minimising pain during intravenous cannulation', *British Medical Journal*, 338 (7692): 422.

Mosiman, W. and Pile, D. (2013) 'Emerging therapies in pediatric pain management', *Journal of Infusion Nursing*, 36 (2): 98–106.

Nilsson, S., Finnström, B. and Kokinsky, E. (2008) 'The FLACC behavioral scale for procedural pain assessment in children aged 5–16 years', *Paediatric Anaesthesia*, 18 (8): 767–74.

Nilsson, S., Hallqvist, C., Sidenvall, B. and Enskär, K. (2011) 'Children's experiences of procedural pain management in conjunction with trauma wound dressings', *Journal of Advanced Nursing*, 67 (7): 1449–57.

Noel, M., Chambers, C.T., McGrath, P.J., Klein, R.M. and Stewart, S.H. (2012) 'The role of state anxiety in children's memories for pain', *Journal of Pediatric Psychology*, 37 (5): 567–79.

O'Brien, L., Taddio, A., Lyszkiewicz, D.A. and Koren, G. (2005) 'A critical review of the topical local anesthetic amethocaine (Ametop®) for pediatric pain', *Pediatric Drugs*, 7 (1): 41–54.

Papa, A. and Zempsky, W. (2010) 'Nurse perceptions of the impact of pediatric peripheral venous access pain on nurse and patient satisfaction: results of a national survey', *Advanced Emergency Nursing Journal*, 32 (3): 226–33.

Pate, J., Blount, R., Cohen, L. and Smith, A. (1996) 'Childhood medical experience and temperament as predictors of adult functioning in medical situations', *Children's Health Care*, 25 (4): 281–98.

Pillai Riddell, R.R., Racine, N.M., Turcotte, K., Uman, L.S., Horton, R.E., Din Osmun, L., Ahola Kohut, S., Hillgrove Stuart, J., Stevens, B. and Gerwitz-Stern, A. (2012) *Non-pharmacological Management of Infant and Young Child Procedural Pain. Cochrane Database of Systematic Reviews 2011*, 10: CD006275. doi: 10.1002/14651858.CD006275.pub2.

Polkki, T., Laukkala, H., Vehvilainen-Julkunen, K. and Pietila, A.M. (2003) 'Factors influencing nurses' use of nonpharmacological pain alleviation methods in paediatric patients', *Scandinavian Journal of Caring Sciences*, 17 (4): 373–83.

Rennick, J.E., Johnston, C.C., Dougherty, G., Platt, R. and Ritchie, J.A. (2002) 'Children's psychological responses after critical illness and exposure to invasive technology', *Journal of Developmental and Behavioral Pediatrics*, 23 (3): 133–44.

Richardson, J., Smith, J.E., McCall, G. and Pilkington, K. (2006) 'Hypnosis for procedure-related pain and distress in pediatric cancer patients: a systematic review of effectiveness and methodology related to hypnosis interventions', *Journal of Pain and Symptom Management*, 31 (1): 70–84.

Sadeghi, T., Mohammadi, N., Shamshiri, M., Bagherzadeh, R. and Hossinkhani, N. (2013) 'Effect of distraction on children's pain during intravenous catheter insertion', *Journal for Specialists in Pediatric Nursing*, 18 (2): 109–14.

Schmitt, Y.S., Hoffman, H.G., Blough, D.K., Patterson, D.R., Jensen, M.P., Soltani, M., Carrougher, G.J., Nakamura, D. and Sharar, S.R. (2011) 'A randomized, controlled trial of immersive virtual reality analgesia, during physical therapy for pediatric burns', *Burns*, 37 (1): 61–8.

Spagrud, L.J., von Baeyer, C.L., Ali, K., Mpofu, C., Fennell, L.P., Friesen, K. and Mitchell, J. (2008) 'Pain, distress, and adult-child interaction during venipuncture in pediatric oncology: an examination of three types of venous access', *Journal of Pain and Symptom Management*, 36 (2): 173–84.

Sparks, L. (2001) 'Taking the "ouch" out of injections for children', *American Journal of Maternal/Child Nursing*, 26 (2): 72–8.

Stevens, B.J., Abbott, L.K., Yamada, J., Harrison, D., Stinson, J., Taddio, A., Barwick, M., Latimer, M., Scott, S.D., Rashotte, J., Campbell, F. and Finley, G.A. (2011) 'Epidemiology and management of painful procedures in children in Canadian hospitals', *Canadian Medical Association Journal*, 183 (7): E403–E410.

Stevens, B.J., Harrison, D., Rashotte, J., Yamada, J., Abbott, L.K., Coburn, G., Stinson, J. and Le May, S. (2012) 'Pain assessment and intensity in hospitalized children in Canada', *The Journal of Pain*, 13 (9): 857–65.

Stephens, B.K., Barkey, M.E. and Hall, H.R. (1999) 'Techniques to comfort children during stressful procedures', *Accident & Emergency Nursing*, 7 (4): 226–36.

Stinson, J., Yamada, J., Dickson, A., Lamba, J. and Stevens, B. (2008) 'Review of systematic reviews on acute procedural pain in children in the hospital setting', *Pain Research & Management*, 13 (1): 51–7.

Taddio, A., Ilerisch, A.L., Ipp, M., Kikuta, A., Shah, V. and Team, H. (2009) 'Physical interventions and injection techniques for reducing injection pain during routine childhood immunizations: systematic review of randomized controlled trials and quasi-randomized controlled trials', *Clinical Therapeutics*, 31: S48–S76.

Uspal, N.G., Marin, J.R., Alpern, E.R. and Zorc, J.J. (2013) 'Factors associated with the use of procedural sedation during incision and drainage procedures at a children's hospital', *The American Journal of Emergency Medicine*, 31 (2): 302–8.

Vaartio, H., Leino-Kilpi, H., Suominen, T. and Puukka, P. (2009) 'Measuring nursing advocacy in procedural pain care – development and validation of an instrument', *Pain Management Nursing*, 10 (4): 206–19.

Vaartio, H., Leino-Kilpi, H., Suominen, T. and Puukka, P. (2008) 'The content of advocacy in procedural pain care – patients' and nurses' perspectives', *Journal of Advanced Nursing*, 64 (5): 504–13.

Walco, G.A. (2008) 'Needle pain in children: contextual factors', *Pediatrics*, 122 (Supplement 3): S125–S129.

Windich-Biermeier, A., Sjoberg, I., Dale, J.C., Eshelman, D. and Guzzetta, C.E. (2007) 'Effects of distraction on pain, fear, and distress during venous port access and venipuncture in children and adolescents with cancer', *Journal of Pediatric Oncology Nursing*, 24 (1): 8–19.

Chapter 4

Pain in Sickle Cell Disease

Vivian's and Fauzana's stories

Vivian Kagendo's story

Vivian Kagendo now 5 years old was born in Meru, Kenya. She was the second child in a family of two. Vivian had no unique problems during her first year. Like other children in her environment, she completed the routine childhood immunisations and started moving around and playing with other children.

At one-and-a-half years of age, her mother noticed that her child was 'not as fast as the other children, and did not want to play with the mother and her siblings like before'. Vivian was also uncomfortable sitting in the 'pottie' unlike before. After talking with her husband again, they decided to get advice from the local health centre.

The health providers examined Vivian and found nothing abnormal. They did blood tests which did not review any infection. However, they noticed that she had not achieved the correct weight as per the standard for her age. She was given some medicine for worms and referred for nutritional counselling within the health centre. She complied and received the counselling together with other women. That day she went home unsatisfied.

Two weeks passed and nothing improved in Vivian's health. She had even started complaining of pains in her hands, feet and even more on the chest. The child was becoming weak and her colour was changing. Vivian's mother decided to take her to the district hospital about 15 km away. It was here that Vivian was diagnosed as having sickle cell disease. She had moderate anaemia and an infection. However, she was not in crisis. Vivian was treated to the satisfaction of her parents.

They were given medicine and went home. Vivian's first appointment was two weeks from the day of diagnosis. This was not to be. Three days after diagnosis, the pain became worse. She cried and told her mother 'my hands feels as if they are being stabbed inside, my behind is very painful'. The parents panicked.

They rushed her to hospital where she was admitted and put on intravenous fluids, painkillers and antibiotics. On the second day of admission, the pain had reduced but the doctors decided to transfuse blood to Vivian. Everything went well and she went home after five days. The mother was advised on good nutrition, bed rest, giving of medications and prevention of infections.

After hospital admission, Vivian became weak and withdrawn, the parents noticed. The pain sites increased from the lower back, legs and the wrist joints to involve the chest and she started experiencing difficulty in breathing. She would develop fever and difficulty breathing and be rushed to the hospital at night. Four months from her admission date, Vivian got into a worse painful crisis. Vivian's mother remembers that day as her worst.

It was a normal day and she went to the farm. The house help went running to call her from the farm. Vivian was screaming with pain and sweating profusely. She did not want to be touched since every part of her was extremely painful. She was speaking some unusual words which did not make sense. Again, the mother rushed her to the hospital. Fortunately, the staff in the hospital knew the child and put her on treatment immediately. She received strong painkillers and intravenous fluids.

After four days of admission, she was discharged home again with more instructions to prevent painful crises. Vivian's parents are following the medical advice well and the painful episodes are infrequent.

Fauzana Nakigosi's story

I was born 15 years ago, my mum tells me she thought I wouldn't make it because of the caution I was in right from the beginning of my journey. I was born in a little country that had low knowledge about sickle cells. When people saw me they felt sorry for my mum, most of them really didn't believe I would grow any older. My mum doubted it too but because she cared she never gave up on me. My birth brought a lot of difficulties and changes to my family.

But what made it worse was the fact that no one knew about the illness, most people thought my mum was cast and others thought it was witchcraft. My early childhood was the most difficult of my whole life but I can't tell you a lot about that because I started understanding what sickle cell is and mastered pain when I was about four. This is when I actually knew what was going on and probably in the most painful stages of my entire life. When I started school I didn't do very well because I spent like half a year without school either at home in pain or in hospital in more pain. Because I was young I used to cry for the whole of the night and the whole of the day in most cases: the pain was tripled because I didn't have them strong pain relievers so I had to hack the pain until it stopped. That wasn't all, in school I was separated from the normal students, I wasn't allow to do most things and the other kids took that chance and made fun of me in any way possible, not only the kids but even some teachers who thought I was too anorectic.

I moved to London when I was ten and this was the change of my life. A brand new life was provided. A life where pain is not a worry any more, a life where I don't physically pay for my treatment, and the most important thing a life where people understand what sickle cell disease is, people who care and try their best to help. At the beginning of my journey everyone thought I didn't have anywhere to go, now I have hope: I don't think I am going to die or that I can't make it because there is help and with the right help anyone can make it: if I have hope with everything I went through at quite a young age I definitely believe anyone can with the right people. Now I am not worried about pain because I know that there is lots of help out there.

Introduction

It is estimated that there are between 12,000 and 15,000 people with sickle cell disease in the UK, and the incidence is rising (NICE 2012). The main cause of pain for children and young people with sickle cell disease is a vaso-occlusive episode (VOE) or what is often known as sickle cell crisis. The pain involved is the most frequent cause of seeking health care professionals help (Edwards et al. 2005). Nurses caring for children in crisis need to have knowledge of the pathophysiology of the stages of crisis and how they impact on the child or young person. This knowledge will enhance the nurse's ability to meet the individual needs of a child in what can amount to severe pain and will enable the nurse to advise the family on measures to take to reduce the risk of further crises, thus providing the family with a greater sense of control. In both of the stories there is a feeling of being in control in relation to sickle cell disease. Fauzana feels that having moved to London her pain is something that she does not have to worry about as she has confidence in the health professionals that care for her. In Vivian's story, although the diagnosis was not straightforward, by the end of the story her parents were following the advice provided by the health professionals which has meant a reduction in sickle cell crises and therefore the avoidance of pain. The two stories demonstrate how effective support can give control to families and instil confidence in their ability to cope with sickle cell disease.

What happens in painful vaso-occlusive episodes?

Painful crisis results from avascular necrosis of the bone marrow (Jacob et al. 2005).

The changes that occur in the bone marrow are necrosis; increased calcium turnover; decreased bone marrow blood flow; fibrosis, which may become permanent; infarction; oedema; increased fat; and erythropoiesis. Necrotic bone marrow, fat, and spicules of bone may occur as emboli in the small vessels of the brain, lungs, or kidneys. During crises patients experience severe back pain, chest tightness, dyspnoea and a decrease in arterial oxygen tension. They may show systemic signs of embolisation involving the respiratory, renal, and central nervous system. Ischaemia, infarction and inflammation may be responsible for initiating the painful crisis.

These signs reflect the accumulation of inflammatory mediators, such as bradykinin and substance P, that are known to cause local pain, vasodilation, extravasation of fluids, and oedema.

There are four phases in a vaso-occlusive episode which determine the severity of pain experienced by a child.

1. Prodromal phase. The prodromal phase typically lasts up to 24 hours involving numbness, aches, and paraesthesia (pins and needles) in different areas.
2. Infarctive phase. Pain escalates to a maximum level with the following changes occurring in the blood: a decrease in the deformability of erythrocytes; an increase in the percentage of dense cells in the circulation, which increases the likelihood of trapping of deformed (sickle-shaped) erythrocytes. The pain increases gradually in severity and reaches a peak by the second or third day of the crisis.
3. Post-infarctive phase. This phase is also known as the established or inflammatory phase, and can last 4–5 days. Predominant features of this phase include persistence of severe pain and indications of inflammation such as pyrexia, swelling, tenderness and joint effusions.
4. Resolving phase. This phase is also known as the healing, recovery or post-crisis phase, and involves a gradual decrease in pain severity, which may last 1–2 days. Features of this phase include a decrease in the percentage of dense erythrocytes, and a decrease in the number of irreversibly sickled cells. There is a return of haemoglobin and reticulocyte counts to their pre-crisis levels.

Beyer et al. (1999) developed a chronology of pain and comfort in relation to the pain of a vaso-occlusive episode and comfort measures used. These stages provide information for those caring for a child experiencing a sickle cell crisis, and may indicate when to provide early analgesics, to prevent pain escalating to the point of severity often experienced in sickle cell crisis. Eight stages were identified:

- *Baseline*: this is the child's usual state and involves no pain.
- *Prepain*: the child shows no signs of pain but demonstrates other prodromal signs and symptoms of vaso-occlusion, such as yellow eyes and fatigue.
- *Pain starting point*: the child complains of mild achy pain in specific areas which gradually or rapidly increases.
- *Pain acceleration*: involves pain continuing to escalate and spread to more areas of the body. A decreased level of activity and differences in behaviour, appearance and mood is noticed by parents.
- *Peak pain experience*: pain continues to escalate and in some cases children are unable to get relief from the pain. Children describe their pain as drilling, pounding, banging, excruciating, unbearable. Parents sometimes seek help for stronger analgesics and to prevent complications such as pyrexia or respiratory distress. Often the pain was so bad that children had to be admitted to hospital.
- *Pain decrease starting point*: this stage occurs after IV fluids and analgesics which allow the child to sleep for longer periods. The pain at this stage is still sharp and throbbing.
- *Steady pain decline*: this phase is when the child's pain decreases steadily or rapidly. The child's activity levels increase and pain is reported as mild.
- *Pain resolution*: pain is at tolerable levels and the child is discharged home on mild analgesics.

Having knowledge of the various phases of a VOE is very likely to be one aspect of helping to deal with the pain experienced. In both Vivian's and Fauzana's stories there was a feeling of confidence in being able to deal with pain effectively and in Vivian's case a feeling of her parents being in control and able to prevent VOEs from occurring. Hayward (1975) carried out seminal work into the effect information has on patients' experience of pain, concluding that information was a prescription against pain. In the two stories here it would appear that having knowledge of VOEs enabled both families to deal effectively and confidently with pain.

Predisposing factors

Much work has been done on exploring factors that can predispose a child to having a sickle cell crisis. Infections, dehydration, pyrexia and acidosis have been observed to precipitate a crisis, which are also more common in cold and damp periods.

Fosdal and Wojner-Alexandrov (2007) found that factors known to precipitate a crisis were cold, exertion or tiredness, stress or worry, and a more recent study by Cox et al. (2011) involving 1,618 children and adults over a 5-year period in Tanzania found that nutritional status influenced an individual having hospital admissions with sickle cell crisis. In Vivian's story her parents received information on how to care for her so that the incidence of crises was reduced. Many of the predisposing factors above can be influenced by parental support. However, parents need the support of health professionals to develop confidence in their ability to support their child and prevent crises occurring.

Quality of life

Frequent episodes of pain can affect a young person's quality of life by impinging on their daily lives, and preventing them from going to school, or spending time with friends. Valrie et al. (2007) found that high pain severity in sickle cell disease was related to poor sleep quality which in turn results in a lack of concentration, leading to poor educational achievement, in a group that is already vulnerable to disruption in their life as a result of hospital admissions. Another study surveyed children and found that in all domains of quality of life, pain impacted negatively during a hospitalisation and up to seven days post discharge (Brandow et al. 2010). Adolescents were also found to have reduced quality of life if they responded to sickle cell pain by internalising symptoms, resulting in anxiety and depression (Barakat et al. 2008a). It would appear therefore that the management of sickle cell crisis needs to encourage children and young people to verbalise their pain so that it can be dealt with effectively as well as enabling them to develop coping strategies to deal with pain.

Managing a sickle cell crisis

A patient who is treated adequately for pain develops trust in health care professionals (Jacob 2001). In Fauzana's story she has clearly developed a good relationship with the health professionals she sees, which has given her confidence in their ability to manage her pain effectively. This trust has very likely been instrumental in her developing a positive attitude and a belief in her ability to cope with painful crises when they occur. The standard treatment for a painful episode with sickle cell disease is rest, rehydration, treatment of underlying infections or other complications and use of analgesics for pain (Stinson and Naser 2003; NICE 2012). With appropriate home care it is possible to avoid hospitalisation. However, if the pain becomes severe, children often find themselves hospitalised mainly for treatment of their pain.

The American Pain Society (2002) suggests that severe pain should be considered a medical emergency, with timely and aggressive management until the pain is tolerable. However, Jacob et al. (2005) found that the APS guidelines are not always followed in practice; they studied 27 hospitalised children with sickle cell crisis. Children were interviewed and described their pain from the day of admission to the day of discharge. Changes were identified that occur during the evolution of a painful episode, i.e. evolving, inflammatory, and resolving. Pain was found to be sudden or of gradual onset. The study demonstrated that a principle of pain management is that prevention of pain is more effective than trying to deal with established pain, which can be much harder to overcome. Treatment should involve hydration and early aggressive pain management in accident and emergency. The majority of patients with painful episodes were managed on an outpatient basis.

The responsiveness of health professionals to a child in painful sickle cell crisis is pivotal in intervening in the pain and preventing it from escalating (Rees et al. 2003). Such responsiveness can be expected at specialist centres which have staff who are experienced and knowledgeable in treating painful sickle cell crisis. Fauzana has the support of a specialist service, which may go some way to explain her confidence in their care. Another crucial support mechanism is the care she and Vivian receive at home. However, many children and young people will attend their local hospital which may not be a specialist service. Studies have been conducted to explore how to standardise and improve the management of sickle cell crisis. Frei-Jones et al. (2009) found that by educating health care professionals and developing standardised prescription charts, the readmission rates for children with sickle cell disease were reduced. A similar approach is needed in accident and emergency departments where many children are seen in severe pain with sickle cell crisis. Shenoi et al. (2011) studied the experience of 150 children and young people seen in an accident and emergency department and found that the median time from arrival to analgesic administration was 90 minutes. Only those children who arrived in severe pain received analgesia more quickly, i.e. within 60 minutes of arrival in the department. When the department was busy, children had to wait longer for analgesics. The reason children arrive in accident and emergency in severe pain is because most sickle cell pain is managed at home and going to hospital is often a last resort.

Managing a sickle cell crisis at home

Most sickle cell crises (60–90 per cent) are managed at home by parents in an attempt to avoid hospital admission. Yoon and Black (2006) surveyed 63 caregivers who had children or adolescents with sickle cell disease, to explore how they managed the pain of sickle cell crisis. The most frequent analgesia used was ibuprofen or acetaminophen with codeine. Complementary therapies were also used by parents to help reduce pain. The use of complementary therapies was significantly higher with children or young people who were receiving more than one analgesic regularly. Many of the caregivers were willing to try various types of complementary therapies to manage their child's pain. Beyer and Simmons (2004) explored the home treatment of pain for children and adolescents with sickle cell disease and found that parents and caregivers made considerable efforts on behalf of their children to avoid painful episodes. This involved keeping a normal routine, 'catching' the pain, getting their minds off the pain, helping the child get through the episode and staying out of hospital. Parents helped their children to cope with pain by using methods to modify mood, anxiety and tension level to relax and calm their child, and reduce muscle tension. Many caregivers admitted that they did everything they could at home, not only to make the child feel better but also to avoid having to go to hospital.

In Fauzana's story she describes her move to London resulting in her being surrounded by people who care and try their best to help. Her belief in the support available to her means that her attitude to pain has changed and she no longer worries about it. Both Fuazana's and Vivian's families appear to have developed systems that work for them.

This situation poses the question as to how to replicate what Vivian's and Fauzana's families have developed. One element that is clearly having a positive impact is the notion of a locus of control developed by Rotter, an American psychologist. Locus of control refers to the extent to which individuals believe that they can control events that affect them. Individuals with a high internal locus of control believe that events result primarily from their own behaviour and actions. Those with a high external locus of control believe that powerful others, fate, or chance primarily determine events. Those with a high internal locus of control have better control of their behaviour and are more likely to attempt to influence other people. They are more likely to assume that their efforts will be successful, which perhaps reflects Fauzana's belief in her ability to cope with pain. They are more active in seeking information and knowledge concerning their situation than externals (Rotter 1966). Vivian's and Fauzana's families are coping well with their sickle cell disease and appear to have a sense of control, which is founded in the belief that if they experience a VOE the appropriate help and support will be there to get effective pain relief and manage the episode confidently. An understanding of locus of control and how to promote an internal locus of control could be used to develop support for parents in the form of a home management regime.

Levers-Landis et al. (2001) found that assisting their child in avoiding the triggers for a painful sickle cell crisis and helping their child to cope with pain are both considerable stressors for caregivers. An earlier study by Hill (1994) studied pain prevention strategies used at home: these included administering medications, monitoring food and fluid, avoiding stress, restricting activities, and preventing over-exertion, overheating and chilling. The study suggested that families only sought medical care when all their strategies for home management had been exhausted. In so doing children and young people would often arrive at hospital in severe pain, which presents real challenges to health care professionals in delivering effective pain relief. The dilemma for parents is to make the judgement about when to seek medical treatment without letting the pain escalate to the point where it is severe and therefore more difficult to relieve, balanced with treating the pain at home in the hope of avoiding a hospital admission.

Barakat et al. (2008b) explored the correlation of pain rating agreement between adolescents with sickle cell disease and their caregivers. They found that there was only moderate consistency in pain ratings between parents and adolescents. Such a finding may go some way to explaining how pain can escalate to a severe level needing hospitalisation. If parents and adolescents had a mechanism to communicate more effectively about increasing pain, there would be more opportunity to alleviate the pain before it becomes severe. One method of communication that has shown promise is the use of smartphones to use an e-diary recording episodes of pain (Jacob et al. 2012). Adolescents completed an e-diary with 80 per cent accuracy, suggesting their use to provide timely and effective pain management and improve communication between patients and health care providers.

The need for continuous improvement

In 2008 The National Enquiry into Patient Outcome and Death (NEPOD) (Lucas and Treasure 2008) studied all heamaglobinopathy deaths in the UK over a two-year period. There were 55 deaths: 41 in hospital, and 14 in the community. Of these there were six deaths of children who had sickle cell disease. The report pointed out that although good pain management is a key requirement for the care of sickle cell patients, there are many complicating factors for both nurses and patients. A lack of knowledge regarding acute pain management was noted as was the lack of evidence of a formal assessment or documentation of pain. As a result of their findings the NEPOD made a number of recommendations, one of which was that there should be a regular assessment of acute pain. It was suggested that the use of a 'track and trigger' system would greatly enhance better pain control. This type of system involves tracking a patient's observations, in this case pain or respiratory rate, which, if abnormal, would trigger an appropriate intervention (Lawson et al. 2007). The conclusion of the enquiry was that expert advice should be sought early when dealing with a deteriorating patient who has sickle cell disease. Of the 26 sites studied only four had a care pathway for heamaglobinopathy patients. The lack of a care pathway is likely to lead to delays in providing children in painful sickle cell crisis with early pain intervention with appropriately strong analgesics. The NEPOD report demonstrated the need for clear, easy to follow guidelines for dealing with the pain of sickle cell crisis.

Guidelines

There are a number of guidelines available outlining how children and adults should be cared for during sickle cell crises. The American Pain Society (1999) developed guidelines for the management of sickle cell crisis, as did Rees et al. (2003) who produced guidelines based on the literature and protocols available at the time. More recently the Royal College of Nursing (2011) developed a set of competencies as a framework for nursing staff, to guide the care of both adults and children. These guidelines were developed partly in response to findings of the 2008 National Enquiry into Patient Outcome and Death from heamaglobinopathies in the UK (Lucas and Treasure 2008). One competence focuses specifically on pain, stipulating that nurses should work with the patient and family to manage their pain. The guide provides details on what nurses at different levels should know and the care they should provide. Ward nurses are required to have knowledge of the following (Royal College of Nursing 2011):

Pathophysiology of acute and chronic pain in sickle cell disease:

- Pain complications associated with sickle cell disease such as priapism and acute chest syndrome.
- Psychosocial and environmental factors that influence sickle cell pain.
- Age and developmental factors that influence pain.
- Cognitive behavioural therapy for the management of pain.

Nurses should also be able to meet the following performance criteria:

- Safely administers analgesic regimes including nurse- and or patient-controlled analgesia.
- Recognises major complications of sickle cell disease and makes appropriate emergency referrals.
- Communicates and advises pain management strategies to patients and families.
- Differentiates between acute and chronic pain.

Nurses should also ensure patient safety when administering opiates and know when to refer to pain management specialists.

The National Institute for Health and Clinical Excellence (NICE 2012) has produced guidance structured around six key points for health care professionals who care for people in sickle cell crisis in hospital (see Figure 4.1).

It is recognised that some hospitals see large numbers of patients with sickle cell disease, and have established protocols and experienced staff (Rees et al. 2003). However, most hospitals see only a handful of patients each year. The likelihood therefore is that in the latter, patients are more likely to be cared for by inexperienced staff, lacking in both knowledge and confidence in dealing effectively with a child in sickle cell crisis. Guidelines such as those by the Royal College of Nursing (2011) and NICE (2012) can play an important role in providing support for such nurses, to enable them to deal effectively with a child in crisis or refer on to a more experienced member of staff.

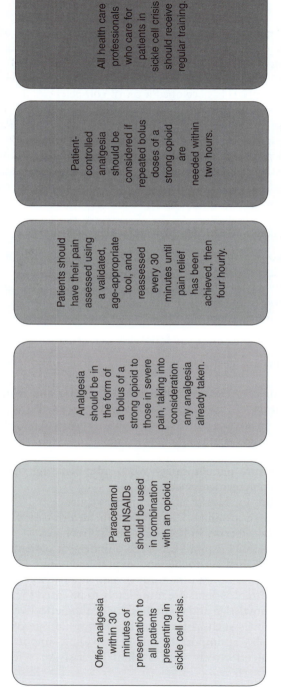

Figure 4.1 Key points for healthcare professionals who care for people in sickle cell crisis in hospital
Developed from NICE (2012)

Despite the availability of guidelines, children admitted in sickle cell crisis have been found to have moderate to high pain intensity throughout their hospital admission (Vijenthira et al. 2012). Suggestions for improvement include improved pain assessment and documentation using valid pain tools, more aggressive multi-modal management of peak sickle cell crisis pain, and better education and support for pain management at home.

Conclusion

Children with sickle cell disease should not be treated just to prevent complications, the aim should be to provide a good quality of life (Ware 2010). This chapter has outlined the trajectory of a sickle cell crisis along with the management of such crises, underpinned with the relevant available guidelines. There is a wealth of knowledge on how to treat pain in sickle cell crisis, however what appears to be missing is the link between home care and hospital care. There is a need for advanced nurse practitioners in the community to have the ability to prescribe strong enough analgesics that can be administered in the home to prevent the escalation of vaso-occlusive episode pain and subsequently reduce the frequency of hospitalisations and therefore improve quality of life for children and young people and the lives of their families.

Key Points

- There are between 12,000 and 15,000 people with sickle cell disease in the UK and the incidence is rising.
- The pain involved in a sickle cell crisis is the most common complaint in sickle cell disease.
- There are recognised predisposing factors to a sickle cell crisis.
- Standard treatment for a painful episode is rest, rehydration, treatment of underlying infections and use of analgesics for pain.
- Most sickle cell crises are managed at home by parents in an attempt to avoid a hospital admission.
- The American Pain Society and NICE have developed guidelines, and the Royal College of Nursing has developed a set of competencies as a framework for nurses caring for patients in a sickle cell crisis.

Additional Resources and Reading

- The full guideline developed by NICE (2012) is:
  - *Sickle Cell Acute Painful Episode. Management of an Acute Painful Sickle Cell Episode in Hospital.* Available at http://guidance.nice.org.uk/CG143/Guidance/pdf/English

References

American Pain Society *(1999) Guideline for the Management of Acute and Chronic Pain in Sickle Cell Disease.* Glenview, IL: American Pain Society.

American Pain Society (2002) *Guideline for the Management of Acute and Chronic Pain in Sickle Cell Disease*, 4th edn. Glenview, IL: The American Pain Society.

Barakat, L.P., Patterson, C.A., Daniel, L.C. and Dampier, C. (2008a) 'Quality of life among adolescents with sickle cell disease: mediation of pain by internalizing symptoms and parenting stress', *Health and Quality of Life Outcomes*, 6 (60):1–9.

Barakat, L.P., Simon, K., Schwartz, L.A. and Radcliffe, J. (2008b) 'Correlates of pain-rating concordance for adolescents with sickle cell disease and their caregivers', *Clinical Journal of Pain*, 25 (5): 438–46.

Beyer, J.E. and Simmons, L.E. (2004) 'Home treatment of pain for children and adolescents with sickle cell disease', *Pain Management Nursing*, 5 (3): 126–35.

Beyer, J.E., Simmons, L.E., Woods, G.M. and Woods, P.M. (1999) 'A chronology of pain and comfort in children with sickle cell disease', *Archives of Pediatric & Adolescent Medicine*, 153: 913–20.

Brandow, A.M., Brousseau, D.C., Pajewski, N.M. and Panepinto, J.A. (2010) 'Vaso-occlusive painful events in sickle cell disease: impact on child well-being', *Pediatric Blood Cancer*, 54: 92–7.

Cox, S.E., Makani, J., Fulford, A.J., Komba, A.N., Soka, D., Williams,T.N., Newton, C.R., Marsh, K. and Prentice, A.M. (2011) 'Nutritional status, hospitalization and mortality among patients with sickle cell anemia in Tanzania', *Haematologica*, 96 (7): 948–53.

Edwards, C.L., Scales, M.T., Loughlin, C., Bennett, G.G., Harris-Peterson, S., De Castro, L.M., Whitworth, E., Abrams, M., Feliu, M., Johnson, S., Wood, M., Harrison, O. and Killough A. (2005) 'A brief review of the pathophysiology, associated pain, and psychosocial issues in sickle cell disease', *International Journal of Behavioral Medicine*, 12(3): 171–79.

Fosdal, M.B. and Wojner-Alexandrov, A.W. (2007) 'Events of hospitalisation among children with sickle cell disease', *Journal of Pediatric Nursing*, 22 (4): 342–6.

Frei-Jones, M.J., Field, J.J. and DeBaun, M.R. (2009) 'Multi-modal intervention and prospective implementation of standardized sickle cell pain admission orders reduces 30-day readmission rate', *Pediatric Blood Cancer*, 53: 401–5.

Hayward, J. (1975) *Information – A Prescription Against Pain*: *Research Project Report*. London: Royal College of Nursing.

Hill, S.A. (1994) *Managing Sickle Cell Disease in Low-income Families*. Philadelphia, PA: Temple University Press.

Jacob, E. (2001) 'The pain experience of patients with sickle cell anemia', *Pain Management Nursing*, 2: 74–83.

Jacob, E., Beyer, J.E., Miaskowski, C., Savedra, M. Treadwell, M. and Styles, L. (2005) 'Are there phases to the vaso-occlusive painful episode in sickle cell disease?', *Journal of Pain and Symptom Management*, 29: 392–400.

Jacob, E., Stinson, J., Duran, J., Gupta, A., Gerla, M., Ann Lewis, M. and Zeltzer, L. (2012) 'Usability testing of a Smartphone for accessing a web-based e-diary for self-monitoring of pain and symptoms in sickle cell disease', *Journal of Pediatric Hematology/Oncology*, 34 (5): 326–35.

Lawson, M., Stone, A., King, D. and Davison, A. (2007) 'The use of track and trigger systems on general medical wards', *Critical Care*, 11 (Supplement 2): 443.

Levers-Landis, C.E., Brown, R., Drotar, D., Bunke, V., Lambert, R. and Walker, A.A. (2001) 'Situational analysis of parenting problems for caregivers of children with sickle cell syndromes', *Journal of Developmental and Behavioral Pediatrics*, 22 (3): 169–78.

Lucas, S. and Treasure, T. (2008) *A Sickle Crisis. National Enquiry into Patient Outcome and Death*. London: NCEPOD.

NICE (2012) *Sickle Cell Acute Painful Episode: Management of an Acute Painful Sickle Cell Episode in Hospital*. Manchester: National Institute for Health and Clinical Excellence.

Rees, D.C, Olujohungbe, A.D., Parker, N.E., Stephens, A.D., Telfer, P. and Wright, J. (2003) 'Guidelines for the management of the acute painful crisis in sickle cell disease', *British Journal of Haematology*, 120: 744–52.

Rotter, J.B. (1966) 'Generalized expectancies for internal versus external control of reinforcement', *Psychological Monographs*, 80, No. 609.

Royal College of Nursing (2011) *Caring for People with Sickle Cell Disease and Thalasseamia Guidelines: A Framework for Nursing Staff*. London: Royal College of Nursing.

Shenoi, R., Ma, L., Syblik, D. and Yusuf, S. (2011) 'Emergency department crowding and analgesic delay in pediatric sickle cell pain crises', *Pediatric Emergency Care*, 27 (10): 911–17.

Stinson, J., and Naser B. (2003) 'Pain management in children with sickle cell disease', *Pediatric Drugs*, 5(4): 229–41.

Valrie, C.R., Gil, K.M., Redding-Lallinger, R. and Daeschner, C. (2007) 'The influence of pain and stress on sleep in children with sickle cell disease', *Children's Healthcare*, 36 (4): 335–53.

Vijenthira, A., Stinson, J., Friedman, J., Palozzi, L., Taddio, A., Scolnik, D., Victor, C., Kirby-Allen, M. and Campbell, F. (2012) 'Benchmarking pain outcomes for children with sickle cell disease hospitalized in a tertiary referral pediatric hospital', *Pain Research & Management*, 17 (4): 291–6.

Ware, R.E. (2010) 'How I use hydroxyurea to treat young patients with sickle cell anemia', *Blood*, 115 (26): 5300–11.

Yoon, S.L. and Black, S. (2006) 'Comprehensive, integrative management of pain for patients with sickle-cell disease', *Journal of Alternative and Complementary Medicine*, 12 (10): 995–1001.

Chapter 5

Parents Managing their Children's Pain

Noah's, Ollie's and Ruari's Stories

Noah's story

I am 5 years old. I went into mummy's and daddy's room last night as I had a tummy ache. I told mummy and daddy 'my tummy hurts lots and lots and it makes me want to cry'. I went to mummy's room because my mummy makes me better by giving me medicine and she rubs my tummy better. Sometimes rubbing it helps, if I do not think about it. I do not know how long it hurts. It hurts all the time. It hurts here (he points everywhere in his tummy and in no specific spot).

[Note: Noah's tummy ache resolves and in the morning he is fine.]

Kayla's and Ollie's Story

We admitted a five-year-old boy called Ollie to the ward. Ollie was accompanied to the ward by his mother, Kayla. According to Kayla, he had an eight hour history of abdominal pain which started at 4.00 a.m. in the morning. Kayla was awoken in the middle of the night hearing him crying, this was unusual behaviour for Ollie. Kayla gave him oral paracetamol and took him to bed with her. However, his pain did not really subside, so she brought him to A&E.

On admission he was pyrexial (temp 38.2°c), pulse rate 128 bpm – pulse full and bounding, his respiration rate was 30 bpm. He was being comforted by Kayla in her arms but he was whimpering all the time. Kayla explained that he couldn't settle in one place. She had also said 'if he holds his breath it seems to ease the pain'. I noticed that his face looked tight and not relaxed, he was curling himself in a ball, he was rubbing his abdomen in a non-specific place and he looked flushed.

Investigations included an abdominal and chest x-ray which were negative. A urine sample showed leukocytes and nitrates. Pain relief was oral paracetamol (250 mg) 4 hourly. This controlled Ollie's pain when given at 4–6 hourly intervals. Kayla said watching *Shrek*, his favourite film, helped to ease Ollie's pain. Following repeat clean catch urinalysis, a urinary tract infection was diagnosed.

Anne's and Ruari's story

As a qualified general and sick children's nurse, you would assume I had acquired a lot of the education, skills and experience required to rear my own three children without any significant trauma. However, my three children would beg to differ with that assertion. Indeed they have been known to say that the only way that they would be allowed have a day off school would be if they stopped breathing. My usual treatment for ills and complaints is a glass of water, rest, and in extreme circumstances, paracetamol.

Bearing my introduction in mind, my story relates to Ruari, my 12–year-old son. One sunny evening while playing a Gaelic football match, in the last minute of the game, he put his hand up to catch a ball, and in doing so, he injured his arm. Ruari fell to the ground holding his injured arm, indicating severe pain. He was pale and clammy. As our side had lost the match and it was a warm summer's evening, I tended to think it was due to the loss of the match, combined with the heat of the day, and possible dehydration that caused the furore, and not because Ruari might actually be hurt.

However, following the 'magical' water treatment along with prerequisite ice pack application, both the pain and complaints continued relentlessly, so this time I did bring him to the local hospital's A&E department, where Ruari gave an Oscar-winning performance that would put the cream of Hollywood to shame. The arm was x-rayed, and a fractured radius was confirmed.

Once Ruari was given this information and subsequently viewed the x-ray films, his pain was immediately relieved, even prior to a 'back-slab' being applied. In Ruari's case, here I was, very clearly shown that once I did acknowledge the injury, and was shown that there was indeed a fracture, that very acknowledgement was the only form of analgesia he required. As a mother, and a nurse, I felt very guilty over the event. I would be very well served to remember that 'pain is whatever the person experiencing it says it is'. To have one's pain acknowledged is often the first step in dealing with that pain and its likely eventual relief.

Introduction

Noah's and Ollie's stories are fairly unremarkable stories of pain. Noah's story, in particular, is such a commonplace occurrence that it is a pain story that could easily be overlooked. Every parent of a young child will have had to deal with their child's tummy aches, headaches, earaches and other aches and pains; at all hours of the day and often at night. To most health care professionals, Noah's and Ollie's stories are fairly routine and lacking in drama. However, they reflect the 'what' and 'how' and 'where' of most children's pain experiences. For the children and their parents they can be anything but a routine experience.

The vast majority of children's pain is dealt with by their parents at home, without any recourse to external help. Children expect and trust their parents to be able to 'make the pain go away'. By the time a parent brings their child to a health care professional they will almost always have tried to manage their child's pain using their own resources, and they will almost always be worried, tired and stressed from trying and failing to 'make it better'.

The literature that underpins parents' decision-making in relation to minor ailments and symptoms is relatively small and pain is just one of a number of symptoms, such as fever or respiratory illness, which triggers parents to seek professional health care advice. Health care professionals come into contact with parents of children both in their roles as professionals (e.g., in clinics and surgeries) as well as in their off-duty role when they asked for their advice about what to do. Health care professionals who are parents also have to deal with the everyday tummy aches and pains from cuts and falls that their children experience. Anne's story shows how, even as a health professional, she managed to connect the cues and clues incorrectly and there was a delay between Ruari's injury and her seeking help.

The word 'everyday' in this chapter denotes the sorts of pains that most parents of children will deal with; the use of the term does not imply that a child will have pain every day.

In this chapter we explore some of the factors influencing and underpinning how parents assess and manage their children's everyday pain, how they manage uncertainty and their decision-making in relation to seeking help. We use 'tummy ache' as the main exemplar, although parents appear to use similar decision-making strategies in other situations where they have to make decisions about their child's illness-related behaviours. We also address health care professionals' responses to parents and how these can shape parents' future decisions.

Two stories, two starting points, at least two outcomes

Noah's and Ollie's stories have similar starting points, although the outcomes are different. Noah's tummy ache settles down, he goes back to bed and back to sleep. He wakes up in the morning none the worse for his middle of the night trip to mummy's and daddy's room. Mummy did make his tummy ache better. Ollie's tummy ache does not resolve and, despite Kayla's efforts to sort it out, he does not settle. Kayla takes Ollie to hospital and he is admitted. He is assessed and the health care professionals check his vital signs (temperature, pulse, respiration) and they undertake routine tests (abdominal x-ray, chest x-ray, urine sample). The clinical information they gain from their observation and investigation of the child (whimpering, curled up, rubbing abdomen, 'negative' x-rays and leukocytes and nitrates in the urine) allows a diagnosis to be made. The health care professionals are able to draw on much more data than Kayla has available to her. They can draw on objective data (test results) as well as more subjective behavioural data to come up with the diagnosis.

Ollie's story, while more dramatic for him and his mother, is still likely to be viewed by health care professionals as a fairly routine episode within the context of children's acute hospital care. Neither Ollie's nor Noah's mother knew where the middle of the night request 'to make it better' would lead them; they both had to act and make decisions about what needed to be done. The real difficulty for parents is that what starts off as a fairly innocuous tummy ache can resolve itself with little more than some reassurance, a comforting hug and perhaps a dose of paracetamol. The same presentation of tummy ache could be the early presentation of a urinary tract infection, as in Ollie's case, or potentially something significantly more serious such as a ruptured appendix or a tumour. The problem for parents is that most of the time they are feeling their way and are not sure what it is they are dealing with.

Parents as first line managers of their children's illness and pain

Parents manage many childhood illness and symptoms such as pain at home (Bruijnzeels et al. 1998; Rogers and Nicolaas 1998) and are 'first in line' to judge the severity of their child's illness and pain and to determine what action to take (Ertmann et al. 2011a: 23). Parents try to understand their child's illness and to make sense of it by drawing on their previous experience, common sense knowledge (Hay et al. 2005) and their intuition (Ertmann et al. 2011a). They tend to assess their child's illness and symptoms in relation to their child's 'normal' health (Cunningham-Burley and Irvine 1987; Neill 2000) and changes to the child's usual behaviour (Neill 2000; Winskill et al. 2011) relying on their interpretation of factors such as bodily expression (Ertmann et al. 2011a). Kelly et al. (2005) note that the common sense model proposed by Leventhal et al. (1997) suggests that individuals understand illness based on their own life experiences and the presenting somatic symptoms. This can be significantly different to the biomedical view of illness, which relies more heavily on the physical effects wrought by the illness or ailment (Sullivan 1997; Robbins et al. 2003).

Assessing and contextualising their child's pain

Although most parents would not necessarily couch their actions in the following clinical terms, they do actually assess, propose preliminary diagnoses, treat, evaluate their actions and consider their child's response to their interventions. They do all of this with no formal training, with limited resources and while being concerned about the child's distress and the cause of their child's illness or pain (see Figure 5.1).

Parents' assess their child's pain through a range of different cues. They observe their child's facial expression to determine if they look relaxed, or if their expression suggests pain. They consider their child's level of activity, the way they are holding their body or protecting part of their body, how still or active they are. They take into account how close or distant their child's behaviours are to their usual behaviour and the degree to which the child is like 'their usual self'. More explicit elements are also assessed, such as the child's verbal expression or self-report of pain as well as any para-verbal expressions such as moans, whimpers and groans. Tears, crying and rocking can all indicate pain, although not all children cry tears if they are in pain.

While nurses and other health care professionals have the advantage of pain assessment tools, parents use a mental checklist based on their intimate, subjective

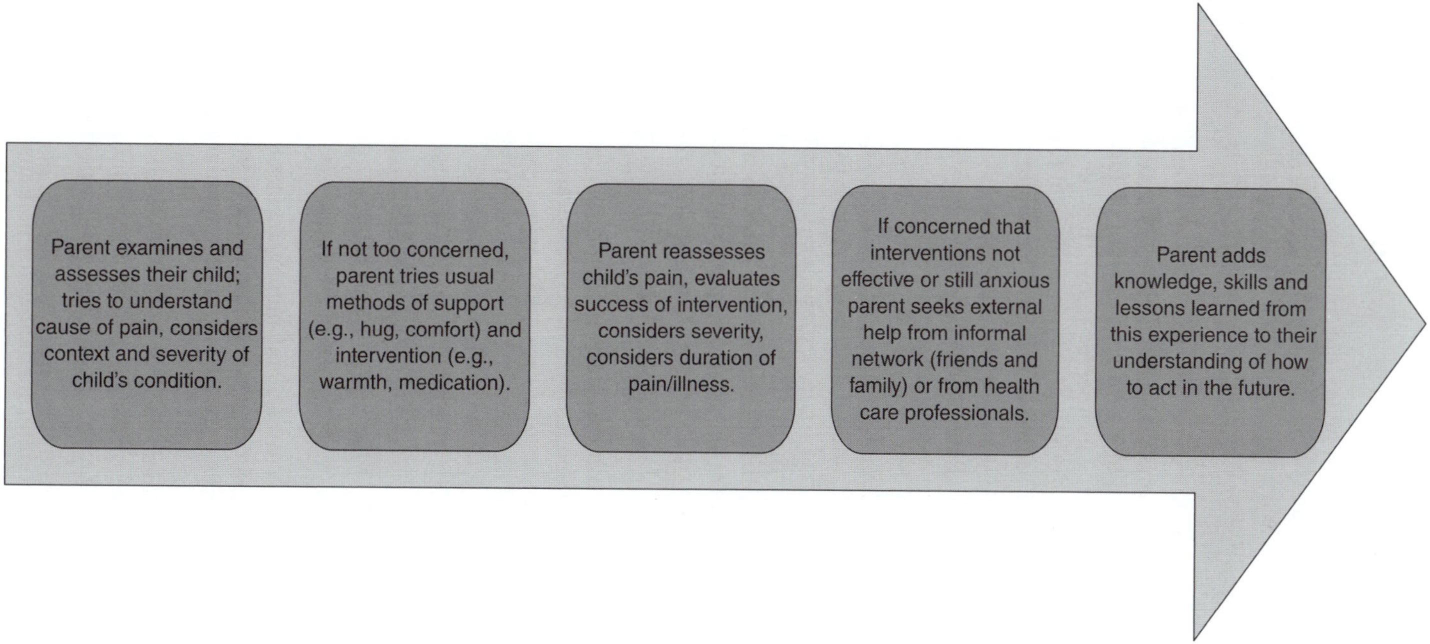

Figure 5.1 Trajectory of parental decision-making

knowledge of their child's usual behaviour and responses to pain. They are invariably right, even though some studies suggest that parents either under-assess or over-assess their child's pain. Where the pain cues are not explicit or where other factors are complicating the picture, parents may well miss the cues or simply not make the right connections. In these circumstances, parents will be their own sternest critics and will feel guilty for missing something that feels obvious once a diagnosis is made. Anne's story for example shows her making plenty of plausible but incorrect connections. Kayla knew that her child was in pain but had no idea what was causing it and there is no reason to expect a mother to know that her child had a urinary tract infection. However, if Ollie gets tummy ache again, then Kayla will have this experience to draw upon and will probably bring the possibility of the pain being caused by another urinary tract infection into consideration.

Parents assess the child's pain using the cues they recognise and understand, matching these with the context to try to explain what is happening and what might be causing their child's pain. For example, if Noah had been to his friend's birthday party, his mother might well put his tummy ache down to the excitement of the party and too much birthday cake, and while she would care for him she would probably not be too perturbed as she had found a plausible explanation for the pain.

Parents have to make pragmatic decisions about their child's report of pain, not least because a child being off sick from school often means that their parent has to either stay at home with them or make alternative child-care arrangements. Anne's story about Ruari may well ring true for many parents and their approach to their children's minor ailments. Although it is unlikely that 'the only way that they would be allowed have a day off school would be if they stopped breathing', it does reflect many parents' determination to play down minor ailments. Night-time complaints of pain can sometimes be managed by a little reassurance, a warm drink and being tucked up into bed. In other cases, if the child's pain does not respond to treatment, this can result in a disturbed night for the parents and child, as was the case for Ollie and Kayla.

Treating 'everyday' pain

Hugs, reassurance, rubbing or stroking the area that is hurting and keeping their child close to them are core to parental management of pain. Children also have strategies to help ease their pain and can be quite active in using pain-reducing strategies. Noah notes that rubbing a hurt away only 'sometimes works' and even though he is only five years old, he accepts he has some responsibility to help his pain management by trying 'not to think about it [pain]'. Ollie also tries to help his pain by rubbing his abdomen. Other strategies that children and parents use are based on distraction techniques, and Kayla talks of how Ollie's pain was eased when he was watching his favourite film, *Shrek*.

Using common over-the-counter medicines for pain management is fairly routine practice by parents as an initial intervention along with parental care practices such as comforting and reassuring. Medicines such as paracetamol and ibuprofen are often used during the period of 'wait and see' (Neill 2000) when parents are monitoring their child for a possible improvement or deterioration in their condition. Trajanovska et al. (2010) note that over-the-counter medicines are used extensively by parents to manage childhood ailments such as pain and Ertmann et al. (2012) found that during the winter nearly all children in their Danish study had been given paracetamol by their parent with the most common reasons being earache and fever. Hameen-Anttila et al. (2011) noted that parents in their study considered prescription medicines to be safe and effective but felt that over-the-counter medicines were less so. Similarly, parents in Carter et al.'s (2013) study found it hard to believe that 'ordinary' medicines such as paracetamol and ibuprofen were good enough medicines for use in the management of pain in hospital. These different beliefs and misconceptions have to be taken into account when giving parents advice about analgesia regimes. Parents have to ensure that they give their child the correct dose at the right intervals and this can be another worry for them when they are already anxious about the child's pain, distress and other behaviours.

Worrying about getting first-line management wrong

Parents worry about the consequences for their child if they get something wrong and fail to spot that their child is seriously ill (Kai 1996b). Parents frequently find it difficult to evaluate their child's illness and thus also find it challenging to know when it is appropriate to seek advice from health care professionals and whether the situation is urgent (Winskill et al. 2011). They often find themselves having to second guess outcomes by asking themselves 'do I, don't I ask for help?' (Neill and Carter 2012). Initially, if needing more information or a source of reassurance or advice, parents may seek help from people such as family and friends within their 'lay network' (Kai 1996a, 1996b); some members of this lay network may include more expert friends or friends/family who are health care professionals (Neill 2000, Neill and Cowley 2010). Parents also access advice from the pharmacist (Cunningham-Burley and Maclean 1987; Cantrill et al. 1996) about which pain medicines they could use or advice about whether they should seek an appointment with their general practitioner.

While reasonably confident about managing minor ('normal') childhood illnesses such as coughs and colds, parents express less confidence and greater uncertainty about managing 'real illnesses' (Neill 2010). Arguably, unexplained pain falls into the category of a potential real illness and, as such, it is likely to trigger the need to manage the uncertainty through accessing professional advice. In these situations of high uncertainty, parents perceive their child's illness as a threat and may be concerned about possible death, disability or chronic illness (Robbins et al. 2003). Neill (2010: 339) talks of the diagnostic, trajectory and symbolic uncertainty engendered when parents are concerned that their child may have a real illness.

Seeking help

Where parents perceive the situation to be problematic and/or are unsure they often seek a second opinion, to either gain reassurance that nothing much is wrong and the child will get better or confirm that there is a problem and that the health care professionals will manage it (Hendry et al. 2005; Winskill et al. 2011).

In Anne's story we see how she was led astray in her assessment and decision-making; the context of the situation meant that she initially misread Ruari's complaints of pain. She ascribed the 'furore' being the result of 'the loss of the match, combined with the heat of the day, and possible dehydration' and although she noted that Ruari went 'pale and clammy' when he fell, she missed making the link to his reports of pain. It was only when her usual interventions of 'the "magical" water treatment along with prerequisite ice pack application' were not effective that she took Ruari to the hospital where a fracture was diagnosed and treated. She explains how Ruari's pain subsided when his injury was acknowledged and the correct treatment was given.

Ertmann et al. (2011a, 2011b) discuss the complexity of decisions to seek medical advice, showing how, as parents become more experienced their threshold for consultation tends to increase. However, Houston and Pickering (2000) found that the threshold could decrease if parents were sensitised if their child had previously experienced a serious illness. The decision to seek medical attention is influenced by many different factors (Neill 2000; Trajanovska et al. 2010; Winskill et al. 2011; Neill and Carter 2012). These factors can broadly be categorised as child-centred, pain-centred, parent-centred and service-centred as can be seen in Figure 5.2.

Parents are often concerned about seeking help too early or too late (Ertmann et al. 2011a); they want to be sure they are 'doing the right thing'(Neill 2010: 333) in seeking help and are worried about being subjected to medical criticism (Neill and Cowley 2010) and made to 'feel silly'(Neill 2010: 340) for having sought medical help. Parents walk a fine line in deciding when the time is right to ask for qualified health care advice. Studies show that they are often made to feel that their decision-making is faulty. While their primary concern is their child's health and well-being, most parents do not want to be perceived as bothering health professionals (Allen et al. 2002) or to generate a track record of being troublesome or time-wasters. Equally they do not want to leave things too late; if this occurs, health professionals are likely to frame their (in)action as being irresponsible if they do not bring their child with a 'real' illness to the health professionals' attention in a timely manner.

Health professionals are often unaware of the extent of internal dialogue (should I, shouldn't I?) that parents have before they take their child with pain to their GP or walk-in centre. Ertmann et al. (2011a: 26) state that 'even the barely ill child that the GP meets has been thoroughly assessed by the parents', and yet parents presenting with a 'barely-ill' child can experience a feeling of professional censure as the child's presenting symptoms are insufficient to be seen – by a health professional – as a 'real illness'. Interestingly, health professionals can face a similar dilemma when confronted by their own 'barely-ill' children and they too quite often take their child to be checked over. Parents simply do not want to overlook signs and symptoms such as pain, which are indicating a dangerous situation. However, this desire to seek help has to be seen in the context of what Neill et al. (2013: 758) talk of as impression

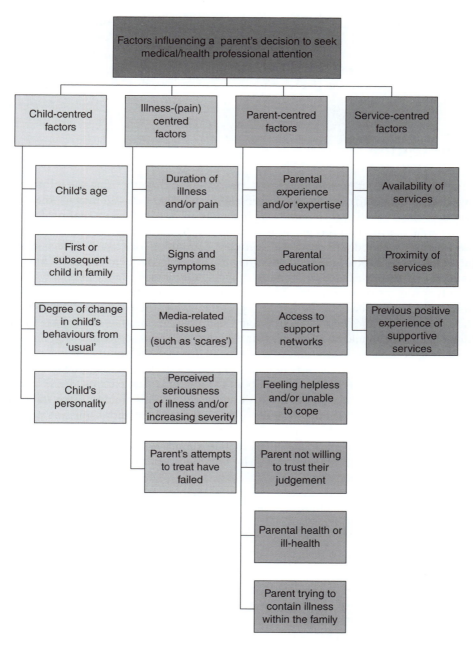

Figure 5.2   Factors influencing a parent's decision to seek medical/health professional attention

management, 'particularly where they feel they may be subject to scrutiny'. Neill et al. further talk of the informal social rules that guide parental actions and which pressure parents to ensure that 'normal or minor illness will be contained within the family whilst medical attention will be sought for 'real' illness' (Neill et al. 2013: 761). Felt or enacted criticism by health professionals can reduce feelings of self-efficacy and shake parents' confidence in their parenting skills. This in turn can shape parents' decisions about whether or not to seek medical help in the future for their child's pain.

Conclusion

Parents have a tough time in identifying, processing and synthesising the information available to them and coming to a decision about whether they can manage the child's pain and illness within their family or if they need to ask for external professional help. Parents have to do this when their child is in pain and distressed and while they are worried and tired. Despite these non-ideal conditions for effective decision-making, most parents are good decision-makers. Noah's mother 'assessed' him and decided that he just needed his 'tummy rubbed', a dose of medicine and he would be fine. This was the right decision and his pain resolved itself by morning. Kayla's initial assessment was similar but she became concerned when these actions did not resolve the situation and she then correctly sought help. Neither mother could have known how the episode would end. Parents fear that they will miss something vital and their child will become seriously ill. Anne spoke of feeling 'very guilty' about ignoring Ruari's pain even though he was fine once the back slab had been applied.

Health professionals need to think about the dilemma that parents face (Neill and Carter 2013) and be supportive about how they deal with children with minor illness. Pain is one of the leading triggers to seek medical help and dismissing parental concerns about a child who professionals determine is barely ill is unforgiveable. We need to gain parents' perspectives so as to gain a more holistic understanding of the child's particular circumstances, their pain and the trajectory of their illness. Engaging parents in a respectful manner that acknowledges their skills and concerns can help promote their confidence and efficacy as parents so that they can both better manage pain and minor illness at home as well as make confident decisions about when they need external help.

Key points

- The vast majority of children's pain is dealt with their parents at home, without any recourse to external help.
- Most children experience a range of different 'everyday' types of pains as part of growing up.
- Parents assess their child's pain using the cues they recognise and understand and match these with the context to try work out the cause of the pain.
- Hugs, reassurance, rubbing or stroking the area that is hurting and keeping their child close to them are core to parental management of pain.

- Using common over-the-counter medicines for pain management is fairly routine practice by parents as an initial intervention.
- Where parents perceive the situation to be problematic and/or are unsure they often seek a second opinion.

Additional Resources and Reading

- The 'My Child is in Pain' web resource includes videos to support parents to manage their child's pain after day case surgery:
  - http://mychildisinpain.org.uk/
- The Spotting the Sick Child website is an interactive tool supporting health professionals to assess the acutely sick child:
  - www.spottingthesickchild.com/?
- Any of the papers by Sarah Neill listed in the references will be a valuable read.
- A good resource (including a slide show) for children and parents about pain is:
  - www.aboutkidshealth.ca/En/ResourceCentres/Pain/AboutPain/Pages/default. aspx

References

Allen, J., Dyas, J. and Jones, M. (2002) 'Minor illness in children: parents' views and use of health services', *British Journal of Community Nursing*, 7 (9): 462–8.

Bruijnzeels, M.A., Foets, M., van der Wouden, J.C., van den Heuvel, W.J. and Prins, A. (1998) 'Everyday symptoms in childhood: occurrence and general practitioner consultation rates', *British Journal of General Practice*, 48 (426): 880–4.

Cantrill, J.A., Johannesson, B., Nicolson, M. and Noyce, P.R. (1996) 'Management of minor ailments in primary schoolchildren in rural and urban areas', *Child: Care, Health & Development*, 22 (3): 167–74.

Carter, B., Bray, L., Blackwell, N. and Franck, L. (2013) *My Child is in Pain Study*. Unpublished report. University of Central Lancashire, Preston.

Cunningham-Burley, S. and Irvine, S. (1987) '"And have you done anything so far?" An examination of lay treatment of children's symptoms', *British Medical Journal*, 295 (6600): 700.

Cunningham-Burley, S. and Maclean, U. (1987) 'The role of the chemist in primary health care for children with minor complaints', *Social Science & Medicine*, 24 (4): 371–7.

Ertmann, R.K., Møller, J.J., Waldorff, F.B., Siersma, V., Reventlow, S. and Söderström, M. (2012) 'The majority of sick children receive paracetamol during the winter', *Danish Medical Journal*, 59 (12): A4555–A4555.

Ertmann, R.K., Reventlow, S. and Soderstrom, M. (2011a) 'Is my child sick? Parents' management of signs of illness and experiences of the medical encounter: parents of recurrently sick children urge for more cooperation', *Scandinavian Journal of Primary Health Care*, 29 (1): 23–7.

Ertmann, R.K., Siersma, V., Reventlow, S. and Söderström, M. (2011b) 'Infants' symptoms of illness assessed by parents: impact and implications', *Scandinavian Journal of Primary Health Care*, 29 (2): 67–74.

Hameen-Anttila, K., Halonen, P., Siponen, S., Holappa, M. and Ahonen, R. (2011) 'Parental attitudes toward medicine use in children in Finland', *International Journal of Clinical Pharmacy*, 33 (5): 849–8.

Hay, A.D., Heron, J. and Ness, A. (2005) 'The prevalence of symptoms and consultations in pre-school children in the Avon Longitudinal Study of Parents and Children (ALSPAC): a prospective cohort study', *Family Practice*, 22 (4): 367.

Hendry, S.J., Beattie, T.F. and Heaney, D. (2005) 'Minor illness and injury: factors influencing attendance at a paediatric accident and emergency department', *Archives of Disease in Childhood*, 90 (6): 629-33.

Houston, A.M. and Pickering, A.J. (2000) '"Do I, don't I call the doctor": a qualitative study of parental perceptions of calling the GP out-of-hours', *Health Expectations*, (4): 234–42.

Kai, J. (1996a) 'Parents' difficulties and information needs in coping with acute illness in pre-school children: a qualitative study', *British Medical Journal*, 313 (7063): 987–90.

Kai, J. (1996b) 'What worries parents when their preschool children are acutely ill, and why: a qualitative study', *British Medical Journal*, 313 (7063): 983–6.

Kelly, K., Leventhal, H., Andrykowski, M., Toppmeyer, D., Much, J., Dermody, J., Marvin, M., Baran, J. and Schwalb, M. (2005) 'Using the common sense model to understand perceived cancer risk in individuals testing for *BRCA1/2* mutations', *Psycho-oncology*, 14 (1): 34–48.

Leventhal, H., Benyamini, Y., Brownlee, S. and et al. (1997) 'Illness representation: theoretical foundations', in J. Weinman and K. Petrie (eds), *Perceptions of Health and Illness*. London: Harwood Publishers, pp. 19–45.

Neill, S. (2000) 'Acute childhood illness at home: the parents' perspective', *Journal of Advanced Nursing*, 31 (4): 821–32.

Neill, S. (2010) 'Containing acute childhood illness within family life: a substantive grounded theory', *Journal of Child Health Care*, 14 (4): 327–44.

Neill, S. and Carter, B. (2012) '"Do I, don't I ask for help?': the perpetual dilemma of parents whose children are ill at home', *Journal of Child Health Care*, 16 (4): 317–19.

Neill, S. and Cowley, S. (2010) 'Felt or enacted criticism theory – a contribution to the understanding of parents' decision making in acute childhood illness', *Pediatric Research*, 68: 641-2.

Neill, S., Cowley, S. and Williams, C. (2013) 'The role of felt or enacted criticism in understanding parent's help seeking in acute childhood illness at home: a grounded theory study', *International Journal of Nursing Studies*, 50(6): 757–67.

Robbins, H., Hundley, V. and Osman, L.M. (2003) 'Minor illness education for parents of young children', *Journal of Advanced Nursing*, 44 (3): 238–47.

Rogers, A. and Nicolaas, G. (1998) 'Understanding the patterns and processes of primary care use: a combined quantitative and qualitative approach', *Sociological Research Online*, 3 (4): U71–U87.

Sullivan, J.M. (1997) 'Learning the baby: a maternal thinking and problem-solving process', *Journal of the Society of Pediatric Nurses*, 2 (1): 21–8.

Trajanovska, M., Manias, E., Cranswick, N. and Johnston, L. (2010) 'Parental management of childhood complaints: over-the-counter medicine use and advice-seeking behaviours', *Journal of Clinical Nursing*, 19 (13–14): 2065–75.

Winskill, R., Keatinge, D. and Hancock, S. (2011) 'Influences on parents' decisions when determining whether their child is sick and what they do about it: a pilot study', *International Journal of Nursing Practice*, 17 (2): 126–32.

Chapter 6

Existential Pain and the Importance of Place and Presence

Erik's Story

Janet's and Erik's Story

This event occurred in the early 1990s when I was a fairly new nurse on a Paediatric Intensive Care Unit (PICU). This event touched me deeply and in a way came to decide my care of all the patients I have cared for after this meeting. I'll tell you from memory as I remember; there is a risk that some things are not really correlated in time but the meaning is the same.

On this particular day I had been responsible for a little boy, 5 years old, who came to us with three chest drains, as he coughed up a large pneumothorax. He was very ill and frail. The doctors had decided that he would not be on a ventilator because they were afraid he would not survive the process. He had cancer for a very long time and his blood counts were very low.

I was told that the boy had already survived two occasions but was now again critically sick; so sick that he was not expected to survive. He had been transferred to us during the early morning hours; all alone, without his parents at his side. I wondered about them, where they were, and if they would come later. To us it was natural that the children that were so severely ill had their parents present all the time and sleeping at their side, in a single room. I was told that his parents had not visited him during the last two weeks as they did not feel good about him being so sick again. They had just got a little baby and the father had failing mental health.

I was dismayed and wondered if any other family member was with him, but no, he was all alone. Burdened, I went into the room to greet this little boy who had to be in a PICU all alone and dying.

Inside the room the lights dimmed and I glimpsed a small skinny boy with tufts of hair on the head. He was so abandoned, alone and vulnerable, yet incredibly strong. He's probably the strongest little patient I have ever cared for. He lay in his bed on his back with three drains in the chest, two on one side and one on the other. He turned his head away to avoid contact and to gain his own space in this medical technology world, where he now found himself.

I greeted him and told him my name and that I would be with him tonight and come back early tomorrow morning. He replied with a small 'hello'. Then he said, still with his face turned away, 'Read for me mom, read Alfie'.

Beside the bed was a book about Alfie and I sat nicely down to read it for him. As I sat there and read, it occurred to me how much at the mercy of other people this poor boy was and how great his desire for his mother was. He created his own world where I, for a moment, was given the role of his mother, even though I'm from the south of Sweden and my accent is inconsistent with his mother's accent. This was a realisation that made me keep reading with tears in my eyes. We could not give him what he longed for or needed the most; the love and closeness of his parents. Ideally, I wanted to take him in my arms and give him that love and closeness, but to do that he must invite me and be willing to accept closeness from another person with whom he had no deeper attachment. What I felt I could do in the situation was to meet his desire to be read to and sit there as a person he wanted just then.

It was incredibly emotionally engaging and touching to care for this boy. During the evening he was lying half asleep and half awake. He wandered in and out of consciousness and presence. When he came to, he said – 'Read for me mom, read Alfie'. And I read. On one of these occasions, quite late at night, he stretched his hand towards me across the blanket, still with his face turned away, and I took it and went on reading *Alfie*. I knew that I could not go out of the room, to 'escape' from him, even though it was very emotionally draining to stay. Here Erik was meeting death alone with such mental strength, despite all the anguish it must have meant for him. I found it emotionally difficult to share this brief moment with him, I understood that I had to put everything else aside and be there and meet him to give good care. By stretching his hand toward me and letting me take it, to touch him, he gave me a confidence. A confidence I did not or could not fail.

Medically, there was not too much to fix around the boy: he was given his pain relief, controls were taken and his thoracic drains controlled, drip replacement of fluid and medications given. The big challenge was to meet him in his loneliness and suffering, trying to satisfy his need for a 'mom' until his mother came. On the evening round, I asked about his parents and if someone had approached them. Someone from the other hospital had been in contact with them prior to the transfer and we were told they would come when they could. This answer was not good and we discussed whether any of us should call them. I do not remember what actually happened.

That night I stayed until he fell asleep. The following day I was early at work and took over his care. The night had passed as the night before. He had been asleep and was awake unregularly. In the morning when I counted fluids, changed the drip and washed him, he looked at me for the first time. He looked straight into my eyes, steady with his blue eyes and he asked – 'Read for me mom, read Alfie'. I sat down at the bedside, holding his hand and read. So the morning passed. He became worse during the day with longer and longer sleep times or moments between consciousness and unconsciousness.

Shortly after lunch his parents came to the PICU. They walked along the wall, two thin people with a baby in their arms. It appeared from their whole body position that they felt unwell and had suffered. I walked up to them and asked if they were the boy's parents, they nodded and asked how their son was. I explained that he longed very much for them and that I had read *Alfie* for him. They told me that it was his favourite book. I asked if they wanted to come in to see and be with him and hold him in their arms, but they did not know if they could. I tried to talk to them. We looked into the room, through the window in the door, and the mother burst into tears and explained that she had never seen him so sick and that she knew that this time he would not manage to get better. I confirmed her feeling and asked her if she could go in for a while because he longed for her. She did not know if she could bear it, because he suffered so, and she wanted to remember him as he was not sick and suffering. We talked a while about the essence of parenthood: to be there for our children, love them to the end, that it was something loving and beautiful and she was the only one who could give her son that. The father pulled away and I did not really reach him. Eventually she followed me into the room to her son. At that point, the father waited with the baby outside.

It was so incredibly emotional when she came through the door. It was like you could have touched upon the emotions that flowed in the room. The boy woke up and said, 'mom, mom you came'. She went up a little hesitant and kissed him. I do not think an eye was dry. The most important thing was that he knew and she knew the love that existed between them. The boy looked considerably relieved, and we helped him up into her arms. There they sat for a good while. Then the doctors came and wanted to talk to the parents. I do not really remember what was said, but afterwards, they came back into the room, this time with the father, and someone had come to take care of the baby. The parents picked up their son in their arms, and shortly afterwards he died in his mother's arms.

Thankfully, I have never before or after met such a lonely and vulnerable child. But the incident has affected me strongly and I have often asked myself what I could have done differently. What should we, as an organisation, have done differently? How could we have supported the family in a better way through this difficult time? I was new to the PICU and maybe a little too cautious on how things should be done. What I took from this experience and promised myself was to never let a child be alone in their illness or situation again. This promise I have kept. It was obvious that, as health care providers, we simply should have sent the whole panorama of support we had access to for this family. We should have done that at soon as it stood clear that they could not share and bear their son's illness. We failed this 5-year-old boy who was dying in the PICU when we left his family to bear this alone, even though they so obviously could not cope. It should go without saying that all children should be able to have one of their parents at their side around the clock when they are hospitalised, regardless of what is required of us to make this possible.

Introduction

It hardly feels necessary to write a chapter based on Janet's story. It stands perfectly well on its own. It makes us think, reflect, reach out, shed a tear and wonder how we would have acted. It makes me want to read 'Alfie' and understand why that story book was Erik's favourite and why it was such a particular comfort to him.

Janet paints an evocative word picture of Erik and how alone he is. She writes of her own feelings as well as her assessment of Erik and his parents. She reminds us that some of the most important things that we can do to ease a child's pain are those things which are fundamentally and intensely human. Janet reaches out to Erik and, when he is ready, Erik reaches back. Janet's story reaches out to us all.

In some senses Janet's story is not an obvious pain story. Janet only uses the word pain once in her story, and this occurs, almost casually, about halfway through. She says, 'Medically, there was not too much to fix around the boy, he was given his pain relief'. She is certainly not dismissive of the technical and medical care he requires. However, her focus is on Erik's suffering which transcends the 'mere' experience of pain. Janet's story is about existential pain and how this affected Erik, his parents, and herself as his nurse. Janet sees Erik's pain as encompassing those elements which can be treated with medication as well as those elements which required her to come to know and be known by the child. She helped to ease Erik's pain by letting him come to know her and to be someone who was a constant in his world. She understands the importance of supporting his parents who were in an unbearable place; the place where their child was dying.

In this chapter we examine the concept of existential pain in terms of suffering and the sense of aloneness, loss and fear that some children can experience. We also examine the concept of being 'at home' and how a PICU is a strange and alienating place. The importance of presence, caring and compassion is explored to show how we can bring comfort and support to children and their families.

Suffering, a sense of place, and finding an anchor

Janet's story is literally set within a PICU, although it takes us well beyond the walls of the unit into an even more disturbing and distressing place.

In brief and disconnected brush strokes, Janet paints a picture of the PICU. We know Erik is in a single room. We know that there is a single bed. We know there is a chair because Janet sits with Erik and we know that he is surrounded by medical technology (drips, monitors, drains). We also know that the single bed is empty and he is alone. We know the lighting is dim. Our imagination and our knowledge of PICU can complete the picture; we know there will be unfamiliar and unexpected noises and smells, unfamiliar people, and uncertainty about what will happen next.

We know that this type of medically dominated environment is almost inevitable if Erik is to receive intensive care. We also know it is an alien and alienating environment and that it is not a good place for Erik. It would be frightening enough for any 5-year-old, let alone a 5-year-old who will have come to know pain, fear and suffering through the treatment he has received for the disease. Initially, apart from the times when Janet – or we hope, another nurse – sits with Erik, he is alone in the PICU environment.

Hospitals tend to be places that evoke negative responses from children: they are all too often associated with loss of power and control, social disconnection, disruption to 'normal' life, fear and separation (Pelander and Leino-Kilpi 2010; Wilson et al. 2010; Ford 2011). Places such as a PICU consist of three main elements: physical, spatial and temporal. PICUs are particularly difficult places within hospitals: they are physically and spatially quite threatening and they are associated with particular meanings such as crisis, impending death, tragedy and loss. While it is perhaps to be expected that they are not easy places for children or their parents, what is less often acknowledged is that they can be difficult places for staff who have to deal with both technologically and emotionally challenging situations. Places such as PICUs challenge children's sense of who they are, their sense of place in the world and their sense of security, particularly their sense of ontological security, their 'confidence … in the continuity of their self-identity and in the constancy of their social and material environments' (Giddens 1990: 92).

The environment of a PICU is about as far away from anything familiar, home-like or comforting for a 5-year-old as can be imagined. Most children will never be able to become attuned to a PICU or feel at home; it is not an easy or familiar enough space to live in. It is worth, perhaps, making a slight detour here to think further about the place – home – where Erik almost certainly longed to be. Home is usually the place that we want to be when we are unwell; the place where we feel most safe. It is a paradox that hospital – the place we go to when we are most unwell, most in need and most in crisis – is so unlike home. Seamon (1979) identifies five prerequisites for a sense of 'at homeness' or feeling of being comfortable and secure, these being: rootedness (a sense of belongingness and familiarity); regeneration (the restorative function of the place); at-easeness (the freedom to be oneself); warmth (an atmosphere that is friendly and supportive); and appropriation (a sense of control). None of these prerequisites is readily available to Erik although it is possible to see him trying to gain a sense of rootedness – perhaps a form of 'borrowed rootedness'[1] – through asking for *Alfie* to be read to him and a sense of control through turning his head away. Janet does her best for him and his parents but for the most part it is not and can never be enough. A PICU is not a place that is conducive to feeling comfortable and secure. Children in PICUs tend to experience high levels of emotional distress and negative psychological sequelae in the short- and long-term (Rennick et al. 2002; Ward-Begnoche 2007; Colville 2008; Rennick and Rashotte 2009). Despite nurses trying to humanise the environment (Gramling 2004), it still remains a deeply disturbing place for children and their parents.

Parents can find a PICU an intimidating and traumatic place (Merk and Merk 2013), not least because of the suffering that is engendered at the thought of the loss of their child (Morais and Costa 2009; Côa and Mandetta Pettengill 2011). Parents are traumatised by their child's illness, the need for hospitalisation, the treatment required, and by some of the major life-changing decisions they have to make (Noyes 1998; Gillian 2008).

Erik is in pain and also alone in a world of loss, fear and aloneness. Erik is suffering. Despite many improvements in drug regimes and pain management some children, like Erik, still experience intractable and escalating pain, distress, dyspnoea, and agitation (Houlahan et al. 2006). This causes suffering for the child, their family and the staff who care for them. Cassell (2004) proposes that suffering reflects an experience that threatens a person's sense of integrity linked to a perception of impending destruction. Boston et al. (2011) note both the range and ambiguity of definitions of existential suffering within the literature and the debilitating nature of existential suffering.

Most of the seminal conceptual work on suffering has focused on adults, with much less work focusing on young children and how suffering re-frames and shifts their life worlds. The loss of control, temporality, isolation, separation and loss of meaning are elements of suffering which have resonance within a discussion of children and suffering. Suffering threatens children's spirituality in terms of how they make meaning of situations (Mueller 2010). An extraordinarily eloquent image comes

---

[1] I am grateful to discussions with Dr Andrew Moore for the notion of 'borrowed rootedness'.

from Rollins's (2005) work with children with cancer in which a 12-year-old girl who had just been diagnosed with a brain tumour drew how she felt (see Figure 6.1). This pencil drawing sums up the sense of loss, separation, and aloneness that is inherent in the pain of existential suffering. The girl draws herself as a tiny figure, lost in the margins of the paper, drawn in the slightest, lightest pencil lines. She creates an image that is almost insubstantial. Her image reaches out and requires a response.

Stanley (2002) talks of how suffering often results in feelings of abandonment; not just through people avoiding contact but also through a decrease in the quality of contact. It would be both too easy and completely wrong to say that Erik's parents had abandoned him; being with him was just excruciating and unbearable for his parents. Without Janet's kind support, they may never have been able to step across the threshold of his PICU room to be with him.

As Erik enters Janet's professional life, he is clearly suffering. He is adrift in a wilderness of experiences, and yet despite this, Erik finds ways of anchoring himself. Janet describes how initially he 'turned his head away to avoid contact and to gain his own space in this medical technology world'. He intentionally and physically tries to remove himself from a place which is painful and frightening. Constrained as he is by 'drips' and 'drains', he is limited by what he can do to escape; all he can do is turn his head. Janet is wise. She respects this movement away from her. She demands nothing from Erik. She greets him and leaves him space to reply and with his face still turned away, he asks 'Read for me mom, read Alfie'. Janet has reached out and Erik has reached back. In his request for Janet to 'read Alfie' he creates an anchor point; an attempt to create a sense of ontological security that will make the place he is in and the suffering he is experiencing a little more bearable.

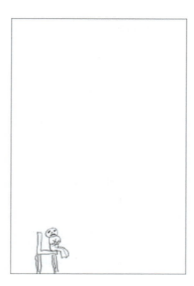

Figure 6.1   Drawing of fear of dying (Rollins 2005)

In the same way that Scarry (1985) talks of pain-resisting language and Frank (2001) talks of how 'aspects of suffering remain unspeakable', Schick Makaroff (2013) acknowledges that many elements of illness are immensely difficult for people to express; she terms these things as 'the unsayable'. While the 'unsayable' for Erik is 'where is my mom?', he is able to ask a nurse to read to him 'like his mom'. Within the limits of the actions available to him, Erik creates a place and space of security for himself with his nurse-mom and his book *Alfie*. *Alfie* acts as Erik's companion, accompanying him and acting as a conduit to allow Erik to gain the contact he so desperately needs from Janet and then from his parents.

Presence, caring and compassion

Janet frames herself 'a fairly new nurse on PICU' and she reflects at the end of the story that maybe she was 'too cautious'. However, through her presence she made a difference to Erik. She talks of feeling 'burdened' by his aloneness and suffering and yet she had the courage to be with this 'small skinny boy with tufts of hair on the head': she helped him through 'unsayable moments' (Schick Makaroff 2013: 482).

Janet chose to be present with Erik and her presence was active and powerful. Through reading Erik his favourite story, Janet was able, at least in a small way, to help reintegrate his sense of self even if she was not able to help him make sense of what he was experiencing. Malone (2003) talks of proximal care in relation to three types of proximity – physical, narrative and moral – as a means of demonstrating presence. Janet was engaging all three aspects of proximity to comfort and support Erik.

The concept of nursing presence is one which has received and continues to receive attention, although most of the literature focuses on care of adults. Finfgeld-Connett's (2008) meta-analysis concludes that caring and nursing presence are, in essence, the same thing. Yet presence, the 'gift of one's self' (Paterson and Zderad 2008), continues to be seen as a core relational aspect of nursing's relational work (McMahon and Christopher 2011). The notion of 'presence' is hard to resist as it suggests a particular way of being with and helping to manage the pain and suffering of the children and families we care for. At its most basic nursing presence is underpinned by three broad elements: 'ways of knowing' (knowing oneself and the other person); 'ways of being' (being there and with people, and being empathetic, courageous, vulnerable, intuitive, in the moment, serene, intuitive, silent, close, sensitive, transcendent, focused, and comfortable with oneself); and 'ways of doing' (advocacy, support, reassurance, connecting, affirming and valuing, accepting the emotional burden, decision-making and commitment) (Stanley 2002; Hain et al. 2007; Finfgeld-Connett 2008; Lindsay et al. 2012).

The shift to 'compassionate care' which is evident within nursing, certainly in the UK (Dewar and Mackay 2010; Commissioning Board Chief Nursing Officer and DH Chief Nursing Adviser 2012; Dewar and Nolan 2013), is in many ways a reworking of presence and 'good, values-based nursing care'. The values and behaviours that are proposed to underpin a culture of compassionate care (Commissioning Board Chief Nursing Officer and DH Chief Nursing Adviser 2012) are described as the 6 Cs (care, compassion, competence, communication, courage, and commitment). The 6 Cs need to be tailored to and enacted in order to provide compassionate care for children who are suffering and/or in pain.

Relationships of care with the child and family need to be built on mutuality (Curley 1997; Schumacher et al. 2008) trust, 'intelligent kindness' (Commissioning Board Chief Nursing Officer and DH Chief Nursing Adviser 2012: 13), empathy and respect. Competence in our care for children who are suffering means we need to draw on our clinical and technological knowledge and expertise. We need to ensure that the care we provide is based both on the best research and evidence and also on our clinical intuition about how we can best intervene for each individual child's pain and distress. Communication is central to creating a sense of connectedness (Stanley 2002) with the children and their families. Communication requires us to listen attentively to what the suffering child and their family are saying or unable to say and to 'be there' for them (Gramling 2004; Murinson et al. 2013; Polikoff and McCabe 2013). Courage comes from personal strength, experience and a vision for how we want to practice. Courage can be enacted in multiple ways such as challenging the status quo and ensuring we are available to the child who is suffering. Building on Malone's (2003) notions of proximal care, we need to be available for the children and families we care for physically, narratively and morally. We also need to 'be available' to each other. Day (2007: 616), writing of courage in critical care nursing, states 'Nurses act courageously when they slow down the efficient machinery of acute care in order to attend to the personal and particular needs of one patient and family.' Commitment involves ensuring that our practice and care are the best they can be for individual patients and through our commitment to nursing itself.

As Dewar (2013: 49) notes compassionate care is about 'the way in which we relate to other human beings when they are vulnerable'. If we are to nurse children like Erik who are suffering we need to be compassionate. We need to be prepared to take personal risks, acknowledge that accompanying them through the end of life is not easy (Lavoie et al. 2008) and accept that we may get hurt by the suffering that we witness. Bearing 'witness to patients' vulnerability and suffering' takes courage (Thorup et al. 2012: 433). Nurses providing end of life (EOL) care in a neonatal intensive care talk of how they were sometimes 'silent and silenced' about their experiences of the end of life care unit (Lindsay et al. 2012: 248) and PICU staff talk of sadness being the pervading response to caring for a dying child (Lee and Dupree 2008). Children's suffering affects us as health professionals and requires us to respond in a variety of ways.

We also have to understand that while holding a child's hand and reading them a story may be the best and most fitting action we can take to relieve pain and suffering, we also have to be prepared to confront things that we think should be done differently. We need to be prepared to act as advocates for children and their families, and be determined in ensuring that the decisions made have taken a child's best interests into account. There is a strong note of regret in Janet's story when she wonders what could have been done differently. Erik's parents should have been offered better support to manage their pain. Looking back, Janet can see how she and her more experienced colleagues might have acted differently, for instance by not passively accepting the absence of Erik's parents. She did ask what was being done but if faced with a similar situation today, she would actively work with his parents to ensure that they had the support they needed to be part of Erik's life in the PICU. Families need to be able to be close to their child. They need to be offered the opportunity and support to touch and hold their child and to be present throughout the dying process (Meert et al. 2008). Families remember health professionals who care with compassion as, unsurprisingly, they find compassion to be supportive during their child's end of life care (Brooten et al. 2013).

Conclusion

Janet's story is of a defining moment; a moment that shifted her understanding of nursing, nursing care, and the nurse she wanted to be. Many of the stories in this book look back on defining moments: profound turning points from which practitioners made decisions that their care would be more proficient and insightful, their knowledge deeper, their advocacy stronger, and their commitment more complete. Caring for children who are suffering requires us to extend the way we care from just physically providing technological care to fully engaging with the life of a suffering child by extending our ways of knowing them (Stein 2003). If we truly care for children in pain we have to learn from the situations we experience first hand as well as those that are shared with us through stories. Reading *Alfie* was crucial to the way in which Janet nursed Erik. *Alfie* created a sense of ontological security for Erik, a point of stability in a situation that was unstable, chaotic, frightening and unpredictable. *Alfie* was a constant in Erik's world, a source of relief; *Alfie* helped to create a sense of 'borrowed rootedness' for Erik. *Alfie* acted as an existential anchor for Erik and Janet understood this.

Janet was deeply touched by caring for this little boy and her story resonates with our own experiences. Janet's claim in the story is that 'we failed this 5-year-old boy'. This may in part be true, but Janet acted well. She was present for Erik and she read *Alfie* to him, even when she was hurting. More importantly she stepped forward to provide support to his parents when they came onto the unit and she stepped back to allow them to be with him, hold him and to be together as a family; to experience some sense of 'at-homeness' in the midst of suffering and loss.

Key Points

- Places such as PICU challenge children's sense of who they are, their sense of place, in the world and their sense of security.
- We need to create a sense of 'at-homeness' for children when they are in hospital and in pain.
- Despite many improvements in pain management some children still experience intractable and escalating pain, distress, dyspnoea, and agitation.
- Suffering often results in feelings of abandonment; not just through people avoiding contact but also through a decrease in the quality of contact.

- Communication requires us to listen attentively to what the suffering child and their family are saying or unable to say and to 'be there' for them.
- Holding a child's hand and reading them a story may be the best and most fitting action we can take to relieve pain and suffering.

Additional Resources and Reading

- Support groups such as The Compassionate Friends can provide advice, support and care for families facing the death of a child or for bereaved families.
  - www.tcf.org.uk/
- The International Children's Palliative Care Network (ICPCN) provides information on palliative care (www.icpcn.org.uk/) and offers e-learning modules.
  - (www.icpcn.org.uk/page.asp?section=0001000100430009&sectionTitle=Pain +assessment+and+management).
- Children can gain an understanding of death and dying from books, e.g.
  - Mills, J.C. and Pillo, C. (2003) *Gentle Willow: A Story for Children about Dying*, 2nd revised edn. Washington, DC: Magination Press.
- Textbooks addressing some of the issues raised in Janet's and Erik's story include:
  - Bearison, D.J. and Granowetter, L. (2012) *The Edge of Medicine: Stories of Dying Children and Their Parents*, 1st edn. Oxford: Oxford University Press.
  - Goldman, A., Hain, R. and Liben, S. (eds) (2012) *Oxford Textbook of Palliative Care for Children*, 2nd edn. Oxford: Oxford University Press.
  - Price, J. and McNeilly, P. (eds) (2009) *Palliative Care for Children and Families: An Interdisciplinary Approach*, 1st edn. Basingstoke: Palgrave Macmillan.

References

Boston, P., Bruce, A. and Schreiber, R. (2011) 'Existential suffering in the palliative care setting: an integrated literature review', *Journal of Pain and Symptom Management*, 41 (3): 604–18.

Brooten, D., Youngblut, J.M., Seagrave, L., Caicedo, C., Hawthorne, D., Hidalgo, I. and Roche, R. (2013) 'Parents' perceptions of health care providers actions around child ICU death: what helped, what did not', *American Journal of Hospice & Palliative Medicine*, 30 (1): 40–9.

Cassell, E.J. (2004) *The Nature of Suffering and the Goals of Medicine/Eric J. Cassell*, 2nd edn. Oxford and New York: Oxford University Press.

Côa, T., and Mandetta Pettengill, M.A. (2011) 'The vulnerability experienced by the family of children hospitalized in a pediatric intensive care unit [Portuguese]', *Revista da Escola de Enfermagem da USP*, 45 (4): 825–32.

Colville, G. (2008) 'The psychologic impact on children of admission to intensive care', *Pediatric Clinics of North America*, 55 (3): 605–17.

Commissioning Board Chief Nursing Officer and DH Chief Nursing Adviser (2012) *Compassion in Practice*. London: Department of Health, NHS Commissioning Board. Available at www.commissioningboard.nhs.uk (accessed 8 August 2013).

Curley, M. (1997) 'Mutuality – an expression of nursing presence', *Journal of Pediatric Nursing*, 12 (4): 208–13.

Day, L. (2007) 'Courage as a virtue necessary to good nursing practice', *American Journal of Critical Care*, 16 (6): 613–16.

Dewar, B. (2013) 'Cultivating compassionate care', *Nursing Standard*, 27 (34): 48–55.

Dewar, B. and Mackay, R. (2010) 'Appreciating and developing compassionate care in an acute hospital setting caring for older people', *International Journal of Older People Nursing*, 5 (4): 299–308.

Dewar, B. and Nolan, M. (2013) 'Caring about caring: developing a model to implement compassionate relationship centred care in an older people care setting', *International Journal of Nursing Studies*, 50 (9): 1247–1258.

Finfgeld-Connett, D. (2008) 'Qualitative comparison and synthesis of nursing presence and caring', *International Journal of Nursing Terminologies & Classifications*, 19 (3): 111–19.

Ford, K. (2011) '"I didn't really like it, but it sounded exciting": admission to hospital for surgery from the perspectives of children', *Journal of Child Health Care*, 15 (4): 250–60.

Frank, A.W. (2001) 'Can we research suffering?', *Qualitative Health Research*, 11 (3): 353–62.

Giddens, A. (1990) *Modernity and Self-Identity: Self and Society in the Late Modern Age.* Stanford, CA: Stanford University Press.

Gillian, C. (2008) 'The psychologic impact on children of admission to intensive care', *The Pediatric Clinics of North America*, 55: 605–16.

Gramling, K.L. (2004) 'A narrative study of nursing art in critical care', *Journal of Holistic Nursing*, 22 (4): 379–98.

Hain, A., Logan, J., Cragg, B. and Van den Berg, R. (2007) 'Presence: coming to know the whole. How expert nurses practice nurse presence in a critical care unit ... Dynamics of Critical Care 2007, Regina, Saskatchewan, October 21–23, 2007', *Dynamics*, 18 (2): 19–20.

Houlahan, K.E., Branowicki, P.A., Mack, J.W., Dinning, C. and McCabe, M. (2006) 'Can end of life care for the pediatric patient suffering with escalating and intractable symptoms be improved?', *Journal of Pediatric Oncology Nursing*, 23 (1): 45–51.

Lavoie, M., Blondeau, D. and De Koninck, T. (2008) 'The dying person: an existential being until the end of life', *Nursing Philosophy*, 9 (2): 89–97.

Lee, K.J. and Dupree, C.Y. (2008) 'Staff experiences with end-of-life care in the pediatric intensive care unit', *Journal of Palliative Medicine*, 11 (7): 986–90.

Lindsay, G., Cross, N. and Ives-Baine, L. (2012) 'Narratives of neonatal intensive care unit nurses: experience with end-of-life care', *Illness, Crisis & Loss*, 20 (3): 239–53.

Malone, R.E. (2003) 'Distal nursing', *Social Science & Medicine*, 56 (11): 2317–26.

McMahon, M.A. and Christopher, K.A. (2011) 'Toward a mid-range theory of nursing presence', *Nursing Forum*, 46 (2): 71–82.

Meert, K.L., Briller, S.H., Schim, S.M. and Thurston, C.S. (2008) 'Exploring parents' environmental needs at the time of a child's death in the pediatric intensive care unit', *Pediatric Critical Care Medicine*, 9 (6): 623–8.

Merk, L. and Merk, R. (2013) 'A parent's perspective on the pediatric intensive care unit: our family's journey', *Pediatric Clinics of North America*, 60 (3): 773–80.

Morais, G. and Costa, S. (2009) 'Existential experience of mothers of hospitalized children in intensive pediatric care unit [Portuguese]', *Revista da Escola de Enfermagem da USP*, 43 (3): 639–46.

Mueller, C.R. (2010) 'Spirituality in children: understanding and developing interventions', *Pediatric Nursing*, 36 (4): 197–203, 208.

Murinson, B.B., Gordin, V., Flynn, S., Driver, L.C., Gallagher, R.M. and Grabois, M. (2013) 'Recommendations for a new curriculum in pain medicine for medical students: toward a career distinguished by competence and compassion', *Pain Medicine*, 14 (3): 345–50.

Noyes, J. (1998) 'A critique of studies exploring the experiences and needs of parents of children admitted to paediatric intensive care units', *Journal of Advanced Nursing*, 28 (0309-2402; 1): 134–41.

Paterson, J. and Zderad,L. (2008) *Humanistic Nursing: (Meta-theoretical Essays on Practice)*, eBook #25020 edn, Project Gutenberg Ebook. Available at www.gutenberg.org/files/25020/25020-8.txt.

Pelander, T. and Leino-Kilpi, H. (2010) 'Children's best and worst experiences during hospitalisation', *Scandinavian Journal of Caring Sciences*, 24 (1471–6712; 0283–9318; 4): 726–33.

Polikoff, L.A. and McCabe, M.E. (2013) 'End-of-life care in the pediatric ICU', *Current Opinion in Pediatrics*, 25 (3): 285–9.

Rennick, J.E. and Rashotte, J. (2009) 'Psychological outcomes in children following pediatric intensive care unit hospitalization: a systematic review of the research', *Journal of Child Health Care*, 13 (2): 128–49.

Rennick, J.E., Johnston, C.C., Dougherty, G., Platt, R. and Ritchie, J.A. (2002) 'Children's psychological responses after critical illness and exposure to invasive technology', *Journal of Developmental and Behavioral Pediatrics*, 23 (3): 133–44.

Rollins, J.A. (2005) "Tell me about it": drawing as a communication tool for children with cancer', *Journal of Pediatric Oncology Nursing*, 22 (4): 203–21.

Scarry, E. (1985) *The Body in Pain: The Making and Unmaking of the World*. New York: Oxford University Press.

Schick Makaroff, K.L. (2013) 'The unsayable: a concept analysis', *Journal of Advanced Nursing*, 69 (2): 481–92.

Schumacher, K.L., Stewart, B.J., Archbold, P.G., Caparro, M., Mutale, F. and Agrawal, S. (2008) 'Effects of caregiving demand, mutuality, and preparedness on family caregiver outcomes during cancer treatment', *Oncology Nursing Forum*, 35 (1): 49–56.

Seamon, D. (1979) *A Geography of the Lifeworld: Movement, Rest, and Encounter*. New York: St Martin's Press.

Stanley, K.J. (2002) 'The healing power of presence: respite from the fear of abandonment', *Oncology Nursing Forum*, 29 (6): 935–40.

Stein, H.F. (2003) 'Ways of knowing in medicine: seeing and beyond', *Families, Systems & Health: The Journal of Collaborative Family Health Care*, 21 (1): 29.

Thorup, C.B., Rundqvist, E., Roberts, C. and Delmar, C. (2012) 'Care as a matter of courage: vulnerability, suffering and ethical formation in nursing care', *Scandinavian Journal of Caring Sciences*, 26 (3): 427–35.

Ward-Begnoche, W. (2007) 'Posttraumatic stress symptoms in the pediatric intensive care unit', *Journal for Specialists in Pediatric Nursing*, 12 (2): 84–92.

Wilson, M.E., Megel, M.E., Enenbach, L. and Carlson, K.L. (2010) 'The voices of children: stories about hospitalization', *Journal of Pediatric Health Care*, 24: 95–102.

Chapter 7

Managing Pain in a PICU

Becky's Story

Becky's story

This 6-year-old child called Becky was day 40 post-bone marrow transplantation (BMT). Her underlying condition was beta thalassemia major. She was cared for in a Paediatric Intensive Care Unit (PICU) after she developed complications post-transplant. Her complications included pulmonary haemorrhage, disseminated intravascular coagulation (DIC) and renal failure.

It is unusual to use pharmacological paralysing agents in intensive care environments, however there are occasions when critically ill children and adults require pharmacological paralysis to treat their lungs effectively with high levels of ventilatory support. When paralysing agents are used it is vital that the child is adequately sedated with adequate analgesia, but this can be challenging because while paralysing agents are in progress there is no accurate method to determine underlying comfort. Vital signs can be interpreted but they are not a sensitive indicator of pain and comfort. It is good practice to stop the paralysing agents at least once in a 24-hour period to fully assess the underlying level of analgesia and sedation.

With Becky's case it was evident that despite escalating doses of fentanyl and midazolam she was not receiving adequate sedation or analgesia. During the period of time when she was not receiving paralysing agents her pain assessments demonstrated that she was in considerable pain. She had previously been treated with high doses of morphine and clonidine, which had proved inadequate. Becky was changed onto remifentanil in combination with midazolam and this combination proved to be more effective.

This case demonstrates how important it is to vigilantly assess pain and analgesia effectiveness whilst children are receiving paralysing agents. The fact that paralysing agents are used so infrequently means we must ensure that clinicians are educated to understand the importance of careful assessment and management of such children from an analgesic and sedation perspective. Sadly the children requiring paralysing agents are amongst the sickest critically ill children, thus the priority of assessment and management of pain and comfort can compete with other assessments and procedures.

Postscript: the pain score used on our PICU patients is: no pain, mild pain/discomfort, moderate pain, severe pain.

Introduction

This story tells of the pain of a critically ill 6-year-old girl in a PICU and the challenges of assessing pain in a paralysed and sedated child. The nurses involved had no accurate method to assess pain in a paralysed and sedated child. While it was clear that Becky was experiencing considerable pain, the nurses could have been misled by the high doses of fentanyl and midazolam, which are powerful analgesics, that Becky had already received. Instead the nurses' persistence in evaluating the effectiveness of the powerful analgesic combinations demonstrated clearly to them that alternative analgesics were required if Becky was to achieve relief of her pain. Finding a solution to the situation was achieved through vigilance in monitoring and adjusting her analgesics. This story demonstrates the challenges of dealing with pain in a critically ill child and the skills required in recognising pain cues despite sedation and the use of paralysing agents.

Pain in critical care

Pain has been found to be a major stressor and patients' worst memory of critical care (Stanik-Hutt 2003). When patients are critically ill the occurrence of pain is high, and a wide array of variables may alter, distort, diminish, or preclude a patient's ability to communicate with caregivers regarding the discomfort (Alspach 2010). Several studies have shown that pain management in critically ill patients is poor and that the seriousness of pain is often misjudged (Carroll et al. 1999).

Critically ill children are frequently exposed to pain which requires skilled assessment and effective treatment. The most reliable resource for assessing pain is the child, but critically ill children are often unable to communicate verbally. Many sedated and intubated patients are unable to communicate their pain level, either verbally or by pointing at visual pain scales, making pain assessment particularly difficult (Herr et al. 2006). At the same time children admitted to critical care may experience moderate to severe pain (Puntillo 2001; Arbour 2008), and there are many factors in critical care that can alter a child's ability to communicate, making pain assessment more difficult (Paulsen-Conger et al. 2011). When children cannot express themselves, physiological and behavioural cues become unique indicators for pain assessment (Solomon 2000). In Becky's story it would not have been unusual for the nurses to accept that as she had been prescribed a combination of two strong analgesics, in escalating doses, that there was no more they could do. However, Becky's pain cues were recognised and acted upon due to the persistence and skill of the nurses.

Unrelieved pain in critical care

Unmanaged or poorly managed pain has been found to have a negative impact on critical care patients. Cousins et al. (2004) found that patients with untreated or insufficiently treated pain have said that they experienced a loss of autonomy, loss of control, and a feeling of not being taken seriously.

The experience of acute pain causes physiologic changes in the patient, making it harder for them to sleep causing tiredness and exhaustion (Lindberg and Engstrom 2011). The need for patients to deal with unrelieved pain themselves means their physiologic resources required for healing and recovery are reduced which can lead to longer hospital stays. Inadequate management of post-operative pain can lead to several other physiological changes, such as increased cardiac activity and reduced ability to cough and breathe adequately. It has also been recognised that insufficient treatment of acute pain can lead to pain continuing to exist after the injury or wound could be expected to have healed and may lead to the patients suffering chronic pain (Manias 2002). In a study by Fortier et al. (2011) of 555 children who had undergone general surgery, 15 per cent developed chronic pain, as a result of persistent post-operative pain.

Nurses in critical care are challenged daily to identify pain in critically ill children. Mattson et al. (2011) studied the experiences of pain in the PICU. Data were collected from 17 experienced nurses describing their perceptions of pain in non-verbal, critically ill, 2–6-year-old children. The study identified two diverse perspectives on pain: measure-orientated and patient-orientated. Nurses identified three categories of pain indicators: changes on measurable parameters; perceived muscular tension; and altered behaviour. It was concluded that nurses need to be vigilant in identifying indicators of pain. Subtle signs of pain are only identified first hand, meaning that nurses have to actively seek to recognise or identify any changes in parameters or behaviour that might indicate pain. In Becky's story the nurses were vigilant in assessing her pain, and did not presume that high doses of powerful analgesics were adequate in dealing with it.

Pain assessment

Pain in critically ill children should be regularly assessed using an appropriate tool (APA 2012) and a therapeutic plan for pain management should be established as a matter of routine and regularly reviewed as a child's condition changes. The first step in pain management is that nurses identify a child's pain. Recognition of pain relies heavily on the expression of the patient as well as interpretation by the caregiver. A number of tools have been developed that measure biobehavioural activity, such as neuroimaging and neuromuscular or behavioural assessment scales (Arif-Rabu et al. 2010).

A considerable amount of work has been undertaken to enable health professionals' access to accurate information on children's pain (Arif-Rabu et al. 2010). The neuromuscular activity of pain has been explored, and although it would be possible to collect such data via electroencephalograms, the use of such a technique is not currently practical and therefore not clinically feasible. Clinical biomarkers of pain are an alternative, which would involve the measurement of, for example, endogenous opioid neuropeptides which have an ability to dampen pain perception or β endorphins which have been associated with pain and stress response (Rittner et al. 2008). However, the use of such biomarkers for pain measurement is complicated by their role in the stress response, and the difficulty in distinguishing between a pain response and a stress response. A more difficult obstacle in their use however is the collection of, for example, cytokines, some of which are contained within the spinal cord (Zhang and An 2007). A third option is to look for behavioural measures of pain, which could involve facial expression, vocal expression or motor behaviours such as movement of the arms and legs. All such behaviour needs to be interpreted by the nurses caring for the child. In Becky's case, non-verbal cues were all that the nurses had in terms of information relating to her pain. Becky was pharmacologically paralysed and therefore the only indicators were physiological markers such as her blood pressure, pulse, or pupil reaction. Once the paralysing agents were removed, for assessment purposes, then non-verbal cues – her limb movement, eye movement, or movement of her mouth around the endotracheal tube – could be used as pain assessment markers. These cues are still problematic because although Becky was sedated she could still be experiencing pain – a real challenge for Becky's nurses.

One of the main challenges for nurses caring for children in a PICU is that many children are unable to communicate verbally, therefore nurses need to be vigilant to non-verbal pain cues. Some of the non-verbal behaviours identified as pain indicators.

Just as verbal reports of pain vary widely among different people, behavioural manifestations may also vary, rendering such observations of single behavioural cues less reliable than others assessed alongside these cues.

For non-verbal patients the American Society for Pain Management Nursing (ASPMN) recommends using multidimensional instruments that are characterised by both behavioural and physiologic indicators of pain (Herr et al. 2006).

Pain assessment tools in critical care

Pain can be triggered by many medical conditions including ischaemia, infections, inflammation, oedema and distension. Other sources of pain for a child like Becky can come from the intravenous lines which are in place – central lines, vascaths (dialysis), urinary catheters, and peripheral lines, as well as a painful throat due to intubation. The first step in dealing with pain is to recognise it. It is necessary to assume that all critically ill patients have pain or are at high risk for pain. Becky is likely to have had generalised pain due to her pulmonary haemorrhage, disseminated intravascular coagulation (DIC) and renal failure. Children like Becky are at a particularly high risk for poor pain management, being unable to vocally communicate, due to being ventilated and during the periods of paralysis she will have no motor movement that can be interpreted as pain cues. Also in Becky's story there was no one site of pain for the nurse to focus on.

The RCN (2009) pain management guidelines emphasise pain prevention, suggesting that nurses should pre-empt pain as it is easier to control pain when you prevent it from gaining a foothold in the first place. Pre-empting pain can be more readily undertaken in relation to procedural or post-operative pain where a specific painful event occurs. In Becky's case her systemic condition was causing her severe pain and would have been very difficult to pre-empt. What may have helped is a tool to measure Becky's pain that is validated for her age group and for use with critically ill or non-verbal children. There has been considerable development in tools that can be used for critically ill patients to assess their pain, two of which are the Finger Span Scale (Merkel 2002) and the COMFORT (Ambuel et al. 1992) scale. Both of these could be used with children of Becky's age.

Finger Span Scale

Merkel (2002) suggests the use of the Finger Span Scale may be particularly useful in children who are critically ill and have difficulty comprehending. Few children lack the physical ability to use the Finger Span Scale (outlined in Figure 7.1), making it easy to incorporate into a routine pain assessment in any setting.

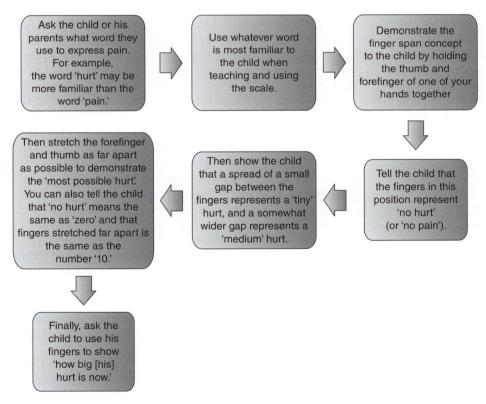

Figure 7.1   Using the Finger Span Scale

Adapted from Merkel (2002)

Pain intensity is determined by estimating the maximum finger span distance the child indicates. This pain intensity estimation can be documented either with numerals (for example, 0 to 10) or the words the child uses.

Merkel (2002) suggests that the Finger Span Scale is just one aspect of a comprehensive pain assessment in a young child. Its use with a behavioural observational scale, such as the FLACC scale (Merkel et al. 1997) will, improve the overall assessment of pain in young children. This scale could only be used once the paralysis has been stopped. It is good practice to stop the paralysis once each day and not to restart until the clinicians are confident that the child is comfortable. This is a challenge because if the child is critically ill this window for opportunity is small. However, during this window of opportunity this scale could be used.

COMFORT Scale

The APA good practice guidelines (APA 2012) suggest the use of the COMFORT Scale for managing pain in children of Becky's age receiving critical care. Managing distress is an essential treatment goal in PICU. Ambuel et al. (1992) developed the COMFORT Scale to assess the psychological distress of critically ill children under the age of 18. Additional research determined that the COMFORT Scale is clinically useful when determining if a child is optimally sedated (Razmus et al. 2003; Wielenga et al. 2004). This tool is considered a pain assessment instrument that provides a method of assessing pain using behavioural or physiological parameters often associated with pain, therefore making it appropriate for use with a non-verbal child such as Becky. Her nurses could use it when the pharmacological agent has worn off.

The original COMFORT scale incorporated eight factors. Of these six were behavioural: alertness, calmness or agitation, respiratory response, physical movement, muscle tension and facial tension. The remaining two factors were physiological: measuring blood pressure and heart rate. Further studies have contributed to the development of the COMFORT Scale in a PICU; Carnevale and Razack (2002) carried out an item analysis of the eight factors with 18 intubated and ventilated children and concluded that the two physiological factors of blood pressure and heart rate demonstrated very little variation in the total the comfort score. They suggested that a modified COMFORT scale could be used, incorporating only the six behavioural factors. Ista et al. (2005) confirmed the finding that the two physiological factors could be omitted without jeopardising the quality of pain assessment and named the modified tool, the COMFORT Behaviour Scale, or COMFORT-B. Further developments were undertaken by Van Dijk et al. (2005), who suggested the use of a visual analogue scale (VAS) alongside the COMFORT-B scale, to allow for the nurses' judgement of the child's pain to be included in the assessment.

Bear and Ward-Smith (2006) demonstrated the interrater reliability of the COMFORT Scale, confirming its appropriateness as a tool to provide assessment data for critically ill children, such as Becky. They stated that assessment should take a full two minutes of observing the child's behavioural cues.

Table 7.1   COMFORT-B scale

Alertness	Calmness/ agitation	Respiratory response (ventilated children)	Cry (non-ventilated children)	Physical movement	Muscle tone	Facial tension
1 Deeply asleep	Calm	No coughing and no spontaneous respiration	Quiet breathing, no crying	No movement	Muscles totally relaxed, no muscle tone	Facial muscle totally relaxed
2 Lightly asleep	Slightly anxious	Spontaneous respiration with little or no response to ventilation	Sobbing or gasping	Occasional, slight movements	Reduced muscle tone	Facial muscle tone normal; no facial muscle tension evident
3 Drowsy	Anxious	Occasional cough or resistance to ventilator	Moaning	Frequent, slight movements	Normal muscle tone	Tension evident in some facial muscles
4 Fully awake and alert	Very anxious	Actively breathes against ventilator or coughs regularly	Crying	Vigorous movement limited to extremities	Increased muscle tone and flexion of fingers and toes	Tension evident throughout facial muscles
5 Hyper alert	Panicky	Fights ventilator, cough or choking	Screaming	Vigorous movements including torso and head	Extreme muscle rigidity and flexion of fingers and toes	Facial muscles contorted and grimacing

Adapted from Ambuel et al. (1992)

Once these observations have been made the nurse assesses the sixth behavioural factor of muscle tone by flexing and extending the child's limbs.

Johansson and Kokinsky (2009) demonstrated the concurrent validity and reliability of the COMFORT-B Scale for assessment of pain and sedation in intubated and ventilated children, concluding that the use of validated scales may improve the assessment and management of pain and sedation in intubated children.

In Becky's story pain assessment was based on four items: no pain, mild pain/discomfort, moderate pain, severe pain. Using the COMFORT-B scale (see Table 7.1) for Becky may have made the challenge of assessing her pain less arduous, because it directs nurses to undertake an assessment of specific behavioural aspects directly related to pain and discomfort. The COMFORT-B Scale could have been used by Becky's nurses on a daily basis when they stopped her paralysing agent to judge her pain. In this case using a pain tool that takes 2–3 minutes appears to be quite feasible. Very frequent pain assessment may render the tool unlikely to be used by busy nurses because it is recognised that ease of use and time are obstacles to nurses using pain assessment tools with children (Simons and Macdonald 2006). Each PICU should evaluate the tool most relevant to their patient population and implement its use.

When established tools are insufficient to evaluate a patient's pain, the following methods of augmenting a pain evaluation should be considered: a pain risk profile; reports from surrogates; and an analgesic trial (Puntillo et al. 2009).

Analgesics

Once nurses establish that a child is in pain the next step is to act to relieve that pain. This can be achieved by using pharmacological methods and/or non-pharmacological methods of pain relief. In Becky's story she had received two different combinations of strong analgesics. She had been receiving morphine and clonidine, which were not having the required analgesic effect, and was then changed to a combination of fentanyl and midazolam, in increasing doses. Despite this strong medication regime Becky was still in considerable pain, requiring the nurses to take an individualised approach, as her response to analgesics was atypical and needed very specific assessment and adjustment in order to arrive at satisfactory pain relief. Only when Becky's analgesics were changed to a combination of remifentanil and midazolam did she gain relief from her pain. Sedation of critically ill children like Becky remains a challenge, mainly due to many variations between individuals and a lack of knowledge of the pharmacodynamics in children. Opioids such as morphine, hydromorphone hydrochloride and fentanyl work within the dorsal horn of the spinal column and in higher areas of the central nervous system to control pain (BNFC 2012). Opioid and non-opioid medications have complementary effects, for example paracetamol and diclofenac are morphine-sparing.

The drugs most commonly used in PICUs are opioids such as morphine or fentanyl, combined with a benzodiazepine such as midazolam or lorazepam (Rigby-Jones et al. 2007). In Becky's case she had been treated with a combination of morphine and clonidine, which was replaced with fentanyl and midazolam with limited success. The third combination was remifentanil and midazolam, and this provided Becky with pain relief. When remifentanil was compared with fentanyl in children aged 3–16 who required mechanical ventilation after spinal surgery, the pain relief achieved was linked with faster recovery in those patients receiving remifentanil (Akinci et al. 2005).

The lack of proven analgesic regimes for children like Becky demonstrates the need for ongoing vigilance and skilled judgement on the part of nurses to continually evaluate their level of comfort.

When managing pain in critically ill children like Becky, it is recommended that effective analgesia should be provided not only through multimodal and pre-emptive analgesia, but also combined with non-pharmacological techniques (Gandhi and Playfor 2010). Becky's nurses managed to provide effective pain relief for her through the use of a pharmacological approach. It may also have been helpful to have considered combining this with a non-pharmacological method to relieve her pain. McDowell (2005) suggests that the use of music therapy can help reduce anxiety and therefore also help in reducing pain. Music has been used in ICU as a method to reduce the negative effect of noise, create a more pleasant environment and reduce both anxiety and pain (Chlan and Tracy 1999). The effect of music in the reduction of pain may be explained by the Gate Control Theory, the basis of which is that when two stimuli are competing for attention, only one 'gets through'. In the case of music therapy, the music stimulus is the one that gets through to the higher centres in the brain. Chlan and Tracy (1999) also suggest that music stimulates the release of endorphins, which contributes to the reduction of pain.

Another non-pharmacological approach that could have been used with Becky is tactile touch. Tactile touch involves effleurage: soft stroking movements along the body, including the face, back, chest, stomach, arms, hands, legs and feet (Taylor 1991). Tactile touch is similar to therapeutic massage which has been recognised for some time for its benefits with cancer patients, as it promotes relaxation and alleviates the perception of pain and anxiety. Henricson et al. (2008) conducted a randomised controlled trial involving a 5-day tactile touch intervention on 44 patients in ICU. The results showed that tactile touch led to significantly lower levels of anxiety. The promotion of relaxation in relation to pain has been recognised as beneficial to post-operative patients (Roykulcharoen and Good 2004; Seers et al. 2008).

The use of either music therapy or tactile touch could have helped to relieve Becky's pain, and might also have helped the nurses in dealing with the stress of challenging and unrelenting pain. Such challenges pose a real threat to a nurses' level of stress and coping.

Nurses and pain in critical care

All critical care nurses share the universality of pain with the children they care for. Alspach (2010) suggests that we have all endured pain and all, intentionally or not, inflicted it, reacted to it, coped with it and recognised its relief. As a result our personal knowledge and experiences with pain may colour our sensitivity and responsiveness when caring for others. Asking a child to explain their pain verbally is considered to be the most reliable method of pain assessment, but there are studies that show that nurses trust their own judgement and experience about how pain is usually manifested after a particular surgery (Simons and Moseley 2009) and do not always trust what the child or young person says about their experience of pain (Schafheutle et al. 2000).

Working in a PICU it is important to be able to recognise signs of pain in patients unable to communicate verbally. Being without pain after surgery implies increased well-being and shorter hospital stays. A factor that influences pain perception is how a patient feels. Pain is influenced by many factors (Eccleston 2001), such as previous experiences of pain, its duration, intensity, extent, what it led to, why the pain arose and if the patient could control it will all determine how an individual experiences and copes with future pain. Lindberg and Engstrom (2011) studied the experiences of critical care nurses dealing with pain and found that the nurses felt that being unable to treat pain successfully was experienced as failing in one's work. Henderson (2001) explored the issue of emotional labour in nursing with 52 nurses in Canada and the UK. Nurses were found to support emotional engagement and considered it as desirable but also felt that too much emotional engagement could render a nurse incapable of doing the job. Nurses believed that nursing demands emotional engagement but that it can be achieved from a detached position. Some nurses in the study saw that they had two identities, one as a nurse and one as a person. Henderson (2001) concluded that in nursing there is a personal reward but also a personal cost to caring that requires emotional engagement.

The issue of emotional engagement can be accentuated when dealing with children in pain especially if, as in Becky's case, the pain was challenging and difficult to relieve. In Becky's story several different attempts were made to adjust her analgesics before she was made comfortable. This meant that nurses assessing her pain were repeatedly finding that they had been unsuccessful, and needed to maintain their motivation in finding an effective combination of analgesics. This situation is likely to have cost the nurses emotionally and could have meant that they disengaged from the situation so as to protect themselves from the distress of feeling powerless in the face of Becky's persistent pain. The cost of caring in nursing was explored by Menzies (1960) in her seminal work on anxiety in nursing which showed how high levels of stress and anxiety impacted on staff turnover and sickness. Menzies found that nurses' anxiety increased when they had to deal with a patient's emotion and as a result a social defence system evolved which manifested itself by nurses retreating from the role or task causing anxiety, and in so doing distancing themselves from patients. This distancing of nurses has been recognised as a defence against anxiety (Allan 2006) and may explain why the management of children's pain has been deemed to be inconsistent (Von Baeyer 2009).

Lindberg and Engstrom (2011) found that nurses viewed their failure to relieve pain and suffering of patients in post-operative care as a failure in nursing. One nurse described it as a personal failure and felt she was a bad nurse when the patients experienced pain despite assiduous attempts to relieve it. In critical care, nurses are faced with double jeopardy: on the one hand their patients are critically ill and therefore more likely to have significant pain, and on the other hand due to their illness or sedation are unable to convey their pain. This critical state and lack of communication makes assessing pain a real challenge, which nurses have to face by being insightful, and persistent in their approach to dealing with pain. Becky's nurses' persistence resulted in them providing effective pain relief. The nurses caring for Becky were experienced, knowledgeable nurses who had undertaken specialist training in caring for children in a PICU. Their level of increased knowledge may have had the double effect of providing them with the confidence to believe in their ability, through persistence, to relieve Becky's pain, which in turn provided them with a level of resistance to what could have been a very anxiety-provoking situation.

Conclusion

Wall and Melzack (1984) contended that pain is much more than a sensation, it is an experience, coloured by many influences that include our immediate circumstances, the urgency of competing priorities, observations of how others central to our lives respond, and learned and observed gender-related responses, as well as ethnic, cultural and at times geographical differences. Pain in critical care is dealt with alongside the need for life-saving interventions, and pain-relieving approaches may therefore become subordinate to such interventions. Nurses have to deal with the competing priorities that caring for a critically ill child like Becky presents. Managing pain in a child who is ventilated requires skill and creativity. Assessing such pain can be facilitated by the use of a validated tool for use with children in intensive care such as the COMFORT-B Scale, and managed by a combination of analgesics complemented by non-pharmacological methods such as tactile touch or music therapy.

Key Points

- Pain has been found to be a major stressor and the worst memory of being in critical care.
- Critically ill children are frequently exposed to pain which means their physiological resources required for healing and recovery are reduced.
- Pain in critically ill children requires skilled assessment by nurses.
- One of the main challenges for nurses assessing pain in critically ill children is their inability to communicate verbally with children.

- There are a number of tools that can be used with children in critical care such as the Comfort B Scale or the Finger Span Scale.
- The management of pain in critically ill children requires multimodal analgesia as well as non-pharmacological techniques.
- The emotional cost of dealing with pain in critically ill children can cause emotional distress in nurses, leading to distancing as a defence mechanism.

Additional Resources and Reading

- You may find the following articles helpful in extending your knowledge of caring for a child in critical care:
  o Gelinas, C. (2010) 'Nurses' evaluations of the feasibility and the clinical utility of the critical-care pain observation tool', *Pain Management Nursing*, 11 (2): 115–25.
  o Huynh, T., Alderson, M. and Thompson, M. (2008) 'Emotional labour underlying caring: an evolutionary concept analysis', *Journal of Advanced Nursing*, 64 (2): 195–208.
  o Small, L., Mazurek Melnyk, B. and Sidora-Arcoleo, K. (2009) 'The effects of gender on the coping outcomes of young children following an unanticipated critical care hospitalisation', *Journal for Specialists in Pediatric Nursing*, 14 (2): 112–22.
  o Ward-Begnoche, W. (2007) 'Posttraumatic stress symptoms in the pediatric intensive care unit', *Journal for Specialists in Pediatric Nursing*, 12 (2): 84–92.

References

Akinci, S.B., Kanbak, M., Guler, A. and Aypur, U. (2005) 'Remifentanil versus fentanyl for short-term analgesia-based sedation in mechanically ventilated postoperative children', *Paediatric Anaesthesia*, 15(10): 870–8.

Allan, H.T. (2006) 'Using participant observation to immerse one in the field – the relevance and importance of ethnography for illuminating the role of emotions in nursing practice', *Journal of Research in Nursing*, 11 (5): 397–407.

Alspach, G. (2010) 'Expanding our understanding and perhaps our empathy, for patients' pain', *Critical Care Nurse*, 30 (3): 11–15.

Ambuel, B., Hamlett, K., Marx, C. et al. (1992) 'Assessing distress in pediatric intensive care environments: the COMFORT scale', *Journal of Pediatric Psychology*, 17: 95–109.

Arbour, R.B. (2008) 'Pain management', in N.C. Molter (ed.), *AACN Protocols for Practice: Creating Healing Environments*. Sudbury, MA: Jones and Bartlett, pp. 149–85.

Arif-Rabu, M., Fischer, D. and Matsuda, Y. (2010) 'Behavioral measures for pain in the pediatric patient', *Pain Management Nursing*, 13(3)157–68.

Association of Paediatric Anaesthetists (APA) (2012) *Good Practice in Postoperative and Procedural Pain*, 2nd edition. London: APA.

Bear, L.A. and Ward-Smith, P. (2006) 'Interrater reliability of the COMFORT scale', *Pediatric Nursing*, 32: 427–34.

BNFC (2012) *British National Formulary for Children*. Available at www.bnf.org (accessed 25 January 2013).

Carnevale, F.A. and Razack, S. (2002) 'An item analysis of the COMFORT scale in a pediatric intensive care unit', *Pediatric Critical Care Medicine*, 3: 177–80.

Carroll, K.C., Atkins, P.J., Herold, G.R., Mlcek, C.A., Shively, M., Clopton, P. and Glaser, D.N. (1999) 'Pain assessment and management in critically ill postoperative and trauma patients: a multisite study', *American Journal of Critical Care*, 82 (2): 105–17.

Chlan, L.L. and Tracy, M.F. (1999) 'Music therapy in critical care: indications and guidelines for intervention', *Critical Care Nurse*, 19 (3): 35–41.

Cousins, M.J., Brennan, E. and Carr, D.B. (2004) 'Pain relief: a universal human right', *Pain*, 112 (1): 1–4.

Eccleston, C. (2001) 'Role of psychology in pain management', *British Journal of Anaesthesia*, 87 (1): 144–52.

Fortier M.A., Chou J., Eva L. Maurer E.L. and Kain Z.N. (2011) 'Acute to chronic post-operative pain in children: preliminary findings', *Journal of Pediatric Surgery*, 46(9): 1700–5.

Gandhi, M. and Playfor, S.D. (2010) 'Managing pain in critically ill children', *Minerva Pediatrica*, 62 (2): 189–202.

Henderson, A. (2001) 'Emotional labor and nursing: an under-appreciated aspect of caring work', *Nursing Inquiry*, 8(2): 130–38.

Henricson, M., Ersson, A., Maatta, S., Segestena, K. and Berglund, A.L. (2008) 'The outcome of tactile touch on stress parameters in intensive care: a randomized controlled trial', *Complementary Therapies in Clinical Practice*, 14: 244–54.

Herr, K., Coyne, P.J., Key, T., McCaffery, M., Merkel, S., Pelosi-Kelly, J. and Wild, L. (2006) 'Pain assessment in the non verbal patient: position statement with clinical practice recommendations', *Pain Management Nursing*, 7 (4): 44–52.

Ista, E., van Dijk, M., Tibboel, D. and de Hoog, M. (2005) 'Assessment of sedation levels in pediatric intensive care patients can be improved by using the COMFORT "behavior" scale', *Pediatric Critical Care Medicine*, 6: 58–63.

Johansson, M. and and Kokinsky, E. (2009) 'The COMFORT behavioural scale and the modified FLACC scale in paediatric intensive care', *Nursing in Critical Care*, 14 (3): 122–30.

Kabes, A.M., Graves, J.K. and Norris, J. (2003) 'Further validation of the nonverbal pain scale in intensive care patients', *Critical Care Nurse*, 29 (1): 59–66.

Lindberg, J. and Engstrom, A. (2011) 'Critical care nurses' experiences: "A good relationship with the parent is a prerequisite for successful pain relief management"', *Pain Management Nursing*, 12 (3): 163–72.

McDowell, B.M. (2005) 'Nontraditional therapies for the PICU – Part 1', *Journal of Specialists in Pediatric Nursing*, 10 (1): 29–32.

Manias, E., Botti, M. and Bucknall, T. (2002) 'Observation of pain assessment and management – the complexities of clinical practice', *Journal of Clinical Nursing*, 11: 724–35.

Mattson, J.Y., Forsner, M. and Arman, M. (2011) 'Uncovering pain in critically ill non-verbal children: nurses' clinical experiences in the paediatric intensive care unit', *Journal of Child Health Care*, 15 (3): 187–98.

Menzies, I.E.P. (1960) 'A case study in the functioning of social systems as a defence against anxiety', *Human Relations*, 13: 95–121.

Merkel, S. (2002) 'Pain assessment in infants and young children: the finger span scale', *American Journal of Nursing*, 102: 55–6.

Merkel, S.I., Voepel-Lewis, T., Shayevitz, J.R. and Malviya, S. (1997) 'The FLACC: a behavioral scale for scoring postoperative pain in young children', *Pediatric Nursing*, 23 (3): 293–7.

Paulsen-Conger, M., Leske, J., Maidl, C., Hanson, A. and Dziadulewicz, L. (2011) 'Comparison of two pain assessment tools in nonverbal critical care patients', *Pain Management Nursing*, 12 (4): 218–24.

Puntillo, K., Pasero, C., Li D., Mularski, R.A., Grap, M.A., Erstad, B.L., Varkey, B., Gilbert, H.C., Medina, J. and Sessler, C.N. (2009) 'Evaluation of pain in ICU patients', *Chest*, 135:1069–74.

Puntillo, K.A., White, C., Morris, A.B., Perdue, S.T., Stanikhutt, J., Thompson, C.L. and Wild, L.R. (2001) 'Patients perceptions and responses to procedural pain: results from Thunder Project II', *Americal Journal of Critical Care*, 10: 238–251.

Razmus, I.S., Clarke,K.A. and Naufel K.Z. (2003) 'Development of a sedation scale for the mechanically ventilated muscle relaxed pediatric critical care patient', *Pediatric Intensive Care Nursing*, 4(1): 7–11.

Rigby-Jones, A.E., Priston, M.J., Sneyd, J.R., McCabe, A.P., Davis, G.I., Tooley, M.A., Thorne, G.C. and Wolf, A.R. (2007) 'Remifentanil–midazolam sedation for paediatric patients receiving mechanical ventilation after cardiac surgery', *British Journal of Anaesthesia*, 99 (2): 252–61.

Rittner, H.L., Brack, A. and Stein, C. (2008) 'Pain and the immune system', *British Journal of Anaesthesia*, 10 (1): 40–4.

Royal College of Nursing (2009) *The Recognition and Assessment of Acute Pain in Children: Update of Full Guideline*. London: Royal College of Nursing.

Roykulcharoen, V. and Good, M. (2004) 'Systematic relaxation to relieve postoperative pain', *Journal of Advanced Nursing*, 48 (2): 140–8.

Schafheutle, E., Cantrill, J.A. and Noyce, P.R. (2000) 'Why is pain management suboptimal on surgical wards?', *Journal of Advanced Nursing*, 33 (6): 728–37.

Seers, K., Crichton, N., Tutton, L., Smith, L. and Saunders, T. (2008) 'Effectiveness of relaxation for postoperative pain and anxiety: randomized controlled trial', *Journal of Advanced Nursing*, 62 (6): 681–8.

Simons, J. and Macdonald, L.M. (2006) 'Changing practice: implementing validated paediatric pain assessment tools', *Journal of Child Health Care*, 10 (2): 160–76.

Simons, J. and Moseley, L. (2009) 'Influences on nurses' scoring of children's post-operative pain', *Journal of Child Health Care*, 13(2): 101–15.

Solomon, P. (2000) 'The clinical utility of pain behaviour measures', *Physical Rehabilitation Medicine*, 12: 193–221.

Stanik-Hutt, J.A. (2003) 'Pain management in the critically ill', *Protocols for Practice*, 23 (2): 99–104.

Taylor, A. (1991) *The Principles and Practice of Physical Therapy*, 3rd edn. Cheltenham: Stanley Thomas.

von Baeyer, C. (2009) 'Children's self-report of pain intensity: what we know, where we are headed', *Pain Research & Management*, 14 (1): 39–45.

van Dijk, M., Peters, J.W., van Deventer, P. and Tibboel, D. (2005) 'The COMFORT behavior scale: a tool for assessing pain and sedation in infants', *American Journal of Nursing*, 105: 33–6.

Wall, P.D. and Melzack, R. (1984) *Handbook of Pain*. Edinburgh: Churchill Livingstone.

Wielenga, J.M., De Vos, R., de Leeuw, R. and De Haan, R.J. (2004) 'COMFORT scale: a reliable and valid method to measure the amount of stress of ventilated preterm infants', *Neonatal Network: The Journal of Neonatal Nursing*. 23(2): 39–44.

Zhang, J.M. and An, J. (2007) 'Cytokines, inflammation and pain', *International Anaesthesiology Clinics*, 45 (2): 27–37.

Chapter 8

Assessing and Managing Pain in a Child who is Cognitively Impaired

Grace's Story

Rosie's and Grace's story

Grace has just had her thirteenth birthday. She hasn't got a diagnosis as such. Grace is classed as profoundly mentally and physically handicapped. And it's sort of a degenerative brain disease – classed as chemical imbalance within her brain – and that's as near as they've come to any kind of diagnosis. She's got brittle bones as well.

Grace has a lot of pain and lots of different pains. I feel that because pain's always been there, there's a lot that she accepts. I think Grace gets headaches and things after her fits. She very rarely cries but she does make a definite reaction to pain. As she's got older she lives with a level of pain which comes from her brittle bones. Grace doesn't scream and cry but every bit of her body will react.

There's times when she's pain free, probably not as much in recent years, because of her physical deterioration and most days are pain days. Some days are bad and she'll have tummy pain, and pain from her spasms and pain from sitting. It's a long list of pains now, it's frightening. When I look back on how she was in the past, when Grace was younger, she'd give me a lot more eye contact, a lot more smiles and things like that. She's still like that sometimes and she has times when she's more responsive to me and will smile more and look more and then I feel that she's happy within herself.

It's very difficult because Grace can't talk or communicate in any way. It's just feelings that you get. I just look at her eyes, the expression in her eyes and the way she's holding herself and things like that if I think she's got pain. I was 'useless' to start with, I never knew whether she had pain or was cross or bored but I've gradually got better. I think Grace has sort of taught me in a way.

When she has pain, Grace just withdraws into herself and the expression in her eyes is like 'Well what are you going to do about how I feel?' Sometimes I don't know for sure if Grace is in pain but I go with my instincts and I'm almost always right now. I didn't used to be but now I just know.

Like the time a few months ago when I took her to the hospital because I knew for sure her leg was broken. And I said to them 'She's greensticked her leg'. And they said 'She couldn't possibly! She'd be screaming her head off crying', but I said 'I'm absolutely positive she has.' The problem is Grace doesn't scream and cry with it. She did the first time she greensticked but now she's done it four times and when I took her to A&E the pain was in her face, it was like she was saying 'Oh I've had this before, this pain. I don't like it.' But she didn't cry and it was hard to convince them [doctors and nurses] there was something wrong and greensticks are hard to pick up on x-rays. But I was absolutely sure and so was my husband because we'd talked before I'd brought her in and then eventually they saw the fracture on the x-ray and it was like 'Oh yes Mrs ... you're right, it's a fracture ... that's got to be painful, how did you know'? And I was saying to myself 'Because she's my daughter and surely you can see the pain in her eyes and her face and her body.'

Introduction

Rosie's story provides a powerful insight into some of the challenges that parents of children like Grace, who have a severe cognitive impairment, face when trying to work out whether their child is in pain. It equally reflects some of the skills and expertise that parents develop over time and how they incorporate these into the everyday care of their child. Rosie's story is full of both certainty – 'I just know' – and uncertainty – 'sometimes, I just don't know for sure'. This sense of balancing between being sure and unsure is a fairly typical experience for parents of children with cognitive impairment.

What is really clear from Rosie's story is how pain assessment is linked with feelings, instincts and some detailed and conscientious detective work. In the absence of Grace being able to talk about her pain, she is reliant on other forms of communication and on other people being sufficiently perceptive at reading this communication. Although Rosie says that 'Grace can't talk or communicate in any way', this is only partially true. Rosie herself goes on to describe in some detail how Grace *does* communicate her pain. Whether Grace's pain communication is intentional is difficult to say but she does communicate pain through her eyes, face and body. The picture that Rosie builds of her daughter's expression of pain is of a child who does not cry or scream and who tends to 'withdraw into herself'. Her expression of pain is quiet and unless we, as professionals, are looking for the pain in her eyes and face, we may miss it.

In this chapter we will explore the epidemiology of pain in children with cognitive impairment. We will also consider the fundamental importance of assessing pain and some of the challenges that relying on proxies creates in ensuring accurate pain assessment. This will be followed by an examination of the main pain assessment tools and a consideration of why children like Grace require different tools from those developed for children without impairment. The chapter will close with an overview of the prevention and management of the typical pains that children with cognitive impairment present with as well as emphasising the importance of working in partnership with the child's parents.

What do we mean by children with cognitive impairment?

There is a varied use of terminology used within the research literature on pain assessment and management to describe the diverse group of children who are so severely cognitively impaired that they are unable to self-report their pain, because they lack the capacity to either verbally communicate their pain or purposefully communicate through other systems.

The terminology used in describing these children often reflects preferences or trends within and between different countries and is sometimes apparently used interchangeably. The terms most frequently used are cognitive impairment (e.g. Breau et al. 2001; Voepel-Lewis et al. 2008; Johansson et al. 2010; Ely et al. 2012; Massaro et al. 2013) and neurological impairment (e.g. Hunt et al. 2003). Some studies talk of profound special needs (Carter et al. 2002), others of children with intellectual disability (e.g. Breau and Burkitt 2009; Solodiuk et al. 2010). Herr et al.'s (2011) position statement on patients who are unable to self-report pain refers to persons with intellectual disability. Other literature uses terminology such as children with severe neurological disability (Hunt et al. 2007) and children with developmental disabilities (e.g. Lotan et al. 2009; Breau and Camfield 2011). These descriptors are often qualified by terms such as severe and profound to reflect the depth of disability or impairment.

The use of terminology in such an interchangeable way is not necessarily a major issue within the literature, providing the authors provide a clear explanation of the group of children they are referring to. There is overlap between the concepts because children with cognitive impairment may also have neurological impairments that can affect their physiology and behaviour (Breau et al. 2001).

Within this chapter, the terminology cognitive impairment is used with the implication that the children experience severe or profound impairment. The children's communicative, social and motor skill functioning is well below that expected of their chronological age. They are a group of children who often have co-morbidities. Many children with cognitive impairment have a seizure disorder, perceptual disorders (such as severe visual and hearing impairments) and physical impairments (such as high levels of spasticity and motor dysfunction) as well as respiratory and feeding problems. Children with cognitive impairment often require full-time care from their parents/caregivers and many may also require high levels of technological and nursing support, medical intervention and often complex drug regimes. Underlying diagnoses include birth asphyxia, cerebral palsy, and neurodegenerative and metabolic disorders.

Incidence of pain in children with cognitive impairment

Children with cognitive impairment have a higher number of pain episodes compared to their healthy peers. Not only do children with cognitive impairment experience the commonplace pains of childhood such as those from falls, toothache and vaccination, they also experience a range of different pains associated with their underlying disorder, other impairments and the prescribed treatments and interventions. Indeed, these children can experience frequent and significant pain, sometimes on an everyday basis (Carter et al. 2002; Breau et al. 2003; Houlihan et al. 2004; Hunt et al. 2004).

Identifying and managing this pain is often challenging for health care professionals and parents and some symptoms will persist even when treatment is instigated (Hauer 2010). Incidence studies are rare, and Breau et al.'s (2003) study is a milestone in identifying the range and extent of pain that children with cognitive impairment experience. Over the course of a year caregivers of 94 severe cognitively impaired children, aged 3–18 years, completed four semi-structured telephone surveys. Although some data were missing, a total of 406 episodes of pain (across all children) occurred during the four weeks the parents were prompted to recall. Children were reported to have pain on 18 per cent (n = 470) of the 2,632 days surveyed. Of the children, 22 per cent were reported as experiencing no pain during the study weeks, but 78 per cent were reported as having experienced at least one pain episode and between 35–52 per cent of children had pain each week. Findings showed that children experienced an average of 9–10 hours of pain per week. These pains were the result of associated illness and co-morbidities. The pain the children experienced had a mean intensity of 6.1 which is clinically significant. The study also found that those children with the fewest abilities were perceived to experience the most pain. The findings from this study identified that pain is clearly a problem for children with cognitive impairment and better clinical management is necessary. Rosie's story reveals that Grace experiences similar causes and levels of pain to the children in Breau et al.'s (2003) study and both Grace's and Rosie's quality of life are affected by Grace's pain.

Other published studies have demonstrated similar findings. Hunt et al. (2004) showed that 20 per cent (n = 27) of the children in their study had daily pain perceived to be of severe or very severe intensity. Stallard et al. (2001) showed that 73.5 per cent (n = 25) of the children had pain on at least one day with 84 per cent (n = 21) having pain on five or more separate days. Twenty-three children were perceived to experience moderate or severe pain, 13 of whom were perceived to experience this level of pain on five or more separate days, and four children were perceived to experience this level of pain for 11 or more days. Similar high levels of pain are found in studies which focus on children from a specific diagnostic group and are evident across a range of disability, as can be seen in Parkinson et al.'s (2010) study of pain prevalence in 806 European children with cerebral palsy. This study included children who could and those who could not self-report and noted a high prevalence of pain, with 73 per cent of parents reporting pain in the previous four weeks.

Types and causes of pain experienced by children with cognitive impairment

Children with cognitive impairment experience a range of different types of pain which arise from diverse sources. Hauer (2010) recognises that children with cognitive impairment are likely to experience different types of pain including nociceptive pain (e.g., from fractures, constipation, dental pain), neuropathic pain (e.g., arising from repeated surgery or injury), visceral hyperalgesia (e.g., related to the gastrointestinal tract) and central pain. Rosie talks of how Grace has 'lots of different pains' including 'headaches', 'tummy pains', pains from 'her brittle bones', 'spasms' and 'pain from sitting'. If we stop and think about what it might feel like to have pain from all these sources on a regular if not daily basis, it suddenly seems to be an impossible burden of pain for anyone to have to live with, let alone a child such as Grace whose life is already complicated by challenges to her health and well-being.

Different studies and writers have generated different ways of categorising the sources of pain in children with cognitive impairment (e.g., Carter et al. 2002;

Table 8.1   Overview of sources of pain experienced by children with cognitive impairment

Pains associated with	Examples of pain experienced
Alterations in gut motility	• Including gastro-oesophageal reflux, vomiting, wind, bowels, constipation and associated with feeding.
Musculo-skeletal problems	• Including pains related to spasticity, muscle spasm, dislocations and fractures (commonly relating to hips, legs, spine and shoulders) and pain generally associated with the child's immobility.
Co-incidental/infection and 'everyday' pains	• Including earache, headache, teething, nappy rash, chest infections, and menstruation pains.
Poorly fitting aids, equipment	• Including inflamed skin at site of feeding tube, traction on tubing, pain associated with wearing splints or supports.
Handling, moving, positioning Accidents and injury Iatrogenic pain	• Including sore ears and other problematic pressure points, discomfort from sitting or being moved.
	• Including pain from falls or injuries.
	• Including pain associated with medical investigations such as endoscopy, physiotherapy, venepuncture, dental care, surgery, medication.

Developed from Carter et al. 2002; Breau et al. 2003; Hunt et al. 2003; Massaro et al. 2013.

Breau et al. 2003; Hunt et al. 2003). Massaro et al. (2013) group pain into the following categories of causation: spasticity; gastro-oesophageal reflux disease; chronic constipation; pathological fractures; stomatological diseases and iatrogenic. Breau et al. (2003) noted pain as being related to accidental, gastrointestinal tract, musculoskeletal, everyday, infection, recurrent, medical, other and unknown. Drawing on these sources, Table 8.1 provides an overview of the types of pain experienced by children with cognitive impairment. Based on Rosie's story, Grace is likely to be experiencing or to have experienced pain associated with each of the sources listed in Table 8.1.

It is important for health care professionals to understand both the type and cause of pain as this creates opportunities to proactively manage the child's pain; wherever possible pain should be prevented rather than treated. Many causes of pain can be pre-empted (APA 2012) or moderated by effective nursing care.

Assessing the pain experienced by children with cognitive impairment

Is there a need for special tools?

Self-report of pain is generally considered to be the gold standard for pain assessment (Stinson et al. 2006). At its best, self-report provides direct person-to-person communication about fundamental aspects, such as the site and severity of a child's pain. However, children with cognitive impairment are unable to report their pain using words and this creates a particular challenge for nurses (McJunkins et al. 2010) and also for parents and carers. As Ely et al. (2012: 402) note 'when self-report of pain intensity is unavailable, clinicians tend to interpret pain behaviors based on experienced, personal attitudes, and beliefs about pain'.

Relying on such highly subjective behaviours is an insufficient response to pain in children who are unable to self-report, and Johansson et al. (2010) identify that this can leave room for misinterpretation. Misinterpretation, as well as what appears to be a dogged determination by medical and nursing staff to ignore Rosie's explanations that her daughter was in pain, show what can happen when personal attitudes and beliefs impede appropriate pain assessment. Rosie explained that Grace does not scream or cry when she has pain and that she tends to 'withdraw into herself'. These responses to pain are atypical of the ways in which children without impairment generally respond to acute pain.

The largest group of children who cannot verbally report pain are babies and pre-verbal children, and their treatment requires tools based on observation of the child's behaviour (von Baeyer and Spagrud 2006). Tools such as FLACC (Merkel et al. 1997; Voepel-Lewis et al. 2001; Manworren and Hynan 2003; Malviya et al. 2006) and COMFORT (Ambuel et al. 1992; van Dijk et al. 2000; Caljouw et al. 2007) are used quite widely. FLACC and COMFORT are recommended measures for procedural and post-operative pain assessment in children with normal or assumed normal cognitive development within the age range of newborn to three years old (APA 2012). Although specific tools have been developed for children with cognitive impairment, many nurses whose caseload does not regularly include children with cognitive impairment are less familiar with these specific tools than with the more generic pain assessment tools that they use on a daily basis.

Initially it might seem reasonable that the tools developed for pre-verbal children with normal cognitive development would be suitable for assessing pain in non-verbal children with severe cognitive impairment. However, there is conflicting evidence on whether behavioural assessment tools developed for the general population of children are effective in assessing the pain of children with cognitive impairment (Voepel-Lewis et al. 2008; Anand et al. 2009). Research by Voepel-Lewis et al. (2008) examined the clinical utility of three pain assessment tools: the revised-Face, Legs, Activity, Cry, Consolability (r-FLACC) tool (Malviya et al. 2006), the Nursing Assessment of Pain Intensity (NAPI) (Stevens 1990; Schade et al.

1996) and the Non-Communicating Children's Pain Checklist-Postoperative Version (NCCPC-PV) (Breau et al. 2002). The findings show that, based on clinicians' ratings, r-FLACC and NAPI had higher clinical utility compared with the NCCPC-PV, which suggests that they might be adopted more easily into clinical practice. However, work by McJunkins et al. (2010) showed that a pain assessment tool specifically developed for cognitively impaired children (NCCPC-PV) was more likely to identify moderate to severe pain than tools such as the Modified Objective Pain Score (MOPS) (Stevens 1990), the Children's Hospital of Eastern Ontario Pain Scale (CHEOPS) (McGrath et al. 1985) and the Visual Analogue Scale (Gallagher et al. 2002) which have been developed for the general population of children. Although only a pilot study, McJunkins et al. (2010: 309) conclude that the use of tools validated for this specific group could result in 'more accurate identification (and resultant treatment) of treatable pain' and that, potentially, this could improve the quality of the children's lives. If Grace's pain had been assessed using a tool validated for children with cognitive impairment it is likely that her pain would have been noticed and its intensity would have been accurately assessed.

Considering the pain burden of children with cognitive impairment, the risks and suffering associated with an inadequate assessment of pain should not be underestimated. It is, therefore, essential that health professionals use assessment tools which have been validated for this group of children, particularly now that there is a relevant and robust best-evidence base to support their use.

Choosing an appropriate and validated tool

Nearly all the tools developed for children with cognitive impairment have been published since the year 2000; this in itself reflects the fact that this group of children have historically been overlooked in terms of pain assessment. However, in recent years specific tools have been developed to assess pain in this diverse group of children. Various reviews of these tools (APA 2012; Ely et al. 2012) have been undertaken to help clinicians identify and use the most appropriate tools for practice. Recently published guidelines (APA 2012) identified five tools (see Table 8.2) that could be recommended for use in this group of children within different settings and situations. They noted that in comparison to tools for non-impaired children there is 'less substantive evidence of reliability, validity, clinical utility, and widespread use within practice settings' (p. 13). However, the field is evolving and the evidence base is becoming much better established. The use of these tools creates an important means of helping to quantify pain intensity (Voepel-Lewis 2011), and although they may remain imperfect instruments, they are an important component of good pain management practice. Pivalizza and Pivalizza (2008: 1233) identify what they propose as being significant deficits in existing pain assessment tools such as the lack of account that the tools generally take in relation to 'significant potential co-morbid behavioral disorders and motor developmental disabilities in the cognitively impaired pediatric population'. They also note the often false assumption of

Table 8.2 Overview of pain tools identified as suitable for use with children and young people with cognitive impairment

Name of tool and author(s)	Intended age group	Intended age group	Scoring	Cut offs[†]
NCCPC-R (Non-Communicating Children's Pain Checklist – Revised) (Breau et al. 2002)	3–18-year-olds	**30 items, seven subscales** **Vocal subscale:** moaning, whining, whimpering (fairly soft); crying (moderately loud); screaming/yelling (very loud); a specific sound or word for pain (for example: a word, cry, or type of laugh). **Eating/sleeping subscale:** eating less, not interested in food; increase in sleep; decrease in sleep. **Social subscale:** not cooperating, cranky, irritable, unhappy; less interaction with others, withdrawn; seeking comfort or physical closeness; being difficult to distract, not able to satisfy or pacify. **Facial subscale:** a furrowed brow, a change in eyes, including squinching of eyes, eyes opened wide, eyes frowning; turning down of mouth, not smiling; lips puckering up, tight, pouting or quivering; clenching or grinding teeth, chewing or thrusting tongue out. **Activity subscale:** not moving, less active, quiet; jumping around, agitated, fidgety. **Body and limbs subscale:** stiff, spastic, tense rigid; gesturing to or touching part of the body that hurts; flinching or moving the body part away, being sensitive to touch, moving the body in specific way to show pain (e.g. head back, arms down, curls up etc.). **Physical signs subscale:** shivering, change in colour, pallor; sweating, perspiring; tears; sharp intake of breath, gasping; breath holding.	0–3, range 0–30 0 = Not present at all during the observation period. 1 = Seen or heard rarely (hardly at all), but is present. 2 = Seen or heard a number of times, but not continuous (not all the time). 3 = Seen or heard often, almost continuous (almost all the time); NA = Not applicable. This child is not capable of performing this action.	Total score of 6 or less indicates a child does not have pain. Total score of 7 or more indicates a child has pain.

Name of tool and author(s)	Intended age group	Intended age group	Scoring	Cut offs[†]
NCCPC-PV (Non-communicating Children's Pain Checklist – post-operative version) (Breau et al. 2002)	3–19-year-olds	**27 items, six subscales** **Vocal subscale:** moaning, whining, whimpering (fairly soft); crying (moderately loud); screaming/yelling (very loud), a specific sound or word for pain (e.g., a word, cry or type of laugh). **Social subscale:** not cooperating, cranky, irritable, unhappy; less interaction with others, withdrawn; seeking comfort or physical closeness; being difficult to distract, not able to satisfy or pacify. **Facial subscale:** a furrowed brow; a change in eyes, including squinching of eyes, eyes opened wide, eyes frowning; turning down of mouth, not smiling; lips puckering up, tight, pouting, or quivering; clenching or grinding teeth, chewing or thrusting tongue out. **Activity subscale:** not moving, less active, quiet; jumping around, agitated, fidgety. **Body and limbs subscale:** floppy; stiff, spastic, tense, rigid; gesturing to or touching part of the body that hurts; protecting, favouring or guarding part of the body that hurts; flinching or moving the body part away, being sensitive to touch; moving the body in a specific way to show pain (e.g. head back, arms down, curls up, etc.). **Physiological subscale:** shivering; change in colour, pallor; sweating, perspiring; tears; sharp intake of breath, gasping; breath holding.	0–3, range 0–27 0 = Not present at all during the observation period. 1 = Seen or heard rarely (hardly at all), but is present. 2 = Seen or heard a number of times, but not continuous (not all the time). 3 = Seen or heard often, almost continuous (almost all the time); NA = Not applicable. This child is not capable of performing this action.	Total score of 6–10 indicates a child has mild pain. Total score of 11 or more indicates a child has moderate to severe pain.

(Continued)

Table 8.2 (Continued)

Name of tool and author(s)	Intended age group	Intended age group	Scoring	Cut offs[†]
PPP (The Paediatric Pain Profile) (Hunt et al. 2004, 2007)	1–18-year-olds	**20 items** 1. Was cheerful (reverse scored) 2. Was sociable or responsive (reverse scored) 3. Appeared withdrawn or depressed 4. Cried/moaned/groaned/screamed or whimpered 5. Was hard to console or comfort 6. Bit self or banged head 7. Was reluctant to eat/difficult to feed (includes nasogastric and gastrostomy feeding) 8. Had disturbed sleep 9. Grimaced/screwed-up face/screwed-up eyes 10. Frowned/had furrowed brow/looked worried 11. Looked frightened (with eyes wide open) 12. Ground teeth or made mouthing movements 13. Was restless/agitated or distressed 14. Tensed/stiffened or spasmed 15. Flexed inwards or drew legs up towards chest 16. Tended to touch or rub particular areas 17. Resisted being moved 18. Pulled away or flinched when touched 19. Twisted and turned/tossed head/writhed or arched 20. Had involuntary or stereotypical movements/was jumpy/startled or had seizures	0–3, range 0–60 3 = Not at all 2 = A little 1 = Quite a lot 0 = A great deal	Scores of 14 or more generally associated with moderate or severe pain.

Name of tool and author(s)	Intended age group	Intended age group	Scoring	Cut offs[†]
Revised FLACC (r-FLACC) (Malviya et al. 2006)	4–19-year-olds	**5 categories** **Face:** 0 = no particular expression or smile; 1 = occasional grimace/frown; withdrawn or disinterested; appears sad or worried; 2 = consistent grimace or frown; frequent/constant quivering chin, clenched jaw; distressed-looking face, expression of fright or panic. Individualised behaviour. **Legs:** 0 = normal position or relaxed; usual tone and motion to limbs; 1 = uneasy, restless, tense; occasional tremors; 2 = kicking, or legs drawn up; marked increase in spasticity, constant tremors or jerking. Individualised behaviour. **Activity:** 0 = lying quietly, normal position, moves easily; regular, rhythmic respirations; 1 = squirming, shifting back and forth, tense or guarded movements, mildly agitated (e.g. head back and forth, aggression), shallow, splinting respirations, intermittent sighs; 2 = arched, rigid or jerking; severe agitation; head banging; shivering (not rigors); breath holding, gasping or sharp intake of breaths, severe splinting. Individualised behaviour. **Cry:** 0 = no cry/verbalisation; 1 = moans or whimpers; occasional complaint; occasional verbal outburst or grunt; 2 = crying steadily, screams or sobs, frequent complaints; repeated outbursts, constant grunting. Individualised behaviour.	0–2, range 0–10	Total score 0–3 indicates a child has mild pain. Total score 4–6 indicates a child has moderate pain. Total score 7–10 indicates a child has severe pain.

(Continued)

Table 8.2 (Continued)

Name of tool and author(s)	Intended age group	Intended age group	Scoring	Cut offs[†]
		Consolability: 0 = content and relaxed; 1 = reassured by occasional touching, hugging or being talked to; distractible; 2 = difficult to console or comfort; pushing away caregiver, resisting care or comfort measures. Individualised behaviour.		
PPPM (Parents Postoperative Pain Measure) (Chambers et al. 2003)	(Parent)	**15 items** 1. Whine or complain more than usual 2. Cry more easily than usual 3. Play less than usual 4. Not do the things they normally do 5. Act more worried than usual 6. Act more quiet than usual 7. Have less energy than usual 8. Refuse to eat 9. Eat less than usual 10. Hold the sore part of their body 11. Try not to bump the sore part 12. Groan or moan more than usual 13. Look more flushed than usual 14. Want to be close to you more 15. Take meds when normally refuses	Yes/No	Cut-off score not confirmed although a previous study (Chambers et al. 1996) suggested a cut-off of 6.

[†] Note: care needs to be taken with cut-offs as they cannot be deemed to be 100% accurate and clinical decisions about pain management should not solely be decided on the pain score.

Developed from the APA (2012) and from the tools themselves

'similarity in the group, whereas reality reflects a diverse population with distinctive characteristics'. The instrument developers (see for example, Hunt et al. 2003) are well aware of potential difficulties and the importance of the clinicians gaining an understanding of the context of the child and his or her surroundings and issues. In addition, there is encouragement to increase knowledge of the child by setting up a baseline of the child's behaviour when well and when in pain and promoting the idea that children may have more than one pain and behave differently with different pains.

In Grace's case, the nurses undertaking the assessment would need to understand Grace's usual behavioural repertoire and ascertain from Rosie how Grace manifests her pain. Importantly, Rosie says, 'Can't you see the pain in her eyes?' Other parents also talk of seeing pain in their child's eyes (Carter et al. 2002). Parents need us, as health care professionals, 'to stop, look and listen' and to take into account the physical and emotional expression of pain.

Choosing the right tool requires consideration of the type of pain, the setting and who is undertaking the assessment. Broadly tools have been developed to be used for procedural/disease-related pain and/or for post-operative pain. Parental involvement supports assessment in all tools but it is central to the Parents Postoperative Pain Measure (PPPM) and the Paediatric Pain Profile (PPP). Figure 8.1 provides an overview of the key tools. In Grace's case, the best choices are likely to be the NCCP-R or the PPP. The PPP has particular value in that it has been designed for on-going use by parents which would facilitate Rosie being able to present Grace's pain history to the staff in the Accident and Emergency department.

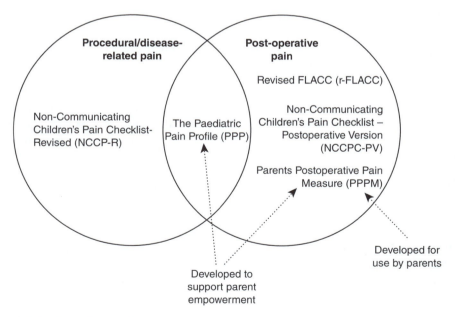

Figure 8.1   Overview of key pain assessment tools for children with cognitive impairment and the type of pain for which they were developed

Many of the tools have been translated into different languages, thus increasing their potential to contribute to pain management on a wider basis. The PPP, for example, has been translated into Urdu, as well as into French, German, Dutch (www.ppprofile.org.uk) and Brazilian-Portuguese (Pasin et al. 2012) while the NCCPC-PV has been translated into Swedish (Johansson et al. 2010).

Once the tool has been chosen, the person using the tool should take care that they understand how to use it. Becoming familiar with and confident in using the tool is fundamental to how effective the tool is in assessing a child's pain. Guidelines for the use of each tool should be followed to ensure that the tool is used correctly.

Involvement of parents in assessment of pain

Studies have demonstrated that the parents of children with cognitive impairment often develop knowledge, skills and sensitivity in determining whether their child is in pain. Therefore it is essential that parents are involved in pain assessment wherever possible as individualising the pain tool may increase the reliability of pain assessments (Voepel-Lewis et al. 2005). Without Rosie's expertise and guidance, health care professionals would not know which specific signs and behaviours to observe Grace for in terms of assessing her pain.

Ely et al.'s (2012) conscientious, quality improvement project recognised the importance of the parental contribution to pain assessment and as a result they developed a caregiver instruction sheet to help promote parent advocacy. Parents benefit from training and support and supporting them in this way may reduce some of the problems identified in the variability in the accuracy of parental reports (Chambers et al. 1998) and parents' variability in underestimating their child's pain. However, Stallard et al. (2002: 148) warn that parental report should not be relied upon as the sole means of determining pain as they 'will probably underestimate the true extent of pain within this vulnerable group'.

The health care professionals should have attended to Rosie's suggested diagnosis that Grace had 'greensticked her legs'. They should also have taken into account Grace's previous history, her diagnosis of brittle bones and Rosie's explanation of Grace's pain behaviours. Hindsight perhaps makes it easy to arrive at a diagnosis, but in Grace's case it would seem that all the information was there before it was confirmed by x-ray. Ignoring Rosie's expertise was at the very least discourteous and, more to the point, clinically foolish.

Preventing and treating the pain of children with cognitive impairment

Managing the pain of children with cognitive impairment remains challenging. In the past, poor pain management practices could be linked to the lack of validated pain assessment tools for this group of children (Breau et al. 2002; Koh et al. 2004).

Table 8.3 Overview of ways of preventing and treating pain experienced by children who have cognitive impairment

Pains associated with	Examples of ways of preventing and treating pain
Alterations in gut motility	• Increasing fluid and dietary fibre intake (Massaro et al. 2013) and prophylactic use of a stool softener or a laxative (Elawad and Sullivan 2001). • Management of gastro-oesophageal reflux through surgical intervention (Massaro et al. 2013).
Musculo-skeletal problems	• Spasticity can be treated with oral or intrathecal baclofen (Massaro et al. 2013) and the use of BoNT-A (botulinum toxin type B). However, there are gaps in the evidence base in term of efficacy, safety and whether the outcomes achieved improve the child's quality of life (Quality Standards Subcommittee of the American Academy of Neurology et al. 2010). • Hip surveillance to ensure early identification of hip displacement in children with cerebral palsy (Hägglund et al. 2007; Elkamil et al. 2011). • Prevention of fracture through prevention of low bone density (Bachrach et al. 2010; Hough et al. 2010).
Co-incidental/'everyday' pains	• Good dental hygiene can prevent problems from dental caries causing toothache. • Earache, headache, teething, and menstruation pains can be managed through simple comforting measures and paracetamol and NSAIDs.
Poorly fitting aids, equipment	• Maintenance of skin integrity at the sites of feeding tubes etc. • Prevention of pain associated with wearing splints or supports.
Handling, moving, positioning	• Careful handling, moving, positioning and regular repositioning of the child.
Accidents and injury	• Ensuring the child's safety and reducing the risk of injury and falls.
Iatrogenic pain	• Individualised treatment plan for child's pain taking into account their prior experience and response to interventions and investigation. • Comforting, reassurance and other measures to be used in conjunction with other therapeutic modalities.

However, this can no longer be used as an excuse: tools are available for use within clinical settings. Some of the problems may partly reflect wider difficulties such as the perceived challenge of implementing change (Chen-Lim et al. 2012), implementing research findings into practice (Kavanagh et al. 2007) and ensuring that pain management 'matters' within organisational priorities (Finley et al. 2005).

Many children experience ongoing and unrelieved pain; prevention is a key management strategy as protecting the child from pain can improve their quality of life. Table 8.3 presents the common sources of pain experienced by children with cognitive impairment and, in each of the domains presented, suggests some measures that can be taken to prevent pain. However, for children with multiple morbidities, there are risks associated with some of the suggested interventions and the evidence base for some interventions is often insufficient (e.g., management of spasticity (Quality Standards Subcommittee of the American Academy of Neurology et al. 2010).

Non-pharmacologic management is an important element of symptom management (Hauer 2010) and parents often routinely use comforting strategies such as stroking, rocking, touching, massaging and repositioning (Carter et al. 2002). These are fundamental elements of an integrated approach to pain management for this diverse group of children and can, in many cases, be incorporated into their daily care.

Children such as Grace need individual assessment and management of their pain by health care professionals who have finely tuned communication and assessment skills and who are able to synthesise information and development strategies to promote the child's quality of life.

Conclusion

It is clear that, despite advances in research, there is still a limited understanding of the pain experienced by children with cognitive impairment (Breau and Camfield 2011) and that assessing and managing their pain can be complex and challenging. However, this is a challenge we need to acknowledge and address in our practice every day. Children like Grace deserve our best attention. The pain load that they carry can be immense but it can be reduced by careful and compassionate care and intervention. The tools that have been designed to be used to assess pain in this diverse group of children provide a structured means for health care professionals to gain an understanding of the child's pain.

Working in partnership with parents is fundamental to nearly every pain situation but it is of particular importance with parents of children with a cognitive impairment. The children's parents become attuned to the nuanced ways in which their child expresses pain. A key responsibility is to closely attend to what parents say about their child's pain. Rosie can 'read' Grace's signs of pain – she explains 'the pain was in her face, it was like she was saying "Oh I've had this before, this pain. I don't like it".' Rosie knew that Grace was in pain because she was observing her and she saw the pain. It was only when the health professionals had hard clinical evidence that they acknowledged that Grace would have a reason to be in pain. Rosie's story ends by saying 'then eventually they saw the fracture on the x-ray and it was like "Oh yes Mrs … you're right, it's a fracture… that's got to be painful, how did you know?" And I was saying to myself "Because she's my daughter and surely you can see the pain in her eyes and her face and her body".' We need to be sure that each time we care for a child with cognitive impairment that we truly do look for the pain in their eyes, face, and body.

Key Points

- Children with cognitive impairment have a higher number of pain episodes compared to their healthy peers.
- Identifying and managing this pain is often challenging for healthcare professionals and parents.
- Children with cognitive impairment experience a range of different types of pain which arise from diverse sources; wherever possible pain shoule be prevented rather than treated.
- Specific tools (e.g., PPP, NCCPC-R, PPPM and FLACC) have been developed to assess pain in this diverse group of children.
- Parents of children with cognitive impairment often develop knowledge, skills and sensitivity in determining whether their child is pain.
- Non pharmacological management is an important element of symptom management.
- Working in partnership with parents is fundamental to nearly every pain situation but it is of particular importance with parents of children with a cognitive impairment.

Additional Resources and Reading

- For more detailed information about the specific assessment:
  - The Paediatric Pain Profile: www.ppprofile.org.uk.
  - The NCCPC-R: http://pediatric-pain.ca/wp-content/uploads/2013/04/NCCPCR_200901.pdf.
  - The NCCPC-PV: http://pediatric-pain.ca/wp-content/uploads/2013/04/NCCPCPV_200901.pdf
  - The PPPM: http://pediatric-pain.ca/our-measures/.
  - FLACC quiz: www.aacn.org/WD/CETests/Media/A1019013.pdf
- The APA (2012) has a sound section on pain assessment and recommended tools for children with cognitive impairment:
  - www.apagbi.org.uk/publications/apa-guidelines
- For an appreciation of working with parents of children with disabilities, read:
  - Fialka, J.M., Feldman, A.K. and Mikus, K.C. (2012) *Parents and Professionals Partnering for Children with Disabilities: A Dance that Matters,* 1st edn. Thousand Oaks, CA: Corwin.

References

Ambuel, B., Hamlett, K.W., Marx, C.M. and Blumer, J.L. (1992) 'Assessing distress in pediatric intensive-care environments – the Comfort Scale', *Journal of Pediatric Psychology*, 17 (1): 95–109.

Anand, K.J.S., Green, A. and McJunkins, A. (2009) 'Pain assessment in cognitively impaired children: a randomized trial of two methods of pain assessment', *Journal of Pediatric Nursing*, 24 (2): e2.

Association of Paediatric Anaesthetists (APA) (2012) *Good Practice in Postoperative and Procedural Pain Management*, 2nd edn, *Pediatric Anesthesia*, 22 (Supplement 1): 1–79.

Bachrach, S.J., Kecskemethy, H.H., Harcke, H.T. and Hossain, J. (2010) 'Decreased fracture incidence after 1 year of pamidronate treatment in children with spastic quadriplegic cerebral palsy', *Developmental Medicine & Child Neurology*, 52(9): 837–42.

Breau, L.M. and Burkitt, C. (2009) 'Assessing pain in children with intellectual disabilities', *Pain Research & Management: The Journal of the Canadian Pain Society (journal de la societe canadienne pour le traitement de la douleur)*, 14 (2): 116–20.

Breau, L.M. and Camfield, C.S. (2011) 'The relation between children's pain behaviour and developmental characteristics: a cross-sectional study', *Developmental Medicine & Child Neurology*, 53 (2): e1–e7.

Breau, L.M., Camfield, C., McGrath, P.J., Rosmus, C. and Finley, G.A. (2001) 'Measuring pain accurately in children with cognitive impairments: refinement of a caregiver scale', *Journal of Pediatrics*, 138 (5): 721–7.

Breau, L.M., Camfield, C.S., McGrath, P.J. and Finley, G.A. (2003) 'The incidence of pain in children with severe cognitive impairments', *Archives of Pediatrics & Adolescent Medicine*, 157: 1219–26.

Breau, L.M., Finley, G.A., McGrath, P.J. and Camfield, C.S. (2002) 'Validation of the non-communicating children's pain checklist-postoperative version', *Anesthesiology*, 96 (3): 528–35.

Caljouw, M., Kloos, M., Olivier, M.Y., Heemskerk, I.W., Pison, W., Stigter, G.D. and Verhoef, A. (2007) 'Measurement of pain in premature infants with a gestational age between 28 to 37 weeks: validation of the adopted COMFORT scale', *Journal of Neonatal Nursing*, 13 (1): 13–18.

Carter, B., McArthur, E. and Cunliffe, M. (2002) 'Dealing with uncertainty: parental assessment of pain in their children with profound special needs', *Journal of Advanced Nursing*, 38 (5): 449–57.

Chambers, C.T., Finley, G.A., McGrath, P.J. and Walsh, T.M. (2003) 'The parents' postoperative pain measure: replication and extension to 2–6-year-old children', *Pain*, 105(3): 437–43.

Chambers, C.T., Reid, C.J., Craig, K.D., McGrath, P.J. and Finley, G.A. (1998) 'Agreement between child and parent reports of pain', *Clinical Journal of Pain*, 14 (4): 336–42.

Chambers, C.T., Reid, C.J., McGrath, P.J. and Finley, G.A (1996) 'Development and preliminary validation of a postoperative pain measure for parents', *Pain*, 68: 307–13.

Chen-Lim, M., Zarnowsky, C., Green, R., Shaffer, S., Holtzer, B. and Ely, E. (2012) 'Optimizing the assessment of pain in children who are cognitively impaired through the quality improvement process', *Journal of Pediatric Nursing*, 27: 750–9.

Elawad, M.A. and Sullivan, P.B. (2001) 'Management of constipation in children with disabilities', *Developmental Medicine & Child Neurology*, 43: 829–32.

Elkamil, A.I., Andersen, G.L., Hägglund, G., Lamvik, T., Skranes, J. and Vik, T. (2011) 'Prevalence of hip dislocation among children with cerebral palsy in regions with and without a surveillance programme: a cross sectional study in Sweden and Norway', *BMC Musculoskeletal Disorders*, 12: 284.

Ely, E., Chen-Lim, M., Zarnowsky, C., Green, R., Shaffer, S. and Holtzer, B. (2012) 'Finding the evidence to change practice for assessing pain in children who are cognitively impaired', *Journal of Pediatric Nursing*, 27 (4): 402.

Finley, G.A., Franck, L., Grunau, R. and von Baeyer, C.L. (2005) 'Why children's pain matters', *Pain: Clinical Updates*, XIII (4): 1–6.

Gallagher, E.J., Bijur, P.E., Latimer, C. and Silver, W. (2002) 'Reliability and validity of a visual analog scale for acute abdominal pain in the ED', *The American Journal of Emergency Medicine*, 20 (4): 287–90.

Hagglund, G., Lauge-Pedersen. H. and Wagner, P. (2007) 'Characteristics of children with hip displacement in cerebral palsy', *BMC Musculoskelet Disorders*, 8: 101.

Hauer, J. (2010) 'Identifying and managing sources of pain and distress in children with neurological impairment', *Pediatric Annals*, 39 (4): 198–205.

Herr, K., Coyne, P.J., McCaffery, M., Manworren, R. and Merkel, S. (2011) 'Pain assessment in the patient unable to self-report: position statement with clinical practice recommendations', *Pain Management Nursing*, 12 (4): 230–50.

Hough, J.P., Boyd, R.N. and Keating, J.L. (2010) 'Systematic review of interventions for low bone mineral density in children with cerebral palsy', *Pediatrics*, 125(3): e670-8. doi: 10.1542/peds.2009-0292.

Houlihan, C.M., O'Donnell, M., Conaway, M. and Stevenson, R.D. (2004) 'Bodily pain and health-related quality of life in children with cerebral palsy', *Developmental Medicine & Child Neurology*, 46 (5): 305–10.

Hunt, A., Goldman, A., Seers, K., Crichton, N., Mastroyannopoulou, K., Moffat, V., Oulton, K. and Brady, M. (2004) 'Clinical validation of the paediatric pain profile', *Developmental Medicine & Child Neurology*, 46 (1): 9–18.

Hunt, A., Mastroyannopoulou, K., Goldman, A. and Seers, K. (2003) 'Not knowing: the problem of pain in children with severe neurological impairment', *International Journal of Nursing Studies*, 40 (2): 171.

Hunt, A., Wisbeach, A., Seers, K., Goldman, A., Crichton, N., Perry, L. and Mastroyannopoulou, K. (2007) 'Development of the paediatric pain profile: role of video analysis and saliva cortisol in validating a tool to assess pain in children with severe neurological disability', *Journal of Pain and Symptom Management*, 33 (3): 276–89.

Johansson, M., Carlberg, E.B. and Jylli, L. (2010) 'Validity and reliability of a Swedish version of the Non-Communicating Children's Pain Checklist – Postoperative Version', *Acta Paediatrica*, 99 (6): 929–33.

Kavanagh, T., Watt-Watson, J. and Stevens, B. (2007) 'An examination of the factors enabling the successful implementation of evidence-based acute pain practices into pediatric nursing', *Children's Health Care*, 36 (3): 303–21.

Koh, J.L., Fanurik, D., Dale Harrison, R., Schmitz, M.L. and Norvell, D. (2004) 'Analgesia following surgery in children with and without cognitive impairment', *Pain*, 111 (3): 239–44.

Lotan, M., Ljunggren, E.A., Johnsen, T.B., Defrin, R., Pick, C.G. and Strand, L.I. (2009) 'A modified version of the non-communicating children pain checklist – revised, adapted to adults with intellectual and developmental disabilities: sensitivity to pain and internal consistency', *The Journal of Pain*, 10 (4): 398–407.

Malviya, S., Voepel-Lewis, T., Burke, C., Merkel, S. and Tait, A.R. (2006) 'The revised FLACC observational pain tool: improved reliability and validity for pain assessment in children with cognitive impairment', *Pediatric Anesthesia*, 16 (3): 258–65.

Manworren, R.C.B. and Hynan, L.S. (2003) 'Clinical validation of FLACC: preverbal patient pain scale. [miscellaneous article]', *Pediatric Nursing*, 29 (2): 140–6.

Massaro, M., Pastore, S., Ventura, A. and Barbi, E. (2013) 'Pain in cognitively impaired children: a focus for general pediatricians', *European Journal of Pediatrics*, 172 (1): 9–14.

McGrath, P.J., Johnson, G., Goodman, J.T., Schillinger, J., Dunn, J. and Chapman, J. (1985) 'CHEOPS: a behavioral scale for rating postoperative pain in children', in H.L. Fields, R. Dubner and F. Cervero (eds), *Advances in Pain Research and Therapy, 9*. New York: Raven Press, pp. 395–402.

McJunkins, A., Green, A. and Anand, K. (2010) 'Pain assessment in cognitively impaired, functionally impaired children: pilot study results', *Journal of Pediatric Nursing*, 25 (4): 307–9.

Merkel, S.I., Voepel-Lewis, T., Shayevitz, J.R. and Malviya, S. (1997) 'The FLACC: a behavioral scale for scoring postoperative pain in young children', *Pediatric Nursing*, 23 (3): 293–7.

Parkinson, K.N., Gibson, L., Dickinson, H.O. and Colver, A.F. (2010) 'Pain in children with cerebral palsy: a cross-sectional multicentre European study', *Acta Paediatrica*, 99 (3): 446–51.

Pasin, S., Avila, F., de Cavata, T., Hunt, A. and Heldt, E. (2012) 'Cross-cultural translation and adaptation to Brazilian Portuguese version of the paediatric pain profile in children with severe cerebral palsy', *Journal of Pain and Symptom Management*, 45 (1): 120–128.

Pivalizza, P.J. and Pivalizza, E.G. (2008) *Pain Assessment Tools for Children with Cognitive Impairment*. Oxford: Wiley-Blackwell.

Quality Standards Subcommittee of the American Academy of Neurology and the Practice Committee of the Child Neurology Society, Delgado, M.R., Hirtz, D., Aisen, M., Ashwal, S., Fehlings, D.L., McLaughlin, J., Morrison, L.A., Shrader, M.W., Tilton, A. and Vargus-Adams, J. (2010) 'Practice parameter: pharmacologic treatment of spasticity in children and adolescents with cerebral palsy (an evidence-based review): report of the Quality Standards Subcommittee of the American Academy of Neurology and the Practice Committee of the Child Neurology Society', *Neurology*, 74 (4): 336–43.

Schade, J.G., Joyce, B.A., Gerkensmeyer, J. and Keck, J.F. (1996) 'Comparison of three preverbal scales for postoperative pain assessment in a diverse pediatric sample', *Journal of Pain and Symptom Management*, 12 (6): 348–59.

Solodiuk, J.C., Scott-Sutherland, J., Meyers, M., Myette, B., Shusterman, C., Karian, V.E., Harris, S.K. and Curley, M.A. (2010) 'Validation of the Individualized Numeric Rating Scale (INRS): a pain assessment tool for nonverbal children with intellectual disability', *Pain*, 150 (2): 231–6.

Stallard, P., Williams, L., Lenton, S. and Velleman, R. (2001) 'Pain in cognitively impaired, non-communicating children', *Archives of Disease in Childhood*, 85 (6): 460–2.

Stallard, P., Williams, L., Velleman, R., Lenton, S. and McGrath, P.J. (2002) 'Behaviors identified by caregivers to detect pain in non-communicating children', *Journal of Pediatric Psychology*, 27 (2): 209–14.

Stevens, B. (1990) 'Development and testing of a pediatric pain management sheet', *Pediatric Nursing*, 16 (6): 543–8.

Stinson, J.N., Kavanagh, T., Yamada, J., Gill, N. and Stevens, B. (2006) 'Systematic review of the psychometric properties, interpretability and feasibility of self-report pain intensity measures for use in clinical trials in children and adolescents', *Pain*, 125 (1–2): 143–57.

van Dijk, M., de Boer, J.B., Koot, H.M., Tibboel, D., Passchier, J. and Duivenvoorden, H.J. (2000) 'The reliability and validity of the COMFORT scale as a postoperative pain instrument in 0 to 3-year-old infants', *Pain*, 84 (2–3): 367–77.

Voepel-Lewis, T. (2011) 'The ongoing quandaries of behavioral pain assessment in children with neurocognitive impairment', *Developmental Medicine & Child Neurology*, 53 (2): 106–7.

Voepel-Lewis, T., Malviya, S. and Tait, A.R. (2005) 'Validity of parent ratings as proxy measures of pain in children with cognitive impairment', *Pain Management Nursing*, 6 (4): 168–74.

Voepel-Lewis, T., Malviya, S., Tait, A.R., Merkel, S., Foster, R. and Krane, E.J. (2008) 'A comparison of the clinical utility of pain assessment tools for children with cognitive impairment', *Anesthesia and Analgesia*, 106 (1): 72–8.

Voepel-Lewis, T.M.S.N., Malviya, S.M.D., Merkel, S.M.S.N. and Tait, A.R.P. (2001) 'Reliability and validity of the FLACC behavioral scale as a measure of pain in cognitively impaired children. [miscellaneous]', *ASA Annual Meeting Abstracts Pediatric Anesthesia*, 95 (3): A1229.

von Baeyer, C.L. and Spagrud, L.J. (2006) 'Systematic review of observational (behavioral) measures of pain for children and adolescents aged 3 to 18 years', *Pain*, 127 (1–2): 140–150.

Chapter 9

Fear, Pain and Illness

Abongile's and Sam's Stories

Rene's and Abongile's Story

I saw Abongile one morning in ICU a few days after his open heart surgery. He was referred to me by one of the student physiotherapists who was convinced at the time that the little boy was in pain because of his non-compliance during chest physiotherapy. Chest physiotherapy is known to be painful and uncomfortable because in essence it requires the patient to cough and expel secretions as soon as possible after surgery. It is an important part of the post-operative treatment of cardiac patients as it is aimed at preventing lung infection.

Abongile refused to cough and nothing in the world could get him to comply with his treatment. I was as confused as the physiotherapist because all steps to minimise pain and discomfort were in place. We all knew that there would be some pain, but that it was a necessary evil and that the chest physiotherapy and coughing were essential. It was only during my third visit that I got the story. Abongile was 'afraid to cough'. He in no uncertain terms asked me 'Do you know anything about "open heart" surgery?' as 'they' (cardiac surgeons) had cut his heart open. Exacerbating the problem was the fact that he'd overheard a doctor describing his heart as 'very weak' to another doctor. (Here we think he could have overheard two medical students on their rotation through the ICU.)

Abongile then went on to tell me that since they had cut his heart open, they 'must have put stitches in it to "sew" it up again' and that 'there were big white bandages around his heart'.

The problem with coughing, he said, was that every time he coughed, his 'heart jumps up and down and that hurts'. And all this jumping up and down cannot be good for his heart, because it is weak and can get tired easily. Because of all the jumping his heart might not be able to hang on to the bandages and that they might come off and that all the stitches might come undone. If that happens he will bleed to death and nobody will notice.

Abongile was convinced that he would die if he coughed, but was willing to compromise. If the doctor could put his heart in the white stuff (I later learned that he was referring to the old fashioned use of Plaster of Paris to splint fractures), then he would cough because then his heart could not 'pop' open.

It took two surgeons and an advanced course in paediatric cardiac anatomy to convince Abongile that coughing was good, and that nothing would pop open any time soon. His recovery was uneventful and he was moved to a general ward a few days later. I never saw Abongile again. I guess his heart is much stronger and that coughing is no more an issue.

Dave's and Sam's story

The following story is built from extracts from Dave's diary and the memories triggered when he re-read his diary as he selected those parts he wanted to share with us. Dave is recalling the start of Sam's story in 1999 when Sam was 12 years old.

1999

Sam develops severe pain in his right leg.

He is, after much disbelief, and inappropriate referral, diagnosed with an extensive internal congenital vascular malformation (CVM). The CVM is causing compressive neuropathy and neuropathic pain. It is (at that time) inoperable.

We are told 'It is not life-threatening, and that is at least a good thing. However, the time may come when Sam will have to choose between life and limb.'

Memory – January 2000

We return from the specialist hospital in London having been told Sam must learn to live with his pain. The family sits and watches the television that evening, Mum, Dad and the three sons, Tom (17), Robert (11) and of course Sam. Time comes for bed, Sam is in pain, and he cannot stand. We get him to the bottom of the stairs and he wails in pain. His Mum cradles from behind, 'Sam, we will get you a stair lift', she strokes his hair. Eventually Tom takes him under his shoulder and I take his legs, as we carry him up stairs he screams, an animal scream, shrieking. Finally in bed, he sobs, we all cry. It was the end of the beginning.

Diary 9-3-2000

Today I crossed a personal hurdle. My once healthy son is now disabled. I am the father of a disabled boy. I have searched in vain for a cure for my son's illness – and I accept now that this is not to be. This makes it easier to move on – in some ways. The cycle of hope and despair when one accepts 'what is'.

Memory – February 2000

Sam experiences florid visual hallucinations as a result of high doses of opiates (codeine). He screams in fear as 'shadow men' come out of the walls to attack him. During this his little brother Robert witnesses this. Sam invents an imaginary Dwarf called Marvin who sits next to him to protect him from the shadow men. Marvin is very real to Sam – he draws us a picture of him, and is surprised we can't see him. In 24 hours the hallucinations disappear. Then we notice that Robert is now unable to go anywhere in the house on his own. Robert has child 'play' counselling for six months before he recovers from this. Robert is today, 22 years old, a graduate of international politics, and still unable to talk about 'that day'.

Spring 2000

Sam is a wheelchair user. School attendance is very erratic. He is day/night inverted. His symptoms are erratic. Parts of a day he may walk, and then he is back in his chair. There is neuropathic pain mixed with sensation loss. None of the medications appear to be helping.

His wheelies in his chair are truly amazing – outside he comes down the hill at about 20 miles an hour! When a pupil at school called him a cripple, he decked him and ran over him in his wheelchair. The medics query 'overlay' depression worsening his symptoms. How does that work in a boy who can be so happy?

Diary 6-6-2000

Sam does not attend school; pain in the morning, improving as usual by the afternoon. Even when pain-free he walks with a pronounced limp. He has a new home tuition teacher who attends this afternoon and he appears to get on with her.

Sam has 'grown' a lot – not just in stature. He has more insight into his difficulties and needs – and in many ways he is now more able to be frustrated and depressed. Yet his sunny personality, his humour and inquisitiveness, overcome.

Midnight – the pain is severe, he reads as usual. Two in the morning, lights out. 'Good night Sam', 'Good night Dad'. Sam is resigned to pain.

Diary 17-7-2000

Sam looks awful today, sad, and pale faced. 'I have a theory Dad, if I go to bed early I can be asleep before the pain starts.'

12.00 Midnight – reading – in pain.

02.00 – reading – in pain.

03.00 – I sit in the dark holding his hand. Finally he sleeps. I am desperate. I need sleep, but can't desert him.

Autumn 2000

Symptoms of numbness appear – his other leg becomes affected. He has migraines. We are passed from one specialist to another across the country. Sam has remissions, lasting days, and then relapses.

Diary 19-9-2000

01.00 – I arrive in his room. The tears flow down his tortured face. We hug, I nearly cry. The pain is inexpressible. We chat, he smiles, and chocolate yogurt helps more than Nabilone. We talk about farting – OK it's crude, but he laughs and grins. It's better than tears.

02.15 – Lights out – he smiles.

Diary 8-11-2000

01.00 – He looks pale, huge bags under his eyes. We talk …

Oh God, Oh God, he looks so ill, my Sam. The gorgeous toddler, the arms around my neck. Sam crushed by pain, he looks like a cancer patient. I can't stand it, it's killing me, I cannot cope or confide. I want to scream, and I want it to go away. But none of that can be, it is not possible. I am 'Dad', but I am not very good at it at the moment.

Introduction

A child's mind is a powerful tool.

   Although its power can be used beneficially to lesson a child's pain, the vividness of children's imaginations can be powerful in summoning up dramatic and frightening scenarios. Additionally, some of the medications used to alleviate pain can cause hallucinations which can take a child to unusual and frightening places. Pain and fear are often intertwined elements of children's experience of hospital and both need to be addressed if pain management is to be successful.

   Rene's story about Abongile and Dave's story about Sam are both extraordinarily evocative. They demand an emotional response from us as readers and as health professionals. Every time I read these stories I feel their strong emotional pull. They each act like a whirlpool; it is impossible not to be physically and emotionally pulled into the story, experiencing something of their fear, their distress, and the emotional turmoil they were experiencing. These stories are distressing to read and distressing to write about. They make me more determined than ever that we should be trying our hardest with every child and family to make them feel safe and secure.

   In this chapter we will explore literature and research relating to children's understanding of health, illness, injury and pain and why Abongile was so distressed and how his distress may have been prevented. We will also look at pain and fear and see how a child's pain does not just affect the child but how it spins out and affects their family and a wider sphere. We will examine how pain can erode a young person's quality of life and how it can strip away a father's ability to protect his son. We will also consider how we can work with children and families who are distressed to help them manage their pain and anxiety.

Children's understanding of health, illness and injury, and pain

Abongile provides a graphic description of his heart being 'cut open' and being surrounded by 'big white bandages' and his heart potentially not being able to 'hang on to the bandages'. He fears that if the bandages 'come off' then 'all the stitches might come undone' and then he 'will bleed to death and nobody will notice'. His description has a clear and consistent internal logic. His fears make sense to him and his decision not to cough is a sensible one based on his perceived sequence of cause and effect. He consciously and deliberately decides to protect his heart by refusing the physiotherapy treatment he thinks will increase his risk of dying. In this story, there is a happy ending. Rene, Abongile's physiotherapist, was conscientious and caring and took time to help Abongile to tell his story. The doctors took his fears seriously and provided him with an alternative, reassuring and scientific explanation that met his particular needs and Abongile was able to overcome his fear and complete his physiotherapy.

As they grow up, children learn about illness, injury and symptoms such as pain by drawing on their own experiences, those of their family and friends, and from other sources such as television and school. These experiences include toothache and bruises and more dramatic episodes such as surgery. When they are very young children learn from picture books which provide information about what to expect as a result of illness (for example, a visit to the doctor) but which often provide very little explanation as to the cause of the illness (Turner 2006). Children's exposure to different influences is inherently diverse. Most children are only ever exposed to minor injury and illness, and even though these can be distressing and intrusive they cannot prepare a child for the sorts of experiences that Abongile, Sam and his siblings faced.

Health care professionals caring for children in pain need an awareness of how children develop their understandings of illness and pain. Reeve and Bell (2009) note that research into children's conceptions of health and illness has been undertaken from a range of different theoretical and conceptual perspectives. Two core academic approaches to considering the development of children's understanding of illness have been proposed: a Piagetian approach or a theory-based approach. Much of the research available is over 20 years old and issues have been raised about the methodological approaches used in these studies. However, even though some of the older research has been contested (Hergenrather and Rabinowitz 1991), it still provides an insight into the ways in which children reason.

Traditionally, a Piagetian approach to cognitive development guided the research that focused on children's understandings of illness, with researchers plotting the development of children's understanding of illness against the four stages outlined in Piaget's theory of development (Myant and Williams 2005). Adopting a Piagetian approach suggests that children's understanding of illness progresses in alignment to their perceptual development. Bibace and Walsh's (1980) research findings articulate six developmentally ordered categories of explanation of illness. Koopman et al.'s (2004) 'Through the Eyes of the Child' (TEC) model provides an alternative set of categories and these, along with the visualisation element, provide an appealing way of considering the development of illness understanding (see Table 9.1).

At nine years old, Abongile would falls within the Piagetian phase of concrete-logical thinking or Bibace and Walsh's (1980) internalisation category. However, there is sufficient detail in his reported story (e.g., his heart is directly connected with blood flow and by implication that it is a pump, and the consequence of his stitches being put under strain is that he would 'bleed to death') to suggest that he could be operating at 'physiologic' which would not usually be achieved until he was around 11 years old. Abongile provides a really interesting example of why age is such a crude delineator; as Crisp et al. (1996) note, the interaction between a child's experience and their age can have a facilitating effect.

A Vygotskian (1979) approach to child development facilitates the consideration of social interactions and cultural factors and their interplay with children's cognitive development. This approach provides an alternative route to researching how children develop an understanding of pain and illness, and more easily accommodates the particular experiences (e.g., previous experience of hospitalisation, medical tests,

Table 9.1 Comparison of key models of cognitive and perceptual development of the child

Theory	Stages of development					
	Senso-motorical, 0–2 years	Pre-operational, 2–7 years		Concrete-operational, 7–11 years		Formal-operational, 11 years	
Piaget (1930), cognitive development						
Bibace and Walsh (1980), Illness Category System	Incomprehension	Phenomenism Child sees illness as a concrete and external and is unable to explain how events cause the illness.	Contagion Child believes that illness is caused by 'magic' or by proximity to people/objects.	Contamination Child thinks illness is caused by contact from a person or thing that has an external effect on their body.	Internalisation Child has vague explanations about an external cause and the illness that is affecting the inside of their body.	Physiological Child can describe how external events have affected the inside of the body and caused their illness.	Psychophysiologic Child able to appreciate that both physiological and physical factors can cause illness.
Through the eyes of the child, the TEC model (Koopman et al. 2004)	Invisible	Distance	Proximity	Contact	Internalisation	Body inside	Body–mind inside

Developed from Koopman et al. (2004)

injury) to which children such as Abongile have been exposed. Acknowledging a child's personal history and experiences (Paterson et al. 1999) alongside an estimation of their cognitive development would seem to be essential if pain management is to be tailored to meet their particular cognitive and perceptual level.

Many researchers now draw on a biological 'theory' approach (Kalish 1999; Buchanan-Barrow et al. 2003, 2004; Sigelman 2012). This is based on the evidence which shows that even young children reason and make predictions based on using naive theories (Wellman and Gelman 1992; Inagaki and Hatano 1996). Buchanan-Barrow et al. (2003: 660) describe a child-theorist as being 'capable of forming and using complex mental structures that function as explanatory systems'. Much of the work has focused on the common diseases and illnesses of childhood (e.g., colds and relatively minor contagious diseases) with much less attention paid to symptoms such as pain or more severe diseases such as cancer (Bares and Gelman 2008). Myant and Williams's (2005: 816) work shows that children as young as 4–5 years are capable of conceptualising some illnesses such as chickenpox in biological terms, although 'these do not become accurate until 9/10 years'. Williams and Binnie (2002: 137) proposed that children in their study 'were drawing on naïve concepts of illness by age 4' and that they had 'a firmly established theory of injury that is also based on a behavioural/mechanistic understanding' which provides them with sufficient information to create correct predictions and explanations.

What is common to nearly all the literature, regardless of its theoretical underpinning, is that children's understanding of illness tends to progress as they get older (Hergenrather and Rabinowitz 1991). They become more aware of psychogenic causes of illness (Notaro et al. 2001), more aware of the influence of time on causes and cures (Raman and Gelman 2007) and develop a more mature understanding of causation and boundaries between self and the world (Burbach and Peterson 1986; Williams and Binnie 2002).

Abongile's theory was based on his direct and indirect experience of his illness, and other factors including his understanding that the surgeons had 'cut his heart open' and that it was 'very weak' and it had 'stitches in it'. The inevitable conclusion was that 'his stitches would come undone' and he 'would bleed to death'. His theory, developed from snippets of overheard conversation and his own knowledge of illness and disease, had an internal logic, and its coherence meant that, for Abongile, it was very convincing. Rene had a hard time trying to counteract such a compelling explanation. As can be seen from the story, Abongile was only convinced after explanations from 'two surgeons and an advanced course in paediatric cardiac anatomy'. The problems that arose for Abongile and the fear that he experienced could have potentially been avoided if he had been better prepared. Since children do create theories that may or may not be misinformed, it is incumbent on health professionals to provide children with clear, individually tailored information about what will happen, checking their understanding and explaining how the professionals will keep them safe.

Returning to the story that Dave told about Sam's pain it is possible to see how Sam, aged 13 years, theorises about his pain. Sam's theory was that 'if I go to bed early I can be asleep before the pain starts', and this reflects some of the bargaining and magical thinking that occurs when people have chronic pain, the sense that 'if I do this, then the pain won't be so bad/will go away'. However, for Sam, his pain never plays fair. Sam finds he cannot cheat pain by going to sleep early. Indeed his pain robs him of the chance to sleep and escape its clutches. Sam's theory is disproved and continues to be disproved at 12 midnight, at 2 a.m. and at 3 a.m. when he is still awake and in pain. For Dave, his son's pain is beyond theorising; he understands that the pain is beyond rationalising.

Most of the studies that have focused on children's concepts of illness have been undertaken in developed countries, with many being undertaken in the USA (Boruchovitch and Mednick 2000), and the majority have been on healthy children. However, of the studies that have been undertaken in developing and/or non-western countries (Berry et al. 1993), the findings suggest that there are strong cross-cultural similarities in the way that children from different cultural backgrounds develop their understanding of illness (Peltzer and Promtussananon 2003) although cultural and/or ethnic influences can exert an effect (Zhu and Liu 2007; Legare and Gelman 2009; Zhu et al. 2009) and words and concepts (e.g., health, illness, pain) may not be readily translated (Onyango-Ouma et al. 2004). Another group of children who has been largely overlooked are those with an intellectual disability. Findings from Drahota and Malcarne's (2008) study show that children with an intellectual disability have significantly different understandings of illness when compared with age-matched children with no disability. However, they have a similar level of sophistication in their understanding compared to developmentally matched children.

Children's fears about pain and being in hospital

Fear in children is a common experience (McMurtry et al. 2011). Within limits, children often relish being a little frightened: many story books deliberately aim to be a bit scary, featuring monsters under the bed and scary creatures, although in young children's books there is usually a happy ending. Being scared but knowing that you are safe, as in the case of a scary story, is a natural part of growing up. However, being scared of something that actually exists and which will actually occur, such as a painful procedure, or being frightened about being in an environment such as a hospital that you cannot control and do not understand, is completely different from make-believe fear or the sort of terror that Sam experienced as part of his hallucinations. Pain-related fear and hospital-related fear are often interlinked and children need to be protected from becoming afraid and supported if they become frightened. Pain-related fear is linked to emotional distress and pain-related disability in children and young people with chronic pain (Simons et al. 2011). The Pediatric Fear Scale developed by Huguet et al. (2011) shows promise in generating evidence to better understand the role of children's pain-related fear and how we can develop enhanced practice.

Despite the move to engage children and young people in the design of new health care settings (Adams et al. 2010) and in the enhancement of existing settings, hospitals can still be stressful and scary places for children (Wilson et al. 2010) as well as their parents. Research shows that strategies which address parental anxiety can be beneficial for both children and parents (Bearden et al. 2012). Separation from family (Coyne 2011), feeling alone (Wilson et al. 2010) and having to deal with a strange, intimidating and unpredictable environment (Wilson et al. 2010; Wennstrom et al. 2008), fear of procedures and/or surgery (Kuivalainen et al. 2012; Fortier et al. 2011), memories of previous pain experiences (Noel et al. 2012) are all stressful. It is therefore unsurprising that anxiety and fear are two of the most commonly reported emotional responses to hospitalisation (Foster and Park 2012). Whereas the aim of hospitalisation is to intervene in a positive manner, the negative experiences can have significant short- and long-term physical, psychosocial and emotional impacts (Ford 2011). The perioperative period is a particularly challenging period for children to deal with and is associated with anxiety and distress and can result in post-operative behaviour changes (Cohen-Salmon 2010). Children in intensive care (Rennick et al. 2011) and other acute settings are at risk from psychological sequelae.

Forsner et al.'s (2009: 523) work on school-aged children's fear of medical care showed that fear was perceived as a threat to the child's existence and was 'like being threatened by a monster'. They describe how the children were 'threatened by medical care' and also how they talked of 'the possibility of breaking the spell of fear'. The monster image is prevalent in young children's descriptions of fear (Boyer and Bergstrom 2011). Children's actual and anticipatory fear stems not just from those things which may seem obvious, such as scary and dangerous equipment like needles and knives and from 'nasty' things like blood, but also from aspects of hospital and being ill which isolate them and make them feel alone. Forsner et al. (2009: 523) describe one girl's anticipatory fear as the expectation that venous blood sampling could go wrong, resulting in the procedure 'destroying something inside my arm'.

Amongst the worst fear-evoking episodes experienced by children in hospital are being outnumbered by health care professionals, and feeling powerless and out of control, isolated and helpless (Pelander et al. 2007; Forsner et al. 2009; Edwards 2010; Salmela et al. 2011).

Children have strengths and are often resilient in the face of adversity. Ford's (2011: 154) work notes that 'positive emotions and experiences serve[d] to ease some of the negative aspects of their experience and constitute[d] an important coping strategy for children'. Polkki et al. (2003) also found that children used self-initiated methods of pain relief such as resting, sleeping and distraction post-operatively. Children in Forsner et al.'s (2009) study also talked about the things they did or needed to help overcome their fear. Being with their parent, being distracted, being in a supportive environment, receiving gentle treatment from staff who spent time with them, being able to share their fear, being respected and being involved in decision-making were among the things that children wanted to be able to access when they were frightened. All of these supportive elements are aspects which should be provided within good nursing care. It is not clear in Abongile's story whether his parents were with him but it is telling that the last part of his story not only involves bleeding to death but *nobody noticing*.

It is unlikely that a child recovering from cardiac surgery will have been left alone, but Abongile's story reflects the perception of aloneness. Children who are frightened and in pain need to be cared for by nurses and other staff who will spend time with them and ensure that they do not feel isolated, alone or ignored.

For much of the time, Sam's pain takes him far beyond the possibility of being rational about it. He is consumed by the pain. He and his family are told that his pain 'is not life-threatening' but while this may be true in the medical sense of the term it nonetheless does threaten his life through its insistent erosion of his quality of life, his well-being, his childhood and his bodily integrity. Sam is overwhelmed and terrified by his pain. It also threatens and hurts his family and they live with him through the cycle of 'hope and despair'. Sam's dad, Dave, talks of his own feelings of fear and despair: 'I can't stand it, it's killing me, I cannot cope or confide. I want to scream, and I want it to go away'.

Despite knowing the cause of his pain, his pain is still incomprehensible and it is beyond understanding. Nothing could prepare Sam and his family for the level of pain he experiences and they manage the best they can to be with Sam and to let him know he is loved and they will not abandon him. Dave explains that despite the fact he can do so little to help, he wants to do what he can, and he says: 'I sit in the dark holding his hand. Finally he sleeps. I am desperate. I need sleep, but can't desert him.'

Children in pain need to know that we will be there for them. Dave's story reflects his own pain-related fears: the fear of not being able to protect his son; the fear of not being 'very good [at] being Dad'; and the fear of watching his son being physically and emotionally changed by pain. Dave also tells us of the terrifying hallucinations that Sam experienced as a result of him taking high doses of codeine. Dave writes of Sam 'screaming in fear as the "shadow men" come out of the walls to attack him' and how Sam invented an 'imaginary Dwarf called Marvin [to] sit next to him to protect him from the shadow men'. The shadow men terrified Sam and that episode continues to have long-lasting ramifications on the family, especially his brother Robert who, at 22 years old, 'is still unable to talk about "that day"'.

Children's understanding about pain

The literature that focuses on children's understanding of pain is a subset of the literature on children's understandings of illness. Seminal research published in the 1980s and 1990s continues to provide a valuable although somewhat inconsistent insight into children's understanding of pain (Lavigne et al. 1986; Gaffney and Dunne 1987; Harbeck and Peterson 1992; Peterson et al. 1993).

Gaffney and Dunne's (1986: 108) study of healthy, Irish school children aged 5–14 years proposed that they acquire their concept of pain in a Piagetian manner, grouping the children's definitions of pain into three composite categories (see Table 9.2). Similar findings were shown in other studies (Harbeck and Peterson 1992). However, this is at odds with Ross and Ross's (1984: 182–3) findings which report the absence of developmental trends and who found 'no developmental transitions similar, for example, to the well-defined stages that have been demonstrated for concepts of illness'.

Table 9.2   Composite, although contested categories

Concrete definitions	Semi-abstract definitions	Abstract definitions
Pain was seen as a 'thing' or an 'it' or 'something' that was defined by its location in the abdomen/tummy/ belly or elsewhere in the body. It was associated with being hurt or sore and with illness or trauma.	Terms were used such as feeling or sensation which also referred to unpleasant physical properties like hurt and sore and to illness or trauma and where synonyms are used such as ache and cramp.	Terms and explanations that cover physiological (nerves, damage), psychological (worry, anxiety, depression) and psychophysiological (suffering) domains were used to explain causation and experience of pain.

Gaffney and Dunne (1986)

Although older children can understand it has warning and protective functions, young children do not perceive pain as having any utility (Harbeck and Peterson 1992). In relation to the causes of pain, children (and adults) tend to be more able to describe why an injection or a skinned knee is painful than what causes a headache to be painful (Harbeck and Peterson 1992). More visible and overtly physical causes are easier to explain and understand.

Experience, per se, of chronic pain does not necessarily result in a more sophisticated understanding. Indeed Berry et al.'s (1993) study of children (aged 6–17 years) with juvenile idiopathic arthritis showed that although there was a developmental progression of understanding, many of the children were functioning below their age-expected level with most of them only operating at a concrete operational level.

Within a Piagetian approach, some authors have explored children's use of immanent justice explanations in which the child believes that the cause of their illness is the result of some form of bad behaviour or transgression on their part (Perrin and Gerrity 1981; Gaffney and Dunne 1986, 1987). Although Kister and Patterson's (1980) findings demonstrated that young children do employ immanent justice in their explanations about illness, other authors find little evidence for it (Myant and Williams 2005; Raman and Winer 2002; Ross and Ross 1984).

Reducing pain-related fear

Every child and their particular situation is unique. The use of guidelines (Australian and New Zealand College of Anaesthetists 2005; APA 2012; Ishizaki et al. 2012), protocol-driven approaches (Bice et al. 2013), and generic preparation via information booklets (Huth et al. 2003) can only really be effective if the health professional tailors the advice, guidance and information to the specific child they are caring for.

Psychological preparation that takes an individualised and holistic approach is needed to mitigate children's and young people's fears about surgery and post-operative recovery (Rullander et al. 2013). This involves taking a child's experience and age into consideration when assessing their understanding (Crisp et al. 1996) rather than simply thinking 'this is a pre-schooler, I will explain using my standard pre-schooler script'. Taking children's health literacy into consideration (Borzekowski 2009; Abrams et al. 2009; DeWalt and Hink 2009) and improving our communication practices means that even young children can feel secure, be empowered and feel confident about what is going to happen to them.

Dialogic practice involves health professionals listening to what children and families are saying, talking with them about their concerns and identifying ways to help them manage pain. The use of peri-operative dialogues (in day case surgery) is proposed as a way of helping to enhance children's sense of control, minimising distress and improving their preparedness for dealing with a situation they find unpredictable and distressing (Wennstrom and Bergh 2008; Wennstrom et al. 2011). However, providing reassurance through dialogue is not as simple as it might seem. McMurtry et al.'s (2007) somewhat counterintuitive findings show that some elements of parental reassurance can increase a child's distress. While the parental intention may be to calm and reassure a child, telling them 'not to worry' can trigger a train of negative thoughts about what should be worrying them (McMurtry 2013) and heighten a child's anxieties (Vacik et al. 2001).

For children like Abongile, who have had cardiac surgery and whose peri-operative care and recovery will involve many procedures such as blood tests, removal of drains and physiotherapy, one novel way of supporting the child and their family is the Heart Beads programme. In this intervention, each child is given a necklace that is personalised with their name and then further personalised through the addition of beads to mark major clinical events (Dengler et al. 2011; Redshaw and Wilson 2012). Each bead tells part of their story of being in hospital, and while it will not necessarily reduce the child's pain it can be used as a touch-point for dialogue, storytelling and preparation. Although Heart Beads is an approach that cannot be rolled out with every child, more modest approaches to help mark a child's experiences can be used by nurses with imagination and creativity.

Managing children's pain-related fear is a challenge for nurses, requiring them to draw on their technical and emotional skills. It requires professionals to be compassionate (Biro 2010; Dewar and Mackay 2010) in their approach to caring for children in pain and to draw on their 'deep humanity' (Forsner et al. 2009: 527). This demands a lot from us as professionals, and some practitioners can feel fearful about caring for children in pain (Ljusegren et al. 2012).

Conclusion

Pain-related fear can and does have short- and long-term impacts on children, their families and the health professionals providing care. While some children recover from a frightening painful episode, other children have to live with lifelong consequences such as needle-phobia and a dread of hospitalisation, which inevitably impacts on their health, well-being and use of health services. We do not know how Abongile's story worked out in the long term. It is not possible to know whether Rene's skilled intervention laid the foundations for Abongile to be able to cope with any future periods of hospitalisation and surgery or if all his future hospital experiences will be traumatic. Good psychological preparation for surgery is vital, and we need a stronger evidence base to support how we should approach this. Individualised preparation must be based on understanding a child's particular experiences, concerns and strengths. This can be achieved through dialogue with the child and tailoring our explanations to meet their needs: we are honour bound to respond to their stories and help manage their pain.

It is good to know that some stories, even painful and awful ones, have happy endings. Dave's story is a 'happy ending' story, although when we left it at the start of the chapter this did not seem to be the way the story would end. Dave's story concludes in 2010, eleven years after Sam developed 'severe pain in his right leg' caused by an 'inoperable' and 'extensive internal congenital vascular malformation (CVM)' that was 'not life-threatening'. During those eleven years the pain did threaten Sam's life. He and his family suffered 'unbearable anguish' and countless episodes of pain, of hope and of despair. Dave's diary in 2010 concludes:

> Sam [aged 22 years] is offered surgery to remove the CVM. Despite huge trepidations he takes the chance. 3 days after the operation the pain has gone. As each day and week passes we cannot believe that it is permanent. What happened cannot be washed away, and scars are there in all of us. Moving from disabled to enabled – a more difficult path than could have perhaps been imagined. It was the beginning of the end.

As Dave says, Sam's story is just beginning.

As health professionals we need to be there for children and their families at every stage of their stories; we also need to be there to prevent pain and fear and to find ways of mitigating fear and promoting well-being. Tailoring our care to meet every child's particular cognitive and perceptual level is a 'big ask', but the alternative is that children experience pain-related fear, and this is not acceptable.

Key Points

- Children learn about illness, injury and symptoms such as pain by drawing on their own experiences as well as those of their family and friends.
- Even young children reason and make predictions based on using naïve theories.
- Children from different cultural backgrounds develop their understanding of illness in similar ways.
- Pain-related and hospital-related fear are often interlinked.

- Children's actual and anticipatory fear stems not just from obvious things (e.g., scary equipment and blood), but also from aspects of hospital and being ill which isolate them and make them feel alone.
- Children have strengths and are often resilient in the face of adversity.
- Although older children can understand pain has warning and protective functions, young children do not perceive pain as having any utility.
- Managing children's pain-related fear requires nurses requiring draw on their technical and emotional skills.

Additional Resources and Reading

- *Pig Heart Boy* is a wonderfully written novel about an adolescent's fears and concerns about dying, heart transplants, and surgery:
  o Blackman, M. (2011) *Pig Heart Boy*. London: Corgi Books.
- A good book on child development:
  o Crowley, K. (2014) *Child Development: A Practical Introduction*, 1st edn. London: Sage.
- A good book on biopsychosocial perspectives:
  o Turner-Cobb, J. (2013) *Child Health Psychology: A Biopsychosocial Perspective*. London: Sage.
- Information about different 'bead schemes':
  o www.childrenshospitaloakland.org/about/documents/MDNewsBeads.pdf
  o Olivia talks about her beads on You Tube. www.youtube.com/watch?v=HKLKnztACnA
- Elliot Krane talks of 'The mystery of chronic pain':
  o www.ted.com/talks/elliot_krane_the_mystery_of_chronic_pain.html

References

Abrams, M.A., Klass, P. and Dreyer, B.P. (2009) 'Health literacy and children: introduction', *Pediatrics*, 124 (Supplement 3): S262–S264.

Adams, A., Theodore, D., Goldenberg, E., McLaren, C. and McKeever, P. (2010) 'Kids in the atrium: comparing architectural intentions and children's experiences in a pediatric hospital lobby', *Social Science & Medicine*, 70 (5): 658–67.

Association of Paediatric Anaesthetists (APA) (2012) *Good Practice in Postoperative and Procedural Pain Management*, 2nd edn, *Pediatric Anesthesia*, 22 (Supplement 1): 1–79.

Australian and New Zealand College of Anaesthetists (2005) *Acute Pain Management: Scientific Evidence*. Melbourne: Australian and New Zealand College of Anaesthetists and Faculty of Pain Medicine.

Bares, C.B. and Gelman, S.A. (2008) 'Knowledge of illness during childhood: making distinctions between cancer and colds', *International Journal of Behavioral Development*, 32 (5): 443–50.

Bearden, D.J., Feinstein, A. and Cohen, L.L. (2012) 'The influence of parent preprocedural anxiety on child procedural pain: mediation by child procedural anxiety', *Journal of Pediatric Psychology*, 37 (6): 680–6.

Berry, S.L., Hayford, J.R., Ross, C.K., Pachman, L.M. and Lavigne, J.V. (1993) 'Conceptions of illness by children with juvenile rheumatoid arthritis: a cognitive developmental approach', *Journal of Pediatric Psychology*, 18 (1): 83–97.

Bibace, R. and Walsh, M.E. (1980) 'Development of children's concepts of illness', *Pediatrics*, 66 (6): 912–17.

Bice, A.A., Gunther, M. and Wyatt, T. (2013) 'Increasing nursing treatment for pediatric procedural pain', *Pain Management Nursing*, in press corrected proof, doi: 10.1016/j. pmn.2012.06.004.

Biro, D. (2010) *The Language of Pain: Finding Words, Compassion, and Relief*. New York: W. W. Norton & Co.

Boruchovitch, E. and Mednick, B.R. (2000) 'Causal attributions in Brazilian children's reasoning about health and illness', *Revista de saude publica*, 34 (5): 484–90.

Borzekowski, D.L.G. (2009) 'Considering children and health literacy: a theoretical approach', *Pediatrics*, 124: S282–S288.

Boyer, P. and Bergstrom, B. (2011) 'Threat-detection in child development: an evolutionary perspective', *Neuroscience & Biobehavioral Reviews*, 35 (4): 1034–41.

Buchanan-Barrow, E., Barrett, M. and Bati, M. (2003) 'Children's understanding of illness: the generalization of illness according to exemplar', *Journal of Health Psychology*, 8 (6): 659–70.

Buchanan-Barrow, E., Barrett, M. and Bati, M. (2004) 'Healthy and chronically-ill children's generalisation of illness to biological and non-biological categories', *Infant and Child Development*, 13 (5): 435–50.

Burbach, D.J. and Peterson, L. (1986) 'Children's concepts of physical illness: a review and critique of the cognitive-developmental literature', *Health Psychology*, 5 (3): 307–25.

Cohen-Salmon, D. (2010) 'Perioperative psychobehavioural changes in children', *Annales Francaises D Anesthesie et de Reanimation*, 29 (4): 289–300.

Coyne, I. (2011) 'Children's experience of hospitalisation and their participation in health-care decision making', in G. Brykczynska and J. Simons (eds), *Ethical and Philosophical Aspects of Nursing Children and Young People*. Oxford: Wiley Blackwell, pp. 127–43.

Crisp, J., Ungerer, J.A. and Goodnow, J.J. (1996) 'The impact of experience on children's understanding of illness', *Journal of Pediatric Psychology*, 21 (1): 57–72.

Dengler, K.A., Scarfe, G., Redshaw, S. and Wilson, V. (2011) 'The heart beads program', *Journal for Specialists in Pediatric Nursing*, 16 (1): 80–4.

DeWalt, D.A. and Hink, A. (2009) 'Health literacy and child health outcomes: a systematic review of the literature', *Pediatrics*, 124 (Supplement 3): S265–S274.

Dewar, B. and Mackay, R. (2010) 'Appreciating and developing compassionate care in an acute hospital setting caring for older people', *International Journal of Older People Nursing*, 5 (4): 299–308.

Drahota, A. and Malcarne, V.L. (2008) 'Concepts of illness in children: a comparison between children with and without intellectual disability', *Intellectual and Developmental Disabilities*, 46 (1): 44–53.

Edwards, M. (2010) *Children's and Young People's Experiences of Being in Hospital: Disruption, Uncertainty, Powerlessness and Restoring Equilibrium*. Preston: University of Central Lancashire.

Ford, K. (2011) '"I didn't really like it, but it sounded exciting": admission to hospital for surgery from the perspectives of children', *Journal of Child Health Care*, 15 (4): 250–60.

Forsner, M., Jansson, L. and Söderberg, A. (2009) 'Afraid of medical care: school-aged children's narratives about medical fear', *Journal of Pediatric Nursing*, 24 (6): 519–28.

Fortier, M.A., Martin, S.R., Chorney, J.M., Mayes, L.C. and Kain, Z.N. (2011) 'Preoperative anxiety in adolescents undergoing surgery: a pilot study', *Pediatric Anesthesia*, 21 (9): 969–73.

Foster, R.L. and Park, J. (2012) 'An integrative review of literature examining psychometric properties of instruments measuring anxiety or fear in hospitalized children', *Pain Management Nursing*, 13: 94–106.

Gaffney, A. and Dunne, E.A. (1986) 'Developmental aspects of children's definitions of pain', *Pain*, 26 (1): 105–17.

Gaffney, A. and Dunne, E.A. (1987) 'Children's understanding of the causality of pain', *Pain*, 29 (1): 91–104.

Harbeck, C. and Peterson, L. (1992) 'Elephants dancing in my head: a developmental approach to children's concepts of specific pains', *Child Development*, 63 (1): 138–49.

Hergenrather, J.R. and Rabinowitz, M. (1991) 'Age-related differences in the organization of children's knowledge of illness', *Developmental Psychology*, 27 (6): 952–9.

Huguet, A., McGrath, P.J. and Pardos, J. (2011) 'Development and preliminary testing of a scale to assess pain-related fear in children and adolescents', *The Journal of Pain*, 12 (8): 840–8.

Huth, M.M., Broome, M.E., Mussatto, K.A. and Morgan, S.W. (2003) 'A study of the effectiveness of a pain management education booklet for parents of children having cardiac surgery', *Pain Management Nursing*, 4 (1): 31–9.

Inagaki, K. and Hatano, G. (1996) 'Young children's recognition of commonalities between animals and plants', *Child Development*, 67 (6): 2823–40.

Ishizaki, Y., Yasujima, H., Takenaka, Y., Shimada, A., Murakami, K., Fukai, Y., Inouwe, N., Oka, T., Maru, M., Wakako, R., Shirakawa, M., Fujita, M., Fujii, Y., Uchida, Y., Ogimi, Y., Kambara, Y., Nagai, A., Nakao, R. and Tanaka, H. (2012) 'Japanese clinical guidelines for chronic pain in children and adolescents', *Pediatrics International*, 54 (1): 1–7.

Kalish, C.W. (1999) 'What young children's understanding of contamination and contagion tells us about their concepts of illness' in M. Siegal, C.C. Petersen, M. Siegal and C.C. Petersen (eds), *Children's Understanding of Biology and Health*. New York: Cambridge University Press, pp. 99–130.

Kister, M.C. and Patterson, C.J. (1980) 'Children's conceptions of the causes of illness: understanding of contagion and use of immanent justice', *Child Development*, 51 (3): 839–46.

Koopman, H.M., Baars, R.M., Chaplin, J. and Zwinderman, K.H. (2004) 'Illness through the eyes of the child: the development of children's understanding of the causes of illness', *Patient Education and Counseling*, 55 (3): 363–70.

Kuivalainen, A., Pitkäniemi, J., Widenius, T., Elonen, E. and Rosenberg, P. (2012) 'Anxiety and pain during bone marrow aspiration and biopsy', *Scandinavian Journal of Pain*, 3 (2): 92–6.

Lavigne, J.V., Schulein, M.J. and Hahn, Y.S. (1986) 'Psychological aspects of painful medical conditions in children. I. Developmental aspects and assessment', *Pain*, 27 (2): 133–46.

Legare, C.H. and Gelman, S.A. (2009) 'South African children's understanding of AIDS and flu: investigating conceptual understanding of cause, treatment and prevention', *Journal of Cognition & Culture*, 9 (3): 333–46.

Ljusegren, G., Johansson, I., Gimbler Berglund, I. and Enskär, K. (2012) 'Nurses' experiences of caring for children in pain', *Child: Care, Health & Development*, 38 (4): 464–70.

McMurtry, C.M. (2013) 'Pediatric needle procedures: parent-child interactions, child fear, and evidence-based treatment', *Canadian Psychology (Psychologie Canadienne)*, 54 (1): 75–9.

McMurtry, C.M., McGrath, P.J., Asp, E. and Chambers, C.T. (2007) 'Parental reassurance and pediatric procedural pain: a linguistic description', *The Journal of Pain*, 8 (2): 95–101.

McMurtry, C.M., Noel, M., Chambers, C.T. and McGrath, P.J. (2011) 'Children's fear during procedural pain: preliminary investigation of the Children's Fear Scale', *Health Psychology*, 30 (6): 780–8.

Myant, K.A. and Williams, J.M. (2005) 'Children's concepts of health and illness: understanding of contagious illnesses, non-contagious illnesses and injuries', *Journal of Health Psychology*, 10 (6): 805–19.

Noel, M., Chambers, C.T., McGrath, P.J., Klein, R.M. and Stewart, S.H. (2012) 'The influence of children's pain memories on subsequent pain experience', *Pain*, 153 (8): 1563–72.

Notaro, P.C., Gelman, S.A. and Zimmerman, M.A. (2001) 'Children's understanding of psychogenic bodily reactions', *Child Development*, 72 (2): 444–59.

Onyango-Ouma, W., Aagaard-Hansen, J. and Jensen, B.B. (2004) 'Changing concepts of health and illness among children of primary school age in Western Kenya', *Health Education Research*, 19 (3): 326–39.

Paterson, J., Moss-Morris, R. and Butler, S.J. (1999) 'The effect of illness experience and demographic factors on children's illness representations', *Psychology & Health*, 14 (1): 117–29.

Pelander, T., Lehtonen, K. and Leino-Kilpi, H. (2007) 'Children in the hospital: elements of quality in drawings', *Journal of Pediatric Nursing*, 22 (4): 333–41.

Peltzer, K. and Promtussananon, S. (2003) 'Black South African children's understanding of health and illness: colds, chicken pox, broken arms and AIDS', *Child Care Health and Development*, 29 (5): 385–93.

Perrin, E.C. and Gerrity, P.S. (1981) 'There's a demon in your belly: children's understanding of illness', *Pediatrics*, 67 (6): 841.

Peterson, L., Moreno, A. and Harbeck-Weber, C. (1993) 'And then it started bleeding: children's and mothers' perceptions and recollections of daily injury events', *Journal of Clinical Child Psychology*, 22: 345–54.

Piaget, J. (1930) *The Child's Conception of Physical Causality*. London: Kegan Paul, Trench, Trubner.

Polkki, T., Pletila, A.M. and Vehvilainen-Julkunen, K. (2003) 'Hospitalized children's descriptions of their experiences with postsurgical pain relieving methods', *International Journal of Nursing Studies*, 40 (1): 33–44.

Raman, L. and Gelman, S.A. (2007) 'Children's recognition of time in the causes and cures of physical and emotional reactions to illnesses and injuries', *The British Journal of Psychology*, 98 (3): 389–410.

Raman, L. and Winer, G.A. (2002) 'Children's and adults' understanding of illness: evidence in support of a coexistence model', *Genetic, Social, and General Psychology Monographs*, 128 (4): 325–55.

Redshaw, S. and Wilson, V. (2012) 'Sibling involvement in childhood chronic heart disease through a bead program', *Journal of Child Health Care*, 16 (1): 53–61.

Reeve, S. and Bell, P. (2009) 'Children's self-documentation and understanding of the concepts "healthy" and "unhealthy"', *International Journal of Science Education*, 31 (14): 1953–74.

Rennick, J.E., Johnston, C., Lambert, S.D., Rashotte, J.M., Schmitz, N., Earle, R.J., Stevens, B.J., Tewfik, T. and Wood-Dauphinee, S. (2011) 'Measuring psychological outcomes following pediatric intensive care unit hospitalization: psychometric analysis of the Children's Critical Illness Impact Scale', *Pediatric Critical Care Medicine*, 12 (6): 635–42.

Ross, D.M. and Ross, S.A. (1984) 'Childhood pain: the school-aged child's viewpoint', *Pain*, 20 (2): 179–191.

Rullander, A., Isberg, S., Karling, M., Jonsson, H. and Lindh, V. (2013) 'Adolescents' experience with scoliosis surgery: a qualitative study', *Pain Management Nursing*, 14 (1): 50–9.

Salmela, M., Aronen, E., T. and Salanterä, S. (2011) 'The experience of hospital-related fears of 4- to 6-year-old children', *Child: Care, Health & Development*, 37 (5): 719–26.

Sigelman, C.K. (2012) 'Age and ethnic differences in cold weather and contagion theories of colds and flu', *Health Education & Behavior*, 39 (1): 67–76.

Simons, L.E., Sieberg, C.B., Carpino, E., Logan, D. and Berde, C. (2011) 'The Fear of Pain Questionnaire (FOPQ): assessment of pain-related fear among children and adolescents with chronic pain', *Journal of Pain*, 12 (6): 677–86.

Turner, J.C. (2006) 'Representations of illness, injury, and health in children's picture books', *Children's Health Care*, 35 (2): 179–89.

Vacik, H.W., Nagy, M.C. and Jessee, P.O. (2001) 'Children's understanding of illness: students' assessments', *Journal of Pediatric Nursing*, 16 (6): 429–37.

Vygotsky, L.S. (1979) *Mind in Society: The Development of High Mental Processes*. Cambridge, MA: Harvard University Press.

Wellman, H.M. and Gelman, S.A. (1992) 'Cognitive development: foundational theories of core domains', *Annual Review of Psychology*, 43 (1): 337.

Wennstrom, B. and Bergh, I. (2008) 'Bodily and verbal expressions of postoperative symptoms in 3- to 6-year-old boys', *Journal of Pediatric Nursing*, 23 (1): 65–76.

Wennstrom, B., Hallberg, L.R.M. and Bergh, I. (2008) 'Use of perioperative dialogues with children undergoing day surgery', *Journal of Advanced Nursing*, 62 (1): 96–106.

Wennstrom, B., Tornhage, C.J., Nasic, S., Hedelin, H. and Bergh, I. (2011) 'The perioperative dialogue reduces postoperative stress in children undergoing day surgery as confirmed by salivary cortisol', *Pediatric Anesthesia*, 21 (10): 1058–65.

Williams, J.M. and Binnie, L.M. (2002) 'Children's concepts of illness: an intervention to improve knowledge', *British Journal of Health Psychology*, 7: 129–47.

Wilson, M.E., Megel, M.E., Enenbach, L. and Carlson, K.L. (2010) 'The voices of children: stories about hospitalization', *Journal of Pediatric Health Care*, 24: 95–102.

Zhu, L. and Liu, G. (2007) 'Preschool children's understanding of illness', *Acta Psychologica Sinica*, 39 (1): 96–103.

Zhu, L., Liu, G. and Tardif, T. (2009) 'Chinese children's explanations for illness', *International Journal of Behavioral Development*, 33 (6): 516–19.

Chapter 10

Acute Pain Developing into Chronic Pain

Ahmet's Story

Ahmet's story

Following surgery for excision of an abscess, a young boy called Ahmet had experienced a very problematic post-operative period. Over the next six months, poor wound healing and pain became a persistent feature in his everyday life. All attempts at pain management met with limited effectiveness and over time this child became quiet and withdrawn, showing signs of physical, emotional and psychological pain.

As part of the Community Children's Nursing Team visiting to perform dressing changes, I decided to reassess this young boy's pain and its management, using new knowledge from a Management of Children's Pain module I was currently undertaking. Using an age-appropriate, multidimensional pain assessment tool (APPT) allowed this young child to differentiate between differing pain sensations and using 'self-report' to accurately describe his pain experience in words that were meaningful to him.

As his nurse, this facilitated much greater clarity and understanding about the complex nature of this young child's pain and highlighted several issues contributing to the ineffective pain management to date. Performing this comprehensive assessment also facilitated recognition that his continued unrelieved pain had evolved into a complex chronic pain problem, which was impacting significantly on many aspects of this boy's life.

Subsequent negotiation resulted in greater involvement by his family and changes by the care team to more appropriate pain management, leading to effective pain relief for this young boy. Central to my learning from this experience is the importance of using an age-appropriate, multidimensional pain tool for accurate assessment and effective management of children's pain.

Introduction

In this story we hear about Ahmet, a 10–year-old boy, who had a minor procedure performed in hospital. One would have expected that within a few days or at most a week he would have been back at school resuming his normal life. However, instead we hear that six months after his minor surgery to drain an abscess he is suffering chronic pain, resulting in changes to his personality leaving him quiet and withdrawn and experiencing significant pain despite ongoing efforts to manage his pain.

All this changed when the Advanced Nurse Practitioner re-evaluated the boy's pain using a multidimensional pain assessment tool. What had started as seemingly straightforward acute post-operative pain had gradually become more complex chronic pain, meaning that his pain required a different approach. The use of a multi-level assessment stimulated effective management of his pain by the care team, and involved his family in a more active way than previously.

The management of Ahmet's pain at home

When Ahmet was hospitalised for surgery for drainage of an abscess, his family would have expected a brief stay in hospital followed by a return to normal activities soon after. Many children undergo day surgery and it has become an efficient way of dealing with minor procedures (Blacoe et al. 2008). Most hospitals have a dedicated day case unit that deals exclusively with day cases from Monday to Friday. However, one prevalent complication of day case surgery is post-operative pain, which has been found to be the most common problem at follow-up after discharge in a paediatric population (Segerdahl et al. 2008).

With the continuing increase in day case surgery there is a need for effective support for parents in managing their child's pain at home. Morgan et al. (2001) found that parents could assess their child's pain but needed support to manage their pain. It has been found that parents do not give enough analgesics to their children post-operatively at home. It is not fully understood why. Fortier et al. (2009) studied the pain management of 261 children at home following tonsillectomy and adenoidectomy. They found that although parents rated nearly all children as having significant pain overall, one quarter of children received no medication or just one medication dose throughout the day. If Ahmet's parents had a similar approach to his pain, it is likely to have contributed to his pain lasting beyond the acute phase. It is clear that parents need targeted support in the initial post-operative period if they are to relieve their child's pain effectively. Initiatives that are effective have been explored. Vincent et al. (2012) conducted a controlled study with 108 children and their parents, in which children and parents were given information and had follow-up sessions on pain management principles which included consequences of unrelieved pain, pain assessment (self-report and behaviour), pharmacological and non-pharmacological treatment of pain, and concerns about analgesics (e.g., side effects and addiction). The result of the intervention was that parents administered more analgesics and managed their children's pain more appropriately. The authors suggest that parents need a lot of support to deal with their child's pain and that written instructions and simple interventions are not enough. An earlier study by Jonas (2003) found that parents managed their child's pain effectively at home when provided with suitable analgesia, information and a follow-up phone call.

Parents' ability to judge their child's pain may be influenced by the perceived threat of the pain. Vervoot et al. (2012) studied the reactions of 62 parents in response to their child's expression of pain. It was found that parents were more sensitive to pain when the perceived threat was high. These findings may explain the lack of involvement of Ahmet's parents in relation to his pain. Ahmet had had a minor procedure which would have been deemed a low threat in relation to pain, not requiring a high level of engagement from his parents. If Ahmet's pain had followed the expected trajectory, his parents apparent lack of active involvement in his pain would not have been an issue of significance. But after six months, with ongoing pain, the inclusion of Ahmet's parents in managing his pain was pivotal in the revised pain management plan.

Studies have explored how to improve the management of children's pain at home. Unsworth et al. (2007) conducted a randomised controlled trial exploring the impact of children using a self-report tool at home following day case surgery. They hypothesised that children who used the tool would receive more analgesia than the control group. The study included 88 children aged between 4 and 12 years of age. However, the findings showed no difference between the two groups. An earlier study by Ling (1996) who studied day case surgery in a district hospital showed that parents were happy to nurse their child at home but frequently needed support from a health care professional to help clarify ambiguous information provided on discharge.

One could ask why the apparently simple process of a child having a minor procedure and sent home with what is expected to be time-limited acute pain is not managed more effectively. The answer could be that what seems simple and straightforward is actually quite complex. Parents are not used to dealing with children in acute post-operative pain, and children may expect their parents to know they are in pain without telling them. At the same time parents are naturally wary of giving analgesics unnecessarily so need to feel their child is in pain before actually administering analgesia. In this way pain is not pre-empted and dealt with quickly, as is recommended by the APA *Good Practice Guidelines* (APA 2012). Instead, children experience unnecessary pain at home.

Qualified professionals can find it challenging to deal with pain effectively, as evidenced by children still experiencing unnecessary pain (Van Hulle et al. 2009), therefore it is not surprising that parents, who may be stressed and anxious about their child's surgery, do not manage to deal with their child's pain effectively at home. One complicating factor in day case surgery is that children often go home pain free, having had analgesia administered in theatre, which leads the parents to believe they do not need anything for pain. This often leads to children having their first experience of post-operative pain at home, with their parents, who do not feel confident in managing their pain, left to cope. Swallow et al. (2000) found that children were as likely to experience their worst pain at home as in hospital, underlining the need for good home care advice for parents on discharge. Jonas's (2003) study involved 100 parents who received a telephone call post discharge from day surgery and found that 79 per cent of parents found the phone call helpful. Most parents expected their child to have pain, and most gave their children analgesia at home, resulting in 48 per cent of children remaining pain free throughout the first 48 hours post-operatively. Although this study demonstrates a simple and apparently effective support mechanism for parents post discharge, 52 per cent of children did experience pain, suggesting that although most parents gave analgesics to their children, this may have been after they waited for the child to complain of pain, rather than pre-empting it.

Acute and chronic pain

Poor management of acute pain can lead to chronic pain. Dunwoody et al. (2008) suggest that untreated acute pain has the potential to produce acute neurohumoral changes, neuronal remodelling and long-lasting psychological and emotional distress which can lead to prolonged chronic pain states. This is supported by Rathmell et al. (2005) who suggest there is a link between poorly controlled post-operative pain and the risk of developing chronic pain. This appears to have happened in Ahmet's case, as his acute unmanaged post-operative pain developed into chronic pain, and six months after his minor procedure to drain an abscess he was in considerable pain which was having a significant impact on his and his family's life.

This phenomenon of acute pain becoming chronic has been recognised and studied in adults for some time but is a new area of research in children's pain. Fortier et al. (2011) conducted a retrospective review of 555 medical records of children who had undergone general surgery: 13 per cent of them developed chronic pain as a result of unrelieved acute pain. No definitions are available in the literature on children's pain management that defines chronic pain after surgery. Page et al. (2013) studied the incidence of chronic post-operative pain in 83 children aged 8–18 years who had undergone major orthopaedic surgery. They found that 22 per cent of children developed chronic post-operative pain, and identified two particular factors that appeared to influence the development of chronic pain post-operatively: children rating their pain 3 or greater on a numerical 0–10 pain scale, and anxiety related to pain. These findings highlight the need for vigilance in the immediate post-operative period in reducing and alleviating pain to prevent it developing into chronic pain, as happened to Ahmet.

Macrae (2008) suggests that chronic pain after surgery is typically pain that develops after a surgical procedure, ranging in length from two days to six months or longer, excludes any pre-operative condition as a potential cause and does not result from another cause such as infection. Severity of acute post-operative pain has been identified as a predictor of the development of chronic pain. It would appear therefore that under-treatment of acute pain in children is likely to predispose them to ongoing pain such as that experienced by Ahmet. The lack of literature on this topic in children, until very recently, may also explain the lack of recognition of Ahmet's pain on the part of the community nurses who visited him at home over a six-month period. The situation was addressed once the Advanced Nurse Practitioner Community approached Ahmet's pain in a different way using the APPT to gain a comprehensive and individualised picture of Ahmet's pain. This was possible because she was confident about her skills and was able to draw on new knowledge.

Defining chronic pain can be difficult as there are a number of interpretations. A short definition is offered by Schecter et al. (2003: 3) suggesting chronic pain is characterised by its prolonged and persistent nature, lasting three months or longer. In relation to the chronic pain experienced by Ahmet an appropriate definition is offered by Wahlstrom (2004: 135) suggesting that 'chronic pain is any pain that persists beyond the usual course of an acute injury or illness, or beyond what is usually expected for recovery'. Ahmet's minor procedure was expected to result in acute pain of a limited duration which should have resolved within a week or two. However, six months after his minor surgery he was experiencing chronic pain.

The effect of chronic pain

How health professionals interact with children experiencing chronic pain has the potential to influence how a child feels about their pain. Dell'Api et al. (2007) found that unsuccessful interactions between children and nurses often led to children becoming disillusioned. In Ahmet's case he had had numerous interactions with community nurses over a six-month period and was still in pain. It is likely that their visits had a negative impact on him due to their ongoing inability to relieve his pain which had gradually developed into chronic pain. Some studies have put the incidence of chronic pain in children at 25 per cent and costing the NHS £4 billion annually (The British Pain Society 2008). There is also a cost to children and their family that cannot be measured in monetary terms. In Ahmet's story after having pain for six months, he was quiet and withdrawn. Jones et al. (2003) found that adolescents with chronic pain problems show less promising long-term health outcomes in regard to functional disability, pain intensity, and depressive symptoms compared to younger children. The danger of not dealing with chronic pain effectively is that Ahmet may have had long-term negative effects due to having to cope with chronic pain.

Lynch et al. (2007) studied the coping styles in children aged 8–12 years experiencing chronic pain and found there were differences between girls and boys in their coping styles. Girls used social support-seeking more than boys, while boys used more behavioural distraction techniques. However, in children with higher pain intensity both boys and girls showed a tendency to report feeling less effective at pain coping. Lynch et al. (2007) suggest that it is possible that experiencing high levels of pain may create feelings of helplessness and lead to perceptions of poor control over pain. On the other hand, children whose coping styles are characterised by low coping confidence may experience heightened pain that is exacerbated by unsuccessful attempts to manage their symptoms. Ahmet appears to have no effective coping strategies, and to be overwhelmed by the effects the chronic pain is having on him. In the story he is described as depressed, having had unrelieved pain for six months. It would appear that the impact of his pain is such that he is not coping with it and is disengaging emotionally, this would appear to be an ineffective coping strategy. Studies have shown that certain actions can help children and young people to cope or not with their pain. Reid et al. (1997) explored the coping strategies of 124 children undergoing day surgery and found that lower levels of emotion-focused avoidance and higher levels of distraction resulted in lower levels of pain. Ahmet does not appear to have had support in developing coping strategies to deal with his pain, and as a result became emotionally withdrawn, which according to Reid et al. (1997) is not likely to help him cope with his pain. These findings are supported by Harding Thomsen et al. (2002) who examined the coping and stress responses of 174 children and adolescents experiencing recurrent abdominal pain and found that disengagement such as escape or inaction-related responses to pain were associated with more somatic symptoms and higher levels of anxiety and depression. These reactions have been described by Lu et al. (2007) as pain-prone coping strategies. In other words these type of reactions actually led to more pain instead of helping the child cope with their pain. These findings may go some way to explain why Ahmet's pain was difficult to relieve over the six months since his operation. Ahmet and his parents needed help in engaging in pain relieving strategies such as distraction, acceptance and positive thinking (Harding Thomsen et al. 2002).

What are the benefits of using a multidimensional tool?

Crandall and Savedra (2005) suggest that misunderstandings about a child's or adolescent's pain may result in mistrust, and under-treatment. There is a need to acknowledge the social and developmental influence that pain has on a child or adolescent. Numerous one-dimensional pain tools are available that have been tested as valid and reliable, however, many of them focus only on pain intensity. Some examples include: the 0–10 Visual Analogue Scale; the Faces Pain Scale (Bieri et al. 1990); Faces scale (Wong and Baker 1988); the Oucher scale (Beyer et al. 1992); and the Word Graphic Rating scale (Tesler et al. 1991). All of these are appropriate to assess pain in a 10-year-old. However, none of them would adequately address the complexity of Ahmet's pain. In his case there was a need for a more complex pain tool to attempt to gain enough information about the multidimensional nature of his pain.

The vast choice of pain assessment tools available to nurses can be quite daunting. There is a need to identify a tool that is validated and appropriate to the child's age and needs. Stinson et al. (2006) conducted a systematic review of 34 validated pain tools and explored their suitability for different age groups. They found that for children over 8 years of age, such as Ahmet, the findings suggested that the Visual Analogue Scale was the tool of choice rather than faces-based tools. This could be due to its ease of use as well as its application as a measure of pain intensity and affect (Goodenough et al. 1999). Stinson et al. (2006) suggest that supplementation of the Visual Analogue Scale with other aspects of pain assessment may increase its effectiveness. Such a suggestion fits well with the Adolescent Pediatric Pain Tool (APPT), which incorporates a word graphic rating scale, a body outline and an extensive word descriptor section. Ahmet's nurse used the APPT to enable a comprehensive assessment of his pain. The information gleaned provided a holistic picture of Ahmet's pain in that he gave his nurse self-report information on not only the intensity of his pain, but also the sensations caused by his pain, how it made him feel, and the pattern of the pain. This level of information then influenced his nurse's choice of analgesic as well as the administration pattern to enable effective relief of his pain. Franck et al. (2002) found that the APPT provides adolescents with a systematic method for describing the characteristics of their pain and provides clinicians with more objective measures for determining the effectiveness of pain-relief interventions.

The three main sections of the APPT developed by Savedra et al. (1989, 1993) are the word graphic rating scale which ranges from 'no pain' to 'worst pain' (2) age appropriate, the body outlines for the front and back of the body and (3) a section including four word categories with specific subcategories to help the young person to build up a rich picture of their pain. The categories are as follows:

- **Sensory words** (n=37) represent thermal, pressure and other sensations or properties of pain.
- **Affective words** (n=11) represent the unpleasant emotional effects of pain.
- **Evaluative words** (n=8) represent the subjective overall intensity of pain.
- **Temporal words** (n=11) indicate the duration and pattern of pain.

To use the tool the young person is asked to use the body outline to indicate the location and extent of their pain (see Figure 10.1), followed by using the word

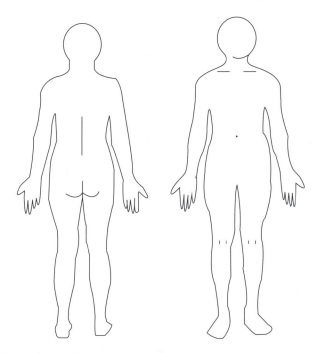

Figure 10.1   Body outline from front and back

graphic scale to indicate the intensity of their pain, and to circle the words from the qualitative word list that describe their current pain. There is also an option to add words that describe their pain.

In this way the APPT is multidimensional and allows the adolescent to provide carers with a comprehensive picture of their pain experience. The tool is validated for use with children and young people aged 8 to 17 years. Crandall and Savedra (2005) found that when using the APPT the qualitative word list provided the most useful information. In Ahmet's story his community children's nurse reports that the use of the APPT 'facilitated much greater clarity and understanding about the complex nature of his pain and highlighted several issues contributing to the ineffective pain management which she could then address'.

The experience of Ahmet's community children's nurse has been backed up by a number of studies on the APPT. It has been found to provide descriptive information about children's and adolescents' reports of pain patterns and quality, and factors influencing pain as well as the psychosocial and functional consequences of pain (Crandall et al. 2002; Franck et al. 2002; Van Cleve et al. 2003).

From Ahmet's story it is clear that measuring pain intensity alone is not adequate when assessing complex pain. When children or adolescents are experiencing complex pain, multidimensional pain assessment is important in their assessment and management. Crandall and Savedra (2005) suggest the APPT provides a mechanism for achieving this. Complex pain can impact on a young person's quality of life, as explored by Gold et al. (2009) who studied the quality of life in 69 children and young people aged 8–18 years and found that children with chronic pain reported a significantly lower quality of life. They suggest that in addition to targeting pain, management interventions should also address emotional health to improve the child's quality of life. The APPT provides nurses with an insight into the emotional impact of pain on children. However, the ease of use of a pain assessment tool is one pivotal determining factor for nurses' use of the tool (Ramitru 2000; Simons and Macdonald 2006), and the APPT by its multifaceted nature could not be described as a tool that is quick to use. Nevertheless nurses should not be put off using this tool for complex pain as Crandall and Savedra (2005), who have worked on the tool's development, suggest a once a day assessment using the APPT is appropriate to assess an adolescent's multidimensional pain experience.

The benefits of taking an individual approach to managing a child's pain

Dell'Api et al. (2007) found that health care professionals' interactions have a tremendous influence on children's perceptions and chronic pain experiences, suggesting that it is essential to provide children with the opportunity to communicate their unique experiences of pain.

The community children's nursing team had been visiting Ahmet at home regularly for six months, carrying out wound dressing changes and trying to deal with his pain. However, it was not until one of the team who had studied a module on pain approached the issue of Ahmet's complex pain with renewed confidence through new knowledge, that the pain was effectively managed. This nurse approached his pain in a holistic way, and gave Ahmet the ability to communicate his complex pain in a way that provided insight into how to address and deal effectively with his pain.

Managing children's pain is challenging and when acute pain becomes chronic the challenge becomes more complex. Habich et al. (2012) evaluated the effectiveness of an evidence-based paediatric pain assessment and management guideline with nurses, parents and children. The new guideline was introduced and evaluations were carried out at three and six months following implementation. Although they found significant increases in pain assessment, the use of the correct tool and also reassessment, no difference was found in nurses' knowledge or attitudes or in parent/family satisfaction in relation to pain management. The findings of this study suggest that improving pain assessment is not enough on its own to improve pain management. The study did not report whether the increased pain assessments led to increased administration of analgesics for pain.

Implications for practice

There are a number of implications for practice in relation to the way that Ahmet's unrelieved acute pain developed into chronic pain. First, if acute post-operative pain lasts past the expected time frame for acute pain it should be reviewed carefully and, where necessary, expert opinion sought. If chronic pain, which can have an overwhelming affect on a child or young person's quality of life, is suspected it should be assessed using a multidimensional pain assessment tool to make a comprehensive assessment. A multidimensional tool such as the Adolescent Pediatric Pain Tool should not be compared to a one-dimensional tool such as a visual analogue scale, as it requires less frequent assessment. In order to ensure pain is managed effectively at home parents should be supported to be involved in their child's pain management.

Conclusion

This chapter has focused on the experience of Ahmet, a 10-year-old boy who developed chronic pain over six months following a minor surgical procedure, and how his community nurse, through holistic pain assessment and management, succeeded in relieving his pain. By evaluating the complexity of Ahmet's situation his nurse recognised the need to change the approach to his pain management which had clearly not been working. She subsequently introduced a different method of pain assessment (the APPT). By having the confidence to tackle his pain practically and differently as well as including Ahmet's parents, his nurse overcame a number of identifiable barriers. She spent valuable time in gaining an understanding of Ahmet's pain in a comprehensive, multidimensional way, and used her knowledge of analgesics to provide effective pain relief. This alone would not have been sufficient in the long run, so the nurse also used her skills in providing support to Ahmet's parents so that they became actively involved in managing his pain effectively.

Key Points

- With the continuing increase in day case surgery there is a need for effective support for parents in managing their child's pain at home.
- Children often go home pain free following day case surgery, leading parents to believe they do not need anything for pain.
- It is recognised that poor pain management of acute pain in children can lead to chronic pain.
- Children whose pain is poorly managed can feel disillusioned and helpless.
- The vast range of pain assessment tools can be quite daunting for nurses.
- Assessing complex pain requires a multidimensional pain assessment tool.

Additional Resources and Reading

- You may want to learn more about the issue of acute pain which is not well managed developing over time into chronic pain. The following two articles focus on this area:
  o Dunwoody, C.J., Krenzischek, D.A., Pasero C., Rathmell J.P. and Polomano R.C. (2008) 'Assessment, physiological monitoring, and consequences of inadequately treated acute pain', *Journal of PeriAnesthesia Nursing*, 23 (1): S15–S27.
  o Fortier, M.A., Chou, J., Maurer, E.L. and Kain, Z.N. (2011) 'Acute to chronic postoperative pain in children: preliminary findings', *Journal of Pediatric Surgery*, 46: 1700–5.

References

Association of Paediatric Anaesthetists (APA) (2012) *Good Practice in Postoperative and Procedural Pain*, 2nd edition. London: APA.

Beyer, J., Denyes, M. and Villarruel, A. (1992) 'The creation validation, and continuing development of the Oucher: a measure of pain intensity in children', *Journal of Pediatric Nursing*, 7: 335–46.

Bieri, D., Reeve, R., Champion, G.D., Addicoat, L. and Ziegler, J. (1990) 'The Faces Pain Scale for the self-assessment of the severity of pain experienced by children: development, initial validation and preliminary investigation for ratio scale properties', *Pain*, 41: 139–50.

Blacoe, D.A., Cunning, E. and Bell, G. (2008) 'Paediatric day-case surgery: an audit of unplanned hospital admission Royal Hospital for Sick Children, Glasgow', *Anaesthesia*, 63: 610–15.

British Pain Society, The (2008) *How Much Does it Cost the NHS in Treatment of Pain?* Available at www.britishpainsociety.org /media_faq.htm (accessed 10 January 2013).

Crandall, M., Miaskowski, C., Kools, S.and Savedra, L. (2002) 'The pain experience of adolescents after acute blunt traumatic injury', *Pain Management Nursing*, 3 (3): 104–14.

Crandall, M. and Savedra, M. (2005) 'Multidimensional assessment using the adolescent pediatric pain tool: a case report', *Journal for Specialists in Pediatric Nursing*, 10 (3): 115–23.

Dell'Api, M., Rennick, J.E. and Rosmus, C. (2007) 'Childhood chronic pain and health professionals interactions: shaping the chronic pain experiences of children', *Journal of Child Health Care*, 11 (4): 269–86.

Dunwoody, C.J., Krenzischek, D.A., Pasero, C., Rathmell, J.P. and Polomano, R.C. (2008) 'Assessment, physiological monitoring, and consequences of inadequately treated acute pain', *Journal of Peri Anesthesia Nursing*, 23 (1): S15–S27.

Fortier, M.A., Chou, J., Maurer, E.L. and Kain, Z.N. (2011) 'Acute to chronic postoperative pain in children: preliminary findings', *Journal of Pediatric Surgery*, 46: 1700–5.

Fortier, M.A., MacLaren, J.E., Martin, S., Perret-Karimi, D. and Kain, Z.N. (2009) 'Pedatric pain after ambulatory surgery: where's the medication?', *Pediatrics*, 124: e588–95.

Franck, L.S., Treadwell, M., Jacob, E. and Vichinsky, E. (2002) 'Assessment of sickle cell pain in children and young adults using the adolescent pediatric pain tool', *Journal of Pain and Symptom Management*, 23 (2): 114–20.

Gold, J.I., Yetwin, A.K., Mahrer, N.E., Carson, M.C., Griffin, A.T., Palmer, S.N. and Joseph, M.H. (2009) 'Pediatric chronic pain and health-related quality of life', *Journal of Pediatric Nursing*, 24 (2): 141–50.

Goodenough, B., Thomas, W., Champion, G., Perrot, D., Taplin, J., von Baeyer, C. and Ziegler, J.B. (1999) 'Unravelling age effects and sex differences in needle pain: ratings of sensory intensity and unpleasantness of venipuncture pain by children and their parents', *Pain*, 80: 179–90.

Habich, M., Wilson, D., Thielk, D., Melles, G.L., Crumlett, H.S., Masterton, J. and McGuire, J. (2012) 'Evaluating the effectiveness of pediatric pain management guidelines', *Journal of Pediatric Nursing*, 27: 336–45.

Harding Thomsen, A., Compas, B.E., Coletti, R.B., Stanger, C., Boyer, M.C. and Konik, B.S. (2002) 'Parents reports of coping and stress responses in children with recurrent abdominal pain', *Journal of Pediatric Psychology*, 27 (3): 215–26.

Jonas, D. (2003) 'Parent's management of their child's pain in the home following day surgery', *Journal of Child Health Care*, 7 (3): 150–62.

Jones, B., Kashikar-Zuck, S., Tessman, C. and Goldschneider, K.R. (2003) 'Six- and twelve-month follow-up data from a pediatric chronic pain program', *Journal of Pain*, 4 (2 Supplement): 100.

Ling, J. (1996) 'Day case provision in a district general hospital', *Paediatric Nursing*, 8 (6): 25–8.

Lu, Q., Tsao, J.I., Myers, C.D., Kim, S.C. and Zeltzer, L.K. (2007) 'Coping predictors of children's laboratory-induced pain tolerance, intensity, and unpleasantness', *The Journal of Pain*, 8 (9): 708–17.

Lynch, A.M., Kashikar-Zuck, S., Goldschneider, K.R. and Jones, B.A. (2007) 'Sex and age differences in coping styles among children with chronic pain', *Journal of Pain and Symptom Management*, 33 (2): 208–16.

Macrae, W.A. (2008) 'Chronic post-surgical pain: 10 years on', *British Journal of Anaesthesia*, 101 (1): 77–86.

Morgan, J., Peden, V., Bhaskar, K., Vater, M. and Choonara, I. (2001) 'Assessment of pain by parents in young children following surgery', *Pediatric Anesthesia*, 11 (4): 449–52.

Page, M.G., Stinson, J., Campbell, F., Isaac, L. and Katz, J. (2013) 'Identification of pain-related psychological risk factors for the development and maintenance of pediatric chronic post-surgical pain', *Journal of Pain Research*, 6: 167–80.

Ramritu, P.L. (2000) 'Use of the oucher numeric and the word graphic scale in children aged 9–14 years with post-operative pain', *Journal of Clinical Nursing*, 9 (5): 763–72.

Rathmell, J.P., Wu, C.L., Sinatra, R.S., Sinatra, R.C., Ballantyne, J.C., Ginsberg, B., Gordon, D.B., Liu, S.S, Perkins, F.M., Reuben, S.S., Rosenquist, R.W. and Viscusi, E.R. (2005) 'Acute post-surgical pain management: a critical appraisal of current practice', *Regional Anesthesia and Pain Medicine*, 31(4, Supplement 1): 1–42.

Reid, G.J., Chambers, C.T., McGrath, P.J. and Finley, G.A. (1997) 'Coping with pain and surgery: children's and parents' perspectives', *International Journal of Behavioural Medicine*, 4 (4): 339–63.

Savedra, M.C. Tesler, M.D., Holzemer, W.I. et al. (1993) *Adolescent Pediatric Pain Tool (APPT) Preliminary User's Manual*. San Francisco, CA: University of California.

Savedra, M.C., Tesler, M.D., Holzemer, W.I. and Wilkie, D. (1989) 'Assessment of postoperative pain in children and adolescents using the Adolescent Pediatric Pain Tool', *Nursing Research*, 42 (1): 5–9.

Schecter, N.L., Berde, C.B. and Yaster, M. (2003) *Pain in Infants, Children and Adolescents: An Overview*. Philadelphia, PA: Lippincott, Williams and Wilkins.

Segerdahl M., Warren-Stomberg M., Rawal N., Brattwall M. and Jakobsson J. (2008) 'Clinical practice and routines for day surgery in Sweden: results from a nation-wide survey', *Acta Anaesthesiologica Scandinavica*, 52(1): 117–24.

Simons, J. and Macdonald, L.M. (2006) 'Changing practice: implementing validated paediatric pain assessment tools', *Journal of Child Health Care*, 10 (2): 160–76.

Stinson, J.N., Kavanagh, P., Yamada, J., Gill, N. and Stevens, B. (2006) 'Systematic review of the psychometric properties, interpretability and feasibility of self-report pain intensity measures for use in clinical trials in children and adolescents', *Pain*, 125 (1–2): 143–57.

Swallow, J., Briggs, M. and Semple, P. (2000) 'Pain at home: children's experience of tonsillectomy', *Journal of Child Health Care*, 4 (3): 93–8.

Tesler, M.D., Savedra, M.C., Holzemer, W.L., Wilkie, D.J., Ward, J.A. and Paul, S.M. (1991) 'The word-graphic rating scale as a measure of children's and adolescents' pain intensity', *Research in Nursing and Health*, 14: 361–71.

Unsworth, V., Fracnck, L.S. and Choonara, I. (2007) 'Parental assessment and management of children's postoperative pain: a randomized clinical trial', *Journal of Child Health Care*, 11 (3): 186–94.

Van Cleve, L., Bossert, E., Beecroft, P., Adlard, K., Alvarez, A. and Savedra, M. (2003) 'The pain experience of children with leukaemia the first year after diagnosis', *Nursing Research*, 53 (1): 1–10.

Vervoot, T., Caes, L., Trost, Z., Notebaert, L. and Goubert, L. (2012) 'Parental attention to their child's pain is modulated by threat-value of pain', *Health Psychology*, 31 (5): 623–31.

Van Hulle, V.C., Wilkie, D.J. and Szalacha, L. (2009) 'Pediatric nurses' cognitive representations of children's pain', *The Journal of Pain*, 11 (9): 854–63.

Vincent, C., Chiappetta, M., Beach, A., Kiolbasa, C., Latta, K., Maloney, R. and Van Roeyen, L.S. (2012) 'Parents' management of children's pain at home after surgery', *Journal for Specialists in Pediatric Nursing*, 17: 108–20.

Wahlstrom, J. (2004) 'The child with chronic pain', *Journal of Specialists in Pediatric Nursing*, 9 (4): 135–38.

Wong, D. and Baker, C. (1988) 'Pain in children: comparison of assessment scales', *Pedatric Nursing*, 14 (1): 9–17.

Chapter 11

Language, Metaphor, Imagery and the Expression of Pain

Tanya Tia's, Shantell's and Hattie's Stories

Tanya Tia's Story

The pain is like poison moving through my veins. I can feel it in my body, sometimes I cry but crying don't help it never does, ... I reach for my tablets the littlest movements in my legs feel like someone has hammered my legs until all my bones have been broken, I grab my tablets and hesitate to take them but in the end I do, but I need something stronger, the pain is still throbbing in my veins, ... I had great killing pains to both of my legs, this was a terrible time I could not walk anywhere and my leg felt like a cupboard full of sparks crushed down on your legs and I felt badly injured and could not move.

Shantell's Story

I am 11 years old and I have chronic back and lower leg pain. I've had my pain since I was born. My legs are hurting so much. My back is hurting so much. My shoulder is hurting so much.

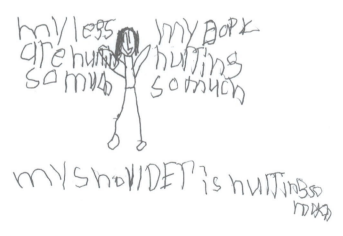

Figure 11.1   Shantell's drawing

Hattie's Story

When I woke up the pain was there. It felt so bad. I didn't know that pain could be like that. It was a terrible pain ... like a monster I couldn't hide from. My mum wasn't there. I wanted to tell someone but I didn't know what to say. I thought if I was quiet, the monster would go away. The nurse asked me if I had pain and I said 'No' and she said 'OK. But tell me if you do get sore' and then I started to cry and she said 'I can help take the pain away' and I cried. I wanted to tell her about the pain but I didn't know what to say. She held my hand and we talked and she helped me explain. I said it was like having a monster pulling your hair. She said my pain sounded bad but she had medicine to get rid of monsters. She gave me some medicine. It didn't work to start with but then it bashed the monster on the nose and the pain got better. When mum got back I told her about the monster and how he'd hurt my tummy.

Introduction

Until pain is expressed it is hidden, known only by the person experiencing it. The act of expression allows the experience of pain to be shared with other people, and through that act of sharing pain can perhaps start to be understood.

Pain can be expressed in many ways. Most commonly we think of pain expression as occurring through words (spoken and written) and through utterances such as whimpers and cries, but it also occurs through gestures, facial expression and body language. Pain can also be expressed through our responses to it, such as fear and distress, and through modalities such as music, art and drama. Bourke (2012) suggests that these are the languages of pain. These different languages of expression can provide a way for a person in pain to try to make their internal experience of pain understandable to other people. However, arguably, none of these modalities does justice to the experience of pain because they often fall short of effectively communicating the essence of the experience of pain.

In this chapter we explore aspects of Tanya Tia's, Hattie's and Shantell's pain by thinking with and about the stories they tell, the language(s) and imagery they use and the impact that their stories have on us. Two of the children – Tanya Tia and Shantell – have chronic pain, while Hattie has acute pain as a result of surgery. All three children present arresting stories of pain using language that calls to us, as health professionals, to care and act.

Tanya Tia, aged 14, shares the pain she experiences in a sickle cell crisis; she 'knows' her pain, she has experienced it before and she knows she will experience it again. This realisation frames her experience and should frame our response to it. How can we possibly ignore pain of the magnitude she describes? How can we not respond and reach out to her, say we believe and will help? Yet in her description of 'reaching', 'grabbing' and 'hesitating to take' her tablets, her cry of pain is framed by her need for us to believe it is real and it is unbelievably bad. Shantell's drawing (Figure 11.1) and the words that accompany it present a strong sense of a world constrained and limited by 'so much' pain and hurt and, to a degree, at odds with her being 11 years old. Her drawing is pared down to the essence of a figure and her words are pared down. Shantell's story evokes a deep sense of sadness, a desire to reach out and break into her world of pain and release her from her hurting. She chooses to use the word 'hurting' to describe her pain and her choice creates a particular resonance and suggests a particular response: a need to comfort and come close, to help and to heal. Hattie's story is different as she does not have the same intimate knowledge of her pain as Tanya Tia and Shantell. One of the things that frightened Hattie about her pain is that she does not know the 'monster', and she was fortunate that her nurses accepted and worked with, rather than dismissed, the monster imagery. Hattie's pain/monster took her to a place she did not understand, one in which she did not know how to respond, and her resolve to be quiet to make the monster go away had an internal logic. The nurse worked with this internal frame of reference and helped her.

The stories that Shantell, Hattie and Tanya Tia tell are ways in which they reach out to us and ask us to care for them. As health professionals, we need to provide children and families with the time, space and support to help to express and communicate their pain. This means that we need to open up the possibility of dialogue so that the children can tell us what their pain is like, how it makes them feel, what it means to them and how we can help. Our actions and response will shape children's immediate and future responses to their pain.

The language(s) of pain

Different philosophical positions exist and existential arguments are presented about the nature of language and pain (Scarry 1985; Herder 2002; Wittgenstein 2009; Ferber 2010). Writers such as Scarry (1985) talk of how language can be broken by pain and that this in turn destroys communication, whereas writers such as Herder (2002) suggest that vocalising pain is a means of reducing it rather than communicating it. Standing apart from theory, both seem to be pragmatically true. However, for most adults and children in pain, these existential arguments and positions are irrelevant: what occupies them is the need to communicate their experience of pain. This can be extraordinarily difficult. However, there are some highly articulate explorations of pain and suffering from people who have experienced and/or are living with pain (e.g., Biro 2010). These first-person narratives can provide astonishingly vivid portraits of what it is to be in pain. However, the difficulty in communicating about pain creates a paradox. Pain is fundamentally something which cannot be easily shared, and yet at the same time it is something that fundamentally *needs* to be shared.

Crying

Even before children have acquired a basic pain vocabulary, they use vocalisations of pain such as crying to communicate their pain. Infants' pain cries are acoustically different to their other cries (e.g., hunger and distress) and pain cries alert caregivers to respond. Other adults such as health professionals can distinguish an infant's pain cry. Work on infants' cries shows that pain cries can be affected by an infant's medical condition and that caregivers' responses can be mediated by factors such as depression (Grunau and Craig 1987; LaGasse et al. 2005; Robb et al. 2011). Many of the infant pain assessment tools such as CRIES (Krechel and Bildner 1995) and FLACC (Merkel et al. 1997) include crying as a component.

  Cries and crying remain a part of the way that we can express pain as children and as adults. The word cry, in the English language, has an active component in that it is associated with the purpose of gaining attention. A 'cry for help' is a means of letting other people know of our pain, suffering or distress, of letting ourselves know of the pain and by vocally externalising it making it less of a threat. However, socialisation tends to mean that crying and the use of utterances such as groans and whimpers become limited to a private rather than a public mode of pain expression. This is true for acute pain, where children soon learn that crying after they have had a minor bump is something that 'only little kids do'. Dubois et al.'s (2008) study found that some children as young as 5 years old exert a form of 'emotional control', preferring silence to crying. Children with chronic pain learn to mask their expression of pain in an attempt to retain their position within friendship groups (Carter 2002). In her story, Tanya Tia tells us that although she cries 'sometimes', 'crying doesn't help'. Tanya Tia's pain takes her to somewhere beyond where crying can help. Scarry (1985) talks of how pain can take us back to a point before language is learned.

Words and utterances

As children start to acquire language, they also start to acquire the capacity to more deliberately describe their pain. This assists parents to respond to their child's pain, teach their child ways to cope and extend their pain vocabulary (Franck et al. 2010).

  In children younger than 18 months old, pain expression is limited using a mix of vocalisations (e.g. 'aargh' or 'ay') or words (e.g., 'ow', 'ouch' and 'oh dear') (Franck et al. 2010) but it is accompanied by behavioural changes and this repertoire means that, with care, parents and health professionals can detect and evaluate the child's pain (Dubois et al. 2008).

  Children's vocalisations develop in alignment with their social and cognitive abilities (Jylli et al. 2006; Dubois et al. 2008). Parents report that their children aged 18–29 months use words such as 'sore', 'hurt', 'poorly' 'bruise' and may be able to link the location of the pain to the pain descriptor (e.g., 'bump head'). The pain language used by children increases in complexity as they get older and they start to use verbs, new descriptors and a more complicated sentence structure. By the age of

2.5–3 years old, children are using 'I' within their pain language (e.g., 'I have an ow') (Franck et al. 2010: 529). By the age of 6 children can use a wider range of words and create more meaningful sentences.

Franck et al. (2010) categorised children's pain words by communicative intent and presented the following categories for 1–6-year-olds:

- Unpleasant sensations: 'got sick', 'yucky' ' 'I've got a sick in my tummy';
- Assistance/treatment requests: vocatives ('mummy I hurt myself); calls for assistance ('make it feel better'); protests ('don't touch it'); specific treatment requests ('I need medicine'); physical comfort ('kiss better');
- Exclamations: 'oh oh', 'oops', 'awww';
- Pain location/visible sign of injury: external ('it's bleeding'); internal ('I've got a nose ache');
- Actions/causes of pain: 'had bump', 'fall down', 'scratching me';
- Reassurances: 'all better'; 'I'm alright', 'I'm brave'.

Wennström and Bergh's (2008: 70) study of the post-operative symptoms of 3–6-year-old boys showed a range of abilities to communicate their pain. Some children were unable to localise their pain but were able to explain 'I feel pain', while some were able to localise their pain 'I have a pain in my willie' and some children spoke of their pain being apart from themselves, 'I'm feeling well but my willie is in pain, it's crying'. It is interesting to note that some children reported that they were 'feeling well' even though they were crying and when asked by the nurse 'why are you crying if you are feeling well?' one child explained 'because my willie is crying'. This little exchange between the nurse and child shows how important it is not to just accept a child's self-report but to see it in the wider context of the other pain cues so as to ensure that the child's pain is well managed. In this same study the boy's pain expression was linked to other factors such as the discovery of a wound 'It's bloody and it hurts'.

Children's pain language reflects many factors, including the type and/or cause of pain (Jylli et al. 2006; Franck et al. 2010), their previous experience of pain and socialisation into a common understanding of frequently used pain words such as pain, ache and hurt (LaFleur and Raway 1999). Jylli et al. (2006) found that with Swedish children aged 6–16 years the words 'terrible', 'aching' and 'sore' were selected more often by children with acute pain (trauma or surgery) than by children with chronic pain (juvenile idiopathic arthritis) and that the older children selected words like 'unbearable' and 'excruciating' to describe their pain. Children with post-operative pain tend to draw on sensory rather than affective words to describe their pain (Jerrett and Evans 1986; Savedra et al. 1993; Jylli et al. 2006). In her story, Tanya Tia uses 'throbbing', 'hammering' and 'crushing' as powerful and graphic sensory words to describe her pain and Hattie talks of 'pulling' as well as using an affective descriptor, 'terrible', to explain how awful her pain made her feel.

Harman et al. (2005: 324) found when children were asked to select words from a list (56 adjectives and adjectival phrases), those with more extensive vocabularies selected fewer words from the list and 'became more careful in their choice of words'. In Franck et al.'s (2010) study the children tended to use words such as 'hurt' and 'poorly' for minor illness-related pain and words like 'ow' 'oh dear' and 'hurt' to describe minor injury-related pain. The words associated with injury emerge before those for illness. Even very young children were reported to 'use language to seek parents' attention and to engage parents in pain relief activities' (Franck et al. 2010: 531).

Figurative expression of pain

Sharing our experience of pain requires us to try to bridge the gap between what we need to say and what we can say. This is difficult in the context of acute pain, and even more evident for people trying to communicate about chronic pain. Biro (2010: 14), talking of why it is important to understand the 'inexpressibility' of (chronic) pain and to generate a 'rhetoric of pain', states that the 'consequences of silence are unacceptable'.

Tanya Tia talks of her legs feeling like a 'cupboard full of sparks' was 'crushed down on them', Shantell's repetition three times of the words 'so much' to describe her 'hurting' and Hattie's description of her 'terrible pain' being 'like a monster' are evocative accounts. The children draw on figurative language such as metaphors and similes in an attempt to both express their pain and impress upon us 'what it is like for them'. Metaphors and other figurative language transpose meaning between the domain of sensation and experience to the domain of symbolic representation (Brodwin 1992).

The use of figurative language is perhaps inevitable, and however evocative the children's descriptions are indirect communications of their pain. Tanya Tia knows that her leg is not actually or literally being crushed by the 'cupboard full of sparks' but out of all the images and descriptions she could have used, this is the description *she* chose to communicate *her* pain *at that time*. No other child will ever experience Tanya Tia's pain or use her specific imagery or feel exactly like she did during that episode of pain. Her description is drawn from her own individual experience. Similarly, even though other children may experience pain as a monster, they will never meet or try to hide from the pain monster that frightened Hattie so much. The use of metaphor helps to fill the void that pain creates and make pain real (Biro 2010). Hattie's, Shantell's and Tanya Tia's descriptions present an uncompromising, albeit indirect, picture of what it felt like to have pain and a plea for us to understand at least something of their experience. It is a plea for us to act. It is a plea for both a human and a professional response.

The indirectness of communication is important to appreciate. Pain exists and then has to be grasped and conceptualised by the person experiencing it before they can choose the words which, for them, come closest to describing it. Scarry (1985: 4) notes pain's resistance to language. The notion of pain being resistant to language is at the heart of many of the difficulties that children and families have in communicating their pain to us and for the problems we face when communicating with them. Much of the problem lies in the fact that the lexicon of pain words in any language is inadequate to sufficiently portray pain experiences. The adjectives available to link with the word pain to describe the type, sensation and affect of pain, for example, are limited. Even when a particular adjective such as 'throbbing' is chosen to describe a pain, it is almost impossible to know what this actually means and what sensation is present. Thus, because the lexicon of words is small, people in pain move quickly on to find other ways of describing their pain through the use of similes or metaphors.

Pain is often personified (e.g., like an animal gnawing) or seen as a weapon (a knife) (Scarry 1985), in terms of weight, colour or agentic descriptions such as a mechanistic description of the body being broken by the pain (Bourke 2012). Pain is therefore described in terms of it being 'like…', 'as if…' or 'as though…'. Tanya Tia does exactly this when she says her pain 'is like poison', 'like someone has hammered my legs until all my bones have been broken' and 'like a cupboard of sparks'. These three images – poison, hammering and sparks - are all used to describe the same pain. She is desperate to make us understand her pain, drawing on different images to ram the message home in different ways. In describing her pain to us, she is also describing her pain to herself; making it real and giving it a presence in the world of words. She brings forth something which we can never fully apprehend and never see (although we can and do see the consequences of pain).

In Tanya Tia's descriptions, the external agents are the poison, the hammer and the cupboard of sparks and the bodily damage is seen as the feeling in her body, the broken bones and the crushing of her leg. The same can be seen with Hattie where the external agent is the monster. Luci, whose story appears elsewhere in the book, describes the pain associated with having her badly grazed knees debrided as if someone had 'got a grater and slit her knee caps off'. In fact for Luci the external agent is so powerful that she entitled her pain story 'The Grater'. As Bourke (2012: 2420) states, 'metaphors do not just describe; they manifest pain'. Viewed from outside the metaphors may seem dramatic, however these metaphors are dramatic because that is their intention.

Without the use of these metaphors, we would have less access to the children's experience. However, the language we use to describe pain does not always perform in an expected manner and it can confuse, mislead and generate unintended meanings.

A visual language of pain

Visual portrayals of pain can help express it in a way that sometimes words cannot do. Historically pain was largely absent within artistic works, although it was evident in Christian iconography of punishment and torture (Hurwitz 2003) and also in the form of images of devils and other agents as causes of pain (Bourke 2012). However, the value of art is increasingly being recognised, particularly within the field of adult chronic pain management, as a way of facilitating people's sense of control, of helping to initiate and improve dialogue between the patient in pain and health professionals (Padfield 2011) and informing and educating health professionals and the public about pain.

For children to be able to effectively communicate about their pain, they need access to language and other modalities and the confidence to use them. In engagement work with children as part of preparation for a study on children's pain literacy, Carter et al. (2013) found that children aged 5–11 years provided richer

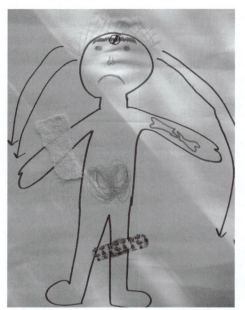
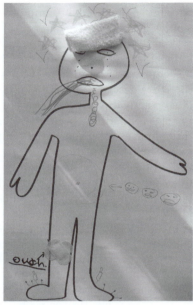
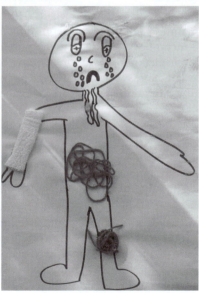

Figures 11.2. a, b, c   Children's collages of their pain

descriptions of the pain they had experienced when they could supplement their verbal description with art work. The children discussed with each other how hard pain was to describe in words but through the use of drawing materials and a range of collage materials (including stickers, glitter, bandages, plasters and lint) they created vibrant representations of their pain that supported their descriptions (see Figure 11.2a, b, and c).

The resulting images are almost at odds with the limited lexicon of words the children initially used. None of these images above suggest pain that could easily be summed up by 'ouch'. Words like 'ouch' – at least to most adult ears – are not inherently powerful. However, if 'ouch' is the only word you have available to use, it is the word you *have* to use to describe the pain when you have 'falled over and got a bump' as well as when you fell from a wall and fractured your arm. As professionals we need to take 'little' words seriously.

Translation

Translation is complex because each sociocultural group and society has a 'set of characteristic idioms' by which people can communicate. Translation of pain words is neither simple nor precise (Migliore 1993) because meanings are culturally, historically and ideologically positioned and influenced by gender, religion and personal experience (Padfield 2011).

The semantics of pain mean words which are readily available and generally understood in one language are either not available or mean something else in another. This is most readily seen when pain assessment tools are translated into other languages (Van Cleve et al. 2001; Collins et al. 2004; Miyamae et al. 2008; Grimm 2011) and especially when the assumption is made that the 'dimensions of pain covered by the source instrument … are transferrable to the target culture' (Strand and Ljunggren 1997: 778). For example, when translating the Paediatric Pain Profile (Hunt et al. 2004) into Brazilian Portuguese, the word 'grimace' could not be easily translated; instead 'makes faces' was the closest phrase that could be translated and used in the tool (Pasin et al. 2012). Translation and interpretation are issues which deserve more attention than can be provided within this chapter and Azize et al. (2011) present a sound overview of the ways in which language and culture can influence a child's expression of pain.

Communicating meanings

Ballantyne (2010: 800) states that clinicians 'tend to work in tangibles' and resort to semi-scientific methods to quantify the components of pain. Health professionals tend to be oriented towards objectivity, to reduce experiences to measurable entities so that they can be more easily charted or documented. This reductionism is perhaps understandable, as it aims to try and structure a subjective experience and to turn it, via a form of shorthand, into something other people will understand. Indeed there is a movement towards the use of standardised pain language to document nursing care so as to create data that will 'identify and monitor trends' (Cavendish 2001: 266) in relation to specific diagnostic groups such as abdominal pain. Although the use of standardisation may have these benefits, the central consideration should be whether the use of standardised language actually assists children to communicate and share their pain. If it does not support communication then it fails as a comprehensive nursing intervention. Toole et al. (2000) propose that children need a list of words to help them describe the quality and severity of their pain. Tools such as the Adolescent Pediatric Pain Tool (Savedra et al. 1993, 1995) use lists of sensory, affective, evaluative and temporal pain descriptors to assess pain intensity. Such lists can facilitate the child to provide a comprehensive description of their pain, although this ultimately depends on the child understanding the words on the list and being able to be selective.

One of the major problems in relation to standardisation lies in the fact that lay people tend to use language in a different way from professionals (Smith 2011). However, studies show that as children (and adults) become more exposed to pain in health care settings they start to adopt the language used by professionals and use 'chart talk' (Skevington 1995; Carter 2002). Barker et al.'s (2009) work focused on the language of adults relating to back pain and they found major differences between the patients' and the professionals' understandings of commonly used words. For example, lay people felt that 'chronic' implied that their 'condition was very severe' or 'constant' and the descriptor 'acute' implied pain was 'severe, in a specific spot or sharp' (Barker et al. 2009: 5). This range of understandings of two of the most commonly used pain-associated words highlights the potential for misunderstanding which can result in patients picking up unnecessarily negative meanings about their pain. Considering the misunderstandings that can occur with words like acute and chronic, professionals need to be aware of the potential challenges for assessments based on standardised lists of word such as 'sharp', 'throbbing', and 'dull'.

Despite the problems inherent in standardisation, standardised lists are, at least, an attempt to move beyond the 'simple' and routine numerical charting of a child's pain intensity which tends to reduce a child's pain to a numerical value while ignoring the experience. Imagine that Shantell, Tanya Tia and Hattie had all scored their pain as 10. All we would know was their pain was awful (the worst possible pain) and that we should do something about it. However, we would not necessarily know what we should do beyond checking a prescription sheet to see what medication we should or could administer. We would not know that Hattie's score of 10 was made up of being too frightened to move because of the pain monster, or that Shantell's score of 10 reflected her legs, shoulders and back 'hurting so much' or that Tanya Tia's score of 10 reflected her pain being 'like poison moving through (her) veins'. The children's words, descriptions and stories tell us so much more. They give us clues about how to nurse and care for these children. Hattie, Shantell and Tanya Tia need our 'nursing presence', our time, our empathy and our skilled technological pharmacological and/or non-pharmacological care and support.

Assigning numerical values to pain is both important and ludicrous. What level of pain on a 0–10 scale equates with having your knees slit off with a grater? How can we expect Tanya Tia to rationally choose a score to reflect the pain of having poison in her body? We absolutely have to listen to children's pain descriptions. We cannot ignore the language that children use. If we do ignore their language, we are ignoring their pain. Wilson et al. (2009: 56) suggest that 'personalized pain descriptors may communicate the pain experience more appropriately' than standardised tools such as the McGill Pain Questionnaire.

Conclusion

Bourke (2012: 2421) talks of the need to pay 'careful attention to the languages of pain' and the ways in which people express their pain through words, images, art, gestures, ritual, utterances, symbols, and performance. Verbal language is both an enormously powerful and an extremely limited tool for communicating pain. It is powerful because it allows children and their families to give voice to the physical, emotional, social and psychological aspects of their pain, and it is limited because words are often insufficient to portray what it is to be in pain. In many situations where a child is trying to convey their pain, they will turn to other experiences or situations that they can use to explain what their pain is like. In her pain story, Tanya Tia explained that 'the littlest movements in my legs feel like someone has hammered my legs until all my bones have been broken'. Her descriptions evoke a response in us, her images convey to us the horror and depth of her pain. Tanya Tia's description of her pain is shocking and real, and her story and the stories of the children we care for cry out for us to understand and care and respond. Anything less than this is indefensible.

Key Points

- Pain can be expressed in many ways.
- Pain is fundamentally something which cannot be easily shared and yet, at the same time it is something that fundamentally *needs* to be shared.
- Cries and crying are part of the way that children and adults can express pain.
- As children start to acquire language, they also start to acquire the capacity to more deliberately describe their pain and often figurative language to express their experience.
- A child's self-report needs to be seen in the wider context of the other pain cues so as to ensure that the child's pain is well managed.
- As professionals we need to take 'little' words seriously.
- Pain is often reduced to a measurable entity – a numerical score – that can be easily documented but this ignores so much of the child's experience.
- Children, young people and their families may use pain language in a different way to professionals.

Additional Resources and Reading

- Visual portrayals of pain provide one means of both expressing and trying to understand pain.
  - Kahlo's images are seen as iconic pain images www.fridakahlo.com/
  - An online exhibition of the work of artists with chronic pain: http://painexhibit.org/
- Further reading about children's acquisition of language:
  - Saxton, M. (2010) *Child Language: Acquisition and Development*, 1st edn. London: Sage.
- A beautiful book by a practising physician whose pain journey started when he was a young doctor:
  - Biro, D. (2010) *The Language of Pain: Finding Words, Compassion, and Relief*. New York: W.W. Norton & Co.
- The British Sign Language (BSL) sign for 'hurt' and a hurt arm and stomach ache can be found at:
  - www.signbsl.com/sign/hurt
- In American Sign Language, the sign is slightly different:
  - http://lifeprint.com/asl101/pages-signs/h/hurt.htm

References

Azize, P.M., Humphreys, A. and Cattani, A. (2011) 'The impact of language on the expression and assessment of pain in children', *Intensive and Critical Care Nursing*, 27 (5): 235–43.

Ballantyne, J.C. (2010) 'Talking pain: review of *The Language of Pain: Finding Words, Compassion, Relief*', *Pain Medicine*, 11 (5): 800.

Barker, K.L., Reid, M. and Minns Lowe, C.J. (2009) 'Divided by a lack of common language? A qualitative study exploring the use of language by health professionals treating back pain', *BMC Musculoskeletal Disorders*, 10: 123.

Biro, D. (2010) *The Language of Pain: Finding Words, Compassion, and Relief*. New York: W.W. Norton & Co.

Bourke, J. (2012) 'Languages of pain', *The Lancet*, 379 (9835): 2420–1.

Brodwin, P.E. (1992) 'Symptoms and social performances: the case of Diane Reden', in M.J. DelVecchio Good, P.E. Brodwin, B.J. Good and A. Kleinman (eds), *Pain as Human Experience: An Anthropological Perspective*. Berkeley, CA: University of California Press, pp. 77–99.

Carter, B. (2002) 'Chronic pain in childhood and the medical encounter: professional ventriloquism and hidden voices', *Qualitative Health Research*, 12 (1): 28–41.

Carter, B., Bray, L., Simons, J. and Satchwell, C. (2013) 'Engaging children in designing a study about children's pain. (Poster)', *Making a Difference for Children and Families*, Children's Nursing Research Unit Conference, Liverpool, UK, 7 May, p. 1.

Cavendish, R. (2001) 'The use of standardized language to describe abdominal pain', *Journal of School Nursing*, 17 (5): 266–73.

Collins, A.S., Gullette, D. and Schnepf, M. (2004) 'Break through language barriers: is your pain assessment lost in translation?', *Nursing Management*, 35 (8): 34.

Dubois, A., Bringuier, S., Capdevilla, X. and Pry, R. (2008) 'Vocal and verbal expression of postoperative pain in preschoolers', *Pain Management Nursing*, 9 (4): 160–5.

Ferber, I. (2010) 'Herder: on pain and the origin of language', *Germanic Review*, 85 (3): 205–23.

Franck, L., Noble, G. and Liossi, C. (2010) 'From tears to words: the development of language to express pain in young children with everyday minor illnesses and injuries', *Child: Care, Health & Development*, 36 (4): 524–33.

Grimm, G.S. (2011) '[The German version of parents' postoperative pain measure (PPPM-D). Validation on children 2–12 years old]', *Schmerz (Berlin, Germany)*, 25 (5): 534.

Grunau, R.V. and Craig, K.D. (1987) 'Pain expression in neonates: facial action and cry', *Pain*, 28 (3): 395–410.

Harman, K., Lindsay, S., Adewami, A. and Smith, P. (2005) 'An investigation of language used by children to describe discomfort expected and experienced during dental treatment', *International Journal of Paediatric Dentistry*, 15 (5): 319–26.

Herder, J.G. (2002) *Philosophical Writings*. Cambridge: Cambridge University Press.

Hunt, A., Goldman, A., Seers, K., Crichton, N., Mastroyannopoulou, K., Moffat, V., Oulton, K. and Brady, M. (2004) 'Clinical validation of the paediatric pain profile', *Developmental Medicine & Child Neurology*, 46 (1): 9–18.

Hurwitz, B. (2003) 'Looking at pain', in D. Padfield (ed.), *Perceptions of Pain*. Stockport: Dewi Lewis Publishing, pp. 7–13.

Jerrett, M. and Evans, K. (1986) 'Children's pain vocabulary', *Journal of Advanced Nursing*, 11 (4): 403–8.

Jylli, L., Broström, E., Hagelberg, S., Stenström, C.H., Olsson, G.L. and Langius-Eklöf, A. (2006) 'Sensory and affective components of pain as recorded with the Pain-O-Meter (POM) among children with acute and chronic pain', *Acta Paediatrica*, 95 (11): 1429–34.

Krechel, S.W. and Bildner, J. (1995) 'Cries – a new neonatal postoperative pain measurement score – initial testing of validity and reliability', *Paediatric Anaesthesia*, 5 (1): 53–61.

LaFleur, C.J. and Raway, B. (1999) 'School-age child and adolescent perception of the pain intensity associated with three word descriptors', *Pediatric Nursing*, 25 (1): 45.

LaGasse, L.L., Neal, A.R. and Lester, B.M. (2005) 'Assessment of infant cry: acoustic cry analysis and parental perception', *Mental Retardation and Developmental Disabilities Research Reviews*, 11 (1): 83–93.

Merkel, S.I., Voepel-Lewis, T., Shayevitz, J.R. and Malviya, S. (1997) 'The FLACC: a behavioral scale for scoring postoperative pain in young children', *Pediatric Nursing*, 23 (3): 293–7.

Migliore, S. (1993) '"NERVES": the role of metaphor in the cultural framing of experience', *Journal of Contemporary Ethnography*, 22 (3): 331–60.

Miyamae, T., Nemoto, A., Imagawa, T., Ohshige, K., Mori, M., Nishimaki, S. and Yokota, S. (2008) 'Cross-cultural adaptation and validation of the Japanese version of the Childhood Health Assessment Questionnaire (CHAQ)', *Modern Rheumatology*, 18 (4): 336–43.

Padfield, D. (2011) '"Representing" the pain of others', *Health*, 15 (3): 241–57.

Pasin, S., Avila, F., de Cavata, T., Hunt, A. and Heldt, E. (2012) 'Cross-cultural translation and adaptation to Brazilian Portuguese version of the paediatric pain profile in children with severe cerebral palsy', *Journal of Pain and Symptom Management*, 45 (1): 120–128.

Robb, M.P., Sinton-White, H. and Kaipa, R. (2011) 'Acoustic estimates of respiration in the pain cries of newborns',*International Journal of Pediatric Otorhinolaryngology*, 75(10: 1265–1270.

Savedra, M.C., Tesler, M.D., Holzemer, W.L. and Brokaw, P. (1995) 'A strategy to assess the temporal dimension of pain in children and adolescents', *Nursing Research*, 44 (5): 272–6.

Savedra, M.C., Holzemer, W.L., Tesler, M.D. and Wilkie, D.J. (1993) 'Assessment of postoperation pain in children and adolescents using the adolescent pediatric pain tool', *Nursing Research*, 42 (1): 5–9.

Scarry, E. (1985) *The Body in Pain. The Making and Unmaking of the World*. New York: Oxford University Press.

Skevington, S.M. (1995) *Psychology of Pain*. Chichester: Wiley .

Smith, C.A. (2011) 'Consumer language, patient language, and thesauri: a review of the literature', *Journal of the Medical Library Association*, 99 (2): 135–44.

Strand, L.I. and Ljunggren, A.E. (1997) 'Different approximations of the McGill Pain Questionnaire in the Norwegian language: a discussion of content validity', *Journal of Advanced Nursing*, 26 (4): 772–9.

Toole, R.J., Lindsay, S.J., Johnstone, S. and Smith, P. (2000) 'An investigation of language used by children to describe discomfort during dental pulp-testing', *International Journal of Paediatric Dentistry*, 10 (3): 221–8.

Van Cleve, L., Muñoz, C., Bossert, E.A. and Savedra, M.C. (2001) 'Children's and adolescents' pain language in Spanish: translation of a measure', *Pain Management Nursing*, 2 (3): 110–18.

Wennstrom, B. and Bergh, I. (2008) 'Bodily and verbal expressions of postoperative symptoms in 3- to 6-year-old boys', *Journal of Pediatric Nursing*, 23 (1): 65–76.

Wilson, D., Williams, M. and Butler, D. (2009) 'Language and the pain experience', *Physiotherapy Research International*, 14 (1): 56–65.

Wittgenstein, L. (2009) *Philosophical Investigations*, 4th edn. Oxford: Wiley Blackwell.

Chapter 12

Minor Injury, Acute Pain, Wounds and What Really Hurts

Luci's Story

Luci's story

The grater

It all started on the same bridge that I walk to school on every day and back at 8:30 and 3:00. Me and my friend Loretta were riding double on the scooter across the flat part of the bridge when we hit a rock. I was standing up by that time! On the other hand Loretta was not and went flying down on the bridge. I couldn't let her go, so I raced after her and cartwheeled over the handle bars.

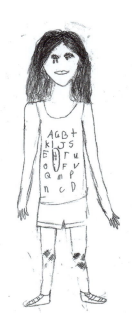

The pain was not there with me until the Dettol came out. I felt like someone had got a grater and slit my knee caps off. When Katie (my sister) got home I was just about in agony! She said I was like Bella from *Twilight* when she got bitten. By the time mum got home with the bandages etc. I was sitting on the couch crying while watching TV.

The worse mistake I made was to let mum put bandages on my leg, the next four days I spent trying to rip off the bandages, it was like trying to rip something off that was stuck on to your leg like a leech. In the end dad took me to the nurse to get it ripped off, the pain was excruciating. Then I had to start again!

PS: Don't let mums put things on your legs, only if the doctor gave it to you!!

By Luci McDougall, aged 10 years

Introduction

Luci's story resonates. It resonates with the excitement of her scooter ride, her friendship with Loretta, the drama of the accident about to happen and the inevitability of her cartwheel over the handlebars. We have to assume that she actually landed from her dramatic cartwheel as her story skips the element that we might reasonably assume is important – the actual injury. However, Lucy feels no need to tell us the pragmatic details of what exactly happened as she moves onto elements of the story that she wants to tell us about: the episodes with the Dettol and the removal of the bandages. Luci's story is dramatic, packed full of warnings and advice, and is probably fairly typical of many minor injuries that children experience. It is interesting to note that even though the fall must have been painful and we can see from her drawing that her knees seem to have borne the brunt of the damage she does not provide any detail about the pain of the injury itself. She says 'the pain was not there till …' At age 10, Luci's story stands as a warning for us to manage the pain associated with injury and wound care as conscientiously and compassionately as possible.

In this chapter we will explore the acute pain associated with minor injuries and why some aspects of treatment can be more noxious than the injury itself. In particular, the pain associated with wound management is explored and suggestions are presented for how good nursing care – including teaching parents about how to care for minor wounds – can help mitigate pain.

Minor injuries and the risks associated with physical activity

Unintentional injuries (accidents) happen. Thinking back to our own childhoods most of us will remember the bumps, bruises, abrasions and grazes that were part and parcel of exploring and interacting with our environment and developing new skills. Most of these episodes were over and done with quickly. Generally all that we needed to help us over the hurt, surprise and distress of the injury was some reassurance that we would be fine and a cuddle from mum or dad.

We tend only to remember the more dramatic events as they create more of an impression and also perhaps a good story. When I was a little girl of around 5 or 6, I fell over while running downhill after my older cousins, landed badly, and ended up falling onto some sharp flinty rock. The ensuing screams from my cousins added to my fright and, worst of all, I realised that Sarah was bleeding. I was distraught and ran back to my parents for help. The right side of my face was covered in blood. As I was frantically trying to get help for Sarah my parents were trying to work out how badly I was hurt. Although my face was sore, it did not really hurt much at the time. I was just very worried for Sarah who was covered in blood. My mum had the sense to 'make Sarah better, before starting to clean my wound'. As it became obvious to me that Sarah – my much-loved doll – was okay, I calmed down. It was only later on that the injury felt really sore. I have two abiding memories: the palpable sense of relief that Sarah was not going to die and how itchy the scabs were as the abrasion healed.

Children have particular risk factors for injury which reflect their developmental stage (e.g., developing coordination and immature risk assessment skills) (Sundblad et al. 2005). This means that they experience many episodes of falls and scrapes as they are growing up. The exact incidence rate of minor injuries in childhood is not clear (Sundblad et al. 2005). Many minor injuries either do not require professional attention or only require modest professional intervention. Luci's actual injury did not require professional intervention. Help was only sought in relation to the dressing. The most robust statistics are collated through hospital-based studies (Hedström et al. 2012) and for many injuries the child does not present at hospital and they are treated by their parents (Boddy and Smith 2008; Howard and Houghton 2012), or by teachers and coaches (Sundblad et al. 2005) who often have no specialist knowledge of wounds, healing or management. Although these injuries are deemed to be at the minor end of the injury continuum and are not a threat to life, they can be painful and distressing for the child and their parents. The ubiquity of minor injuries makes it important that they are not overlooked. Singer et al.'s (2004) study of 654 parents showed that most did not have knowledge about the management of minors wounds and burns, whereas Kendrick and Marsh's (1999) earlier study found that parents felt they knew what to do but were not confident about using that knowledge.

Yet, despite the fact that many injuries are treated at home, around a fifth of children in the UK (approximately 2.3 million children) present at an emergency department with an injury; many of these injuries are wounds or soft tissue injuries (Davies et al. 2003). Hedström et al.'s (2012) study of injury-related visits to an emergency department showed that play (37 per cent) was the most common activity and contusions (24 per cent) and open wound/abrasions (21 per cent) were the two most common types of presenting injury. In Jones and Hammig's (2012) study, soft tissue injuries (contusions, abrasions, haematomas, and strains or sprains) accounted for the majority (57 per cent) of injuries reported. Although physical activity brings risks in terms of activity-related injury, research by Bloemers et al. (2012) shows that physical inactivity itself is a risk factor for physical activity-related injuries in children. The benefits of participation in sports and other physical activities such as a sense of well-being and self-esteem, fun and enjoyment (Verhagen et al. 2009; Collard et al. 2011) almost always will outweigh the consequences of minor injuries especially since: 'physical inactivity is now identified as the fourth leading risk factor for global mortality' (World Health Organization 2010).

Abrasions

Abrasions (or grazes) often seem to be fairly innocuous; they are a commonplace and not overtly dramatic injury but they are often very painful. Children most frequently acquire abrasions from falling and sliding, for example from a fall while they are running or from falling off a bicycle or, in Luci's case, from her scooter. This often means that the wound is dirty with mud, dirt, gravel or other matter. Relative to the size of the child, grazes can cover quite a large surface area and the lower limbs and hands are often sites which children abrade. Areas such as the knee are particularly prone to abrasions and the positioning of the wound over a joint means that this can add to the pain experienced. Most abrasions are superficial, acute wounds in which the protective epidermal layer of the skin has been abraded, exposing nerve endings and which initially leak serous fluid. Some abrasions involve damage to the deeper layers of the skin and while most do not bleed very much, those on the face and head can bleed profusely. Apart from the initial trauma and distress associated with the injury and the potential pain while the wound is healing, abrasions usually cause few problems unless they become infected.

Why wounds hurt

Nociceptive or acute pain is a time-limited, inflammatory response to tissue damage which means that pain reduces as the wound heals, the tissues regenerate and the inflammatory response reduces. Chronic pain, which can be experienced in relation to some wounds, shares some of the mechanisms associated with acute pain but the pathophysiology involves the alteration of pain transmission pathways

Tissue damage, such as Luci's abrasions, initiates nociception. Nociception is the 'neural process of encoding and processing noxious stimuli' and noxious stimuli are 'damaging or potentially damaging stimuli including extremes of temperature, mechanical stimulation, and allogens that provoke an avoidance response' (Dubin and Patapoutian 2010: 3671). Nociception commences with the activation of the primary afferent nociceptors which are widespread in the skin, muscle, connective tissues, blood vessels and viscera (Hudspith et al. 2006). Release of pain and inflammatory mediators such as bradykinin, histamine and prostaglandins provokes transmission of nerve impulses to the dorsal horn of the spinal column and then through to the brainstem, thalamus and the cerebral cortex where the perception of pain occurs. Cutaneous pain is usually sharp and well localised to the area of stimulation (Hudspith et al. 2006). Gate control theory proposes that the 'pain gate' can be closed by the activation of competing signals such as by the stimulation of large diameter (non-pain transmitting) fibres. Anti-inflammatory cytokines also create competition. As Richardson and Upton (2010: 426) note 'it is the balance of all of these different components in generation and transmission that ultimately defines whether or not the individual experiences pain, and if so how much'.

Pain is composed of sensory, cognitive and affective dimensions. The affective dimension has two components: pain unpleasantness which is 'often, although not always, closely linked to the intensity of the painful sensation' and 'secondary pain affect' which includes 'emotional feelings directed toward long-term implications of having pain (e.g., 'suffering')' (Price 2000: 1769).

Luci's pain was compounded by the distress she experienced when her wound was cleaned with the Dettol (she recalls that it felt like someone 'had got a grater and slit my knee caps off') and when her dressings were being removed. Lucy tells us in her story that it was like 'trying to rip something off that was stuck on to your leg like a leech'. In the final paragraph she uses the word 'rip' or 'ripping' several times as she tries to convey the horror of her experience. Her memory of the pain will have an effect on the way that she thinks about, prepares and copes with dressing changes in the future. Looking at her drawing, there are at least five separate grazed areas, each of which may have been dressed separately. If this were the case, Luci has to cope with the removal, cleansing and redressing five times on each occasion, which is possibly what she is referring to when she exclaims 'Then I had to start again!'

Bowers and Barrett (2009: 55) note that 'any technique that features physical contact with the wound has the potential to cause pain'. A range of different factors can be actual or potential causes of wound pain including wound care procedures, wound care products, peri-wound skin integrity, the treatments used, the emotional and social aspects related to the wound, associated disease processes and professional factors (e.g., attitudes, knowledge, skills and communication) (Hollinworth 2005).

Findings from a survey of practitioners from 11 European countries about their primary considerations in relation to dressing changes show that prevention of trauma was ranked as the most important factor and pain prevention was the next most highly ranked (Moffatt et al. 2002). The perceived painfulness of wounds was ranked as follows (from most to least painful): leg ulcers, superficial burns, infected: wounds, pressure ulcers, cuts and abrasions, paediatric wounds, cavity wounds and fungating wounds. The fact that 'paediatric wounds' appears as a particular category when children can and do present with all of the other types of wounds is bizarre, and the fact that their wounds are perceived as being at the less painful end of the ranking reflects a worrying lack of insight and understanding of children's perception of pain and wound care.

Wound management and wound-related pain

The process of wound healing is dynamic (Zaman et al. 2011) and dependent on various factors such as the nature of the injury, pain, absence or presence of infection, health and nutritional status of the child, the general integrity of the skin and the management of the wound itself.

Wound management can be a painful and distressing aspect of a child's care, and compared to other causes of procedural pain such as needle-related pain, much less is known about wound-related pain. This is perhaps surprising as Nilsson et al. (2011) point out that wound dressings generally take a longer time to perform and generate more distress than needle-related procedures. Children are not a special case in terms of finding wound dressings painful and distressing; adults find wound dressing to be (one of the) most painful aspects of having a wound (Hollinworth and Collier 2000).

McCord and Levy (2006) note that much of the evidence base draws on studies on adult populations, and while key elements are transferrable there are some aspects of children's pathophysiology such as skin absorption, metabolism of drugs, healing processes and responses to adhesive products that are sufficiently different to make some aspects of current practice questionable. Practitioners are therefore forced to 'compromise by using wound care products not approved for children' (Ciprandi et al. 2012). Apart from a fairly robust literature on paediatric burns management, there is a surprisingly small literature base to underpin the professional management of children's wounds, despite the fact that 'children are potentially more sensitive and vulnerable to the effects of dressings and greater care must be taken when choosing treatment regimens to manage their wounds' (Meuleneire 2009: 12).

There is almost no research literature that focuses on how parents should manage their children's minor injuries and day-to-day wounds. The most useful literature that parents can access either comes from health care organisations or from commercial companies that manufacture dressings and bandages.

Types of dressings and their effect on pain

Traditionally wound dressings were applied simply to protect the wound bed and their success at doing this was variable. However, much more is both expected and required of contemporary wound dressings. Current dressings aim to 'positively influence the wound environment' (Rippon et al. 2012: 539). Ideal wound dressings have to serve a number of different functions (Thomas 2008). While this perhaps appears complicated, in essence a dressing needs to protect the wound and the peri-wound area from damage, infection and drying out, not irritate the wound or peri-wound skin and be easily removable so that wound healing is not disrupted. One of the previously overlooked issues with wound care and managing wound-related pain was removal of the dressing. Many dressings are secured through the use of adhesives and adhesive tapes; skin stripping or damage to the superficial stratum corneum can occur when these adhesives and adhesive tapes are removed. Denyer (2011: S30) notes that this can lead to 'pain and anticipatory fear'. While Luci's dressing may have provided adequate protection to the wound bed, it was certainly not ideal from her perspective in terms of ease of removal.

Choosing the right dressing requires a knowledgeable practitioner who is able to consider a range of factors including formation of a bacterial barrier, maintenance of wound hydration and optimal wound pH, peri-wound skin protection, and minimisation of pain during application and removal. Dressing-related tissue trauma caused, for example, by the removal of adhesives and tapes and the dressing can result in the patient experiencing more pain, the size of the wound increasing and wound healing being delayed (Cutting 2008).

Although Luci was clearly unimpressed by her mother's first aid techniques or by the problems associated with dressing removal, children commonly prefer wounds to be covered up with a dressing. Having recovered from the fright of an injury or wound, young children will often seek out the comfort of having the wound covered

Table 12.1 Overview of Richardson and Upton's (2010) ten mechanisms underpinning the analgesic effects of dressings

Mechanisms	Brief rationale
Out of sight, out of mind	Reduction of visual stimulus may reduce stress and enhance inhibitory pain pathways.
Dressing as a protector	Physical protection of the wound protects the exposed nerve endings which in turn reduces the triggering of nociceptors.
Moist environment: bathing of nociceptors	The fluid bathing the nociceptor nerve endings may provide an additional protective layer.
Moist environment: control of inflammation and hyperalgesia	Promotion of an environment which facilitates healing and the reduction of inflammation can promote the reduction of pain.
Moist environment: recruitment of analgesic compounds to the wound area	Promotion of an environment which facilitates the recruitment of analgesic compounds (leucocytes and anti-inflammatory cytokines).
Temperature change – generating heat or cooling effects	Dependent on the type of dressing used, the skin temperature around the wound may be increased or decreased and this may be analgesic.
Counter-irritation	Application of a dressing may stimulate the large diameter nerve fibres which could in turn close the pain gates thus reducing pain perception.
Removal of irritant exudate	Some wound exudate can be an irritant, stimulating the local nociceptors, so dressings which reduce exudate irritation may be analgesic.
Sequestration of pro-inflammatory cytokines	Some dressings have been designed to sequester the cytokines which stimulate the inflammatory response.
Direct influence of the dressing material	There is some albeit conflicting evidence suggesting that the dressing material itself (e.g. silicone) may have a direct analgesic effect.

and many manufacturers create colourful plasters which children can 'wear'. Nilsson et al.'s study (2011) noted that children liked to be in control of choosing whether a red or a blue colour plaster was applied. Children, like adults, gain a sense of reassurance from having a wound covered; the removal of the visual stimulus of the damage to the child's body may reduce stress and fear, and in turn also enhance inhibition pathways. Richardson and Upton (2010: 427) refer to this as 'out of sight, out of mind', and they discuss a total of ten mechanisms underpinning why dressings may have an analgesic effect (see Table 12.1), although most of these are only partially understood.

Thomas (2003: 1) identifies two key issues in choice of dressing and subsequent removal: adhesion ('describes the interaction that takes place between the dressing and the intact peri-wound skin') and adherence ('describes the interaction between a dressing and the wound'). Both adhesion and adherence are important in trying to choose a dressing that will have minimal pain and physical and psychological trauma for the child.

Reducing the pain associated with wound management and dressing

Hollinworth (2005) advocates six steps should be adopted when dressing a wound: warming the cleansing solution, removing dressings carefully, using time-out to allow the patient to cope, using atraumatic dressings, applying and removing dressings and bandages correctly, and managing the frequency of dressing changes. These can be adapted for use with children and certainly would have been helpful for Luci.

Preparation and assessment

The child should be informed and appropriately prepared for their wound dressing. This may involve establishing a rapport with the child, careful explanation of what will happen and establishing how the child wants to be involved and what strategies they will use to help avert fear, distress and pain. Nilsson et al. (2011: 1455) note that 'children need to experience security and participation in wound care'. Upton (2009) presents a transactional model to help explain the way in which adults with chronic wounds undertake a primary appraisal (whether the dressing change will be painful/worrying) and a secondary appraisal (whether they feel they can cope with any pain/worry associated with the dressing change). Similar processes are likely to occur in relation to dressing change (and other painful procedures) for children (see Figure 12.1). Understanding such appraisal processes provides nurses with insight into how to try and intervene and promote coping skills and resilience.

One of the key aspects of preparing a child for a dressing change, as with any procedure that might cause pain, is the need for the nurse to be aware of the child's previous experience of the actual or similar procedure, their response and how they coped. Individualising a child's care is essential. Preparation involves considering each step of the process and trying to identify ways in which the child can be protected from pain and/or supported to cope with pain.

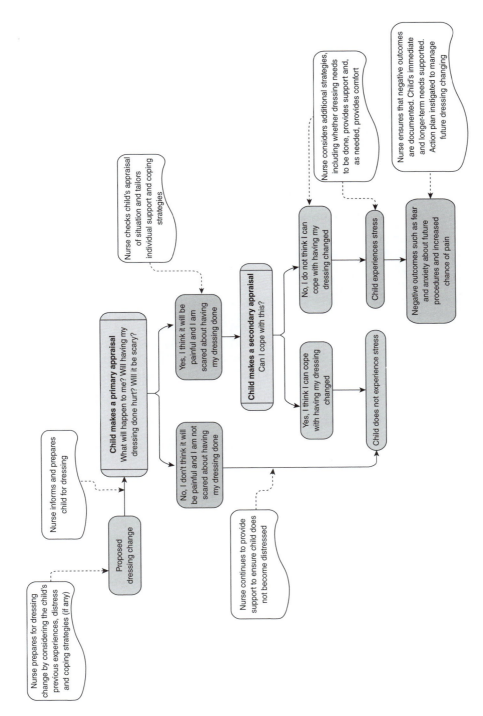

Figure 12.1 Proposed primary and secondary appraisal mechanisms

Pain should be assessed before, during and after the procedure using a validated pain assessment tool that is appropriate to the child; in most cases this choice reflects the child's chronological age (see Table 12.2). Where the child is able to self-report this is the best approach as this facilitates an understanding of their perspective and experience. However, a reliance on chronological age as the sole indicator of a child's capacity to self-report will inevitably generate both false positives and false negatives (APA 2012). Observational measures or tools for assessing pain in children who are cognitively impaired such as Non-Communicating Children's Pain Checklist-Revised (NCCPC-R) or the Paediatric Pain Profile (PPP) are valuable when self-report is not possible (see Table 12.2).

Table 12.2   Recommended measures for procedural and post-operative pain assessment

For children without cognitive impairment (and based on the child's chronological age)	
Child's age	**Measure**
Newborn–3 years	• In this age group, observational measures are indicated: COMFORT (Ambuel et al. 1992; van Dijk et al. 2000; Caljouw et al. 2007); FLACC (Face, Legs, Arms, Cry, and Consolability) (Merkel et al. 1997; Voepel-Lewis et al. 2002, 2003; Manworren and Hynan 2003; Nilsson et al. 2008)
4 years	• FPS-R (Faces Pain Scale-Revised) (Hicks et al. 2001) + COMFORT or FLACC
5–7 years	• FPS-R
7 years +	• Visual analogue scales or Numerical rating scales or FPS-R

For children with cognitive impairment (and based on the child's chronological age)	
Child's age	**Measure**
3–18 years	• NCCPC-R (Non-Communicating Children's Pain Checklist-Revised) (Breau et al. 2000, 2001); NCCPC-PV Non-Communicating Children's Pain Checklist-Postoperative Version) (Breau et al. 2002); Revised FLACC (Malviya et al. 2006)
1–18 years	• PPP (Paediatric Pain Profile) (Hunt et al. 2004, 2007; Pasin et al. 2013)

Developed from APA (2012: 12–13)

Removing the dressing, cleaning the wound and replacing the dressing

Like Luci, many children fear the removal of the sticky tape and plaster because this is the point at which the damaged area is both physically and psychologically exposed; this potentially increases pain, stress and anticipatory fear as it is no longer 'out of sight and out of mind' (Richardson and Upton 2010). Nilsson et al.'s (2011: 1453) study of children aged 5–10 undergoing a trauma wound dressing reports on how the children recognised and valued the clinical competence of the nurse, saying, for example, 'when the bandage was caught the nurse did not just pull, she used the salve'.

Adhesive removers fall into three main categories: alcohol/organic-based solvents, oil-based solvents, and silicone-based removers. While the first two categories of remover can be problematic, the silicone-based removers have many positive attributes as they are gentle, do not dry the skin out, do not leave a residue, do not sting, are inert, cannot be metabolised and are available in different forms (Cutting 2008). Correct technique should be used when removing the adhesive dressing (e.g., vapour permeable dressings should not be pulled off but should be gently stretched parallel to the skin to break the adhesive bond). Denyer's (2011: S34–5) case study of a 10-year-old boy with mild dominant dystrophic epidermolysis bullosa talks of how introducing a silicone medical adhesive remover (SMAR) to painlessly, atraumatically and safely remove the 'everyday plasters' he preferred to use, rather than the more expensive dressings he was prescribed, meant pain-free dressing changes, less distress, less anticipatory fear and less expense.

One of the most painful elements of Luci's experience was having her grazes cleaned with Dettol and debrided (or using her terminology 'grated'). While her mother's intention in using Dettol to clean the wound was meant well it would have been intensely painful. Less irritant cleansing agents mean that this element of wound-related pain can be avoided. Debridement of wounds is often necessary, and unless non-pharmacological and/or pharmacological strategies are used this can be very painful.

Following assessment of the wound and any wound-related pain, the nurse needs to make a careful and considered decision about which is the best dressing to use when re-covering the wound. The decisions made at this point in time are important as they will impact on the healing rate and the amount of wound pain experienced between now and the next dressing change, and will also impact on the child's ability to cope with the next and future dressing changes.

Pharmacological and non-pharmacological strategies to reduce wound pain

It is not clear from Luci's story whether or not she received any pharmacological intervention for her pain, which she describes as 'agony'. It would appear that when her pain was bad, even distraction was not really helping her: she recalls 'sitting on the couch crying while watching TV'.

Although there is little research that specifically focuses on the use of analgesics in the management of pain during a dressing change, pharmacological strategies are an important element in the management of dressing-related wound pain (Nilsson and Renning 2012). However, many non-pharmacological strategies can be used and there is now increasing evidence to underpin their use. Often a best practice approach will see the use of non-pharmacological and pharmacological strategies used together to reduce children's wound-related dressing pain. The strategies chosen depend on factors including the nature of the wound (acute, chronic, minor, major) and the setting in which the dressing is to be undertaken (inpatient, outpatient, emergency department, walk-in centre).

Pharmacological approaches to wound pain management often build on the best evidence in relation to procedural pain management. However, the quality, intensity and duration of pain experienced in relation to dressing-related wound pain are likely to be different from that experienced during needle-related procedures (e.g. cannulation). As with procedural pain, drugs can be used either singly or in combination to good effect. Local anaesthetics such as topical lidocaine adrenaline tetracaine (LAT gel) have good evidence to underpin their use in the repair of lacerations (Eidelman et al. 2011; APA 2012). Non-steroidal anti-inflammatory drugs (such as ibuprofen) and paracetamol can be used to manage mild to moderate pain but need to be administered sufficiently well in advance of the dressing change in order to be effective. Nitrous oxide and oxygen provide rapid onset analgesia (Bruce and Franck 2000) and reduce pain and anxiety during laceration repair (APA 2012). Some children may require opioids to be administered to manage the pain associated with dressing changes. Recommendations within recent good practice guidelines propose that 'potent opioid analgesia given by oral, transmucosal, or nasal routes according to patient preference and availability of suitable preparations should be considered for dressing changes in burned children' (APA 2012: 26).

Non-pharmacological approaches used within procedural pain can be used to help manage a child's dressing-related pain; many of these are based on distraction techniques. Nilsson et al.'s (2011) recent work shows evidence of the effectiveness of both gaming and flavoured lollipops on managing children's pain and distress during wound dressings. Multi-modal sensory-based distraction technology devices have performed well in managing the pain associated with burns dressing when compared with other distraction techniques such as bubbles, television or a PlayStation Portable (Miller et al. 2011). Virtual reality which allows the child to become immersed in a computer-simulated, three-dimensional environment has shown potential in reducing wound-related pain (Van Twillert et al. 2007; Malloy and Milling 2010; Kipping et al. 2012;).

Conclusion

At first it might seem that there is not too much to learn from Luci's story. She was out playing on her scooter, fell off and grazed her knees. However, the emphasis on the story is on how her grazes were managed and her story provides a stern warning for children to be cautious about what they should let their mothers do. However, it could equally stand as a warning for health care professionals.

The key lessons are there for us to take with us to every episode of wound care we are involved in. Wounds and dressings can be painful and we need to think ahead to consider the consequences of any wound-related decisions we make. Choosing the ideal dressing is a complex but important task. Thinking about pain relief is vital at every stage of wound management and it is important that we draw on relevant pain-management strategies to help prevent pain from occurring.

Clinical competency is important as is a holistic approach to the way we care for children, regardless of whether we are dealing with grazed knees or much more significant and long-term wound management.

Key Points

- Pain is composed of sensory, cognitive and affective dimensions.
- Children have particular developmental risk factors for injury.
- Abrasions are a commonplace and often very painful injury.
- Nociceptive pain is a time-limited, inflammatory response to tissue damage.
- Wound management can be a painful and distressing aspect of a child's care.
- Many different factors can be a actual or potential causes of wound pain.
- Children gain a sense of reassurance from having a wound covered but often fear the removal the 'sticky tape' and dressing.
- The child should be informed and appropriately prepared for their wound dressing and the nurse should promote the child's coping skills and resillience.
- Pharamacological and non-pharamacological approaches can be used to help manage a child's dressing-related pain.

Additional Resources and Reading

- For more information about management of minor injuries:
  - Davies, F., Bruce, C.E. and Taylor-Robinson, K.J. (2011) *Emergency Care of Minor Trauma in Children: A Practical Handbook*. London: Hodder & Stoughton Ltd.
- Modules on wound management:
  - www.globalwoundacademy.com/en-GB/
- Non-commercial information about the management of cuts and grazes can be found at:
  - www.nhsinform.co.uk/health-library/articles/c/cuts-and-grazes/treatment
- Wound dressing companies have specific education modules and information for health professionals and parents (and to market their products), e.g.
  - www.molnlycke.com/patient/en/Wound/wounds/Abrasions/#About

References

Ambuel, B., Hamlett, K.W, Marx, C. and Blumer, J.L. (1992) 'Assessing distress in pediatric intensive care environments: the COMFORT scale', *Journal of Pediatric Psychology*, 17 (1): 95–109.

Association of Paediatric Anaesthetists (APA) (2012) '*Good Practice in Postoperative and Procedural Pain Management*, 2nd edn', *Pediatric Anesthesia*, 22 (Supplement 1): 1–79.

Bloemers, F., Collard, D., Paw, M.C.A., Van Mechelen, W., Twisk, J. and Verhagen, E. (2012) 'Physical inactivity is a risk factor for physical activity-related injuries in children', *British Journal of Sports Medicine*, 46 (9): 669–74.

Boddy, J. and Smith, M. (2008) 'Asking the experts: developing and validating parental diaries to assess children's minor injuries', *International Journal of Social Research Methodology*, 11 (1): 63–77.

Bowers, K. and Barrett, S. (2009) 'Wound-related pain: features, assessment and treatment', *Nursing Standard*, 19 (10): 37–46.

Breau, L.M., Camfield, C., McGrath, P.J., Rosmus, C. and Finley, G.A. (2001) 'Measuring pain accurately in children with cognitive impairments: refinement of a caregiver scale', *Journal of Pediatrics*, 138 (5): 721–727.

Breau, L., Finley, G., McGrath, P. and Camfield, C.S. (2002) 'Validation of the non-communicating children's pain checklist-postoperative version', *Anesthesiology*, 96 (3): 528–535.

Breau, L.M., McGrath, P.J., Camfield, C., Rosmus, C. and Finley, G.A. (2000) 'Preliminary validation of an observational pain checklist for persons with cognitive impairments and inability to communicate verbally', *Developmental Medicine and Child Neurology*, 42 (9): 609–616.

Bruce, E. and Franck, L. (2000) 'Self-administered nitrous oxide (entonox) for the management of procedural pain', *Paediatric Nursing*, 12 (7): 15–19.

Caljouw, M.A.A., Kloos, M.A.C., Olivier, M.Y., Heemskerk, I.W., Pison, W.C.R., Stitger, G.D. and Verhoef, A.J.H. (2007) 'Measurement of pain in premature infants with a gestational age between 28 to 37 weeks: validation of the adapted COMFORT Scale', *Journal of Neonatal Nursing*, 13(1): 13–18.

Ciprandi, G., Romanelli, M., Durante, C., Baharestani, M. and Meuli, M. (2012) 'Both skill and sensitivity are needed for paediatric patients', *Wounds International*, 3: 5.

Collard, D.C.M., Verhagen, E.A.L.M., van Mechelen, W., Heymans, M.W., Chin, A. and Paw, M.J.M. (2011) 'Economic burden of physical activity-related injuries in Dutch children aged 10–12', *British Journal of Sports Medicine*, 45 (13): 1058–63.

Cutting, K.F. (2008) 'Impact of adhesive surgical tape and wound dressings on the skin, with reference to skin stripping', *Journal of Wound Care*, 17 (4): 157.

Davies, F.C.W., Robson, W.J. and Smith, A.K. (2003) *Minor Trauma in Children: A Pocket Guide*. Florida: CRC Press.

Denyer, J. (2011) 'Reducing pain during the removal of adhesive and adherent products', *British Journal of Nursing*, 50 (15): S28–35.

van Dijk, M., de Boer, J.B., Koot, H.M., Tibboel, D., Passchier, J. and Duivenvoorden, H.J. (2000) 'The reliability and validity of the COMFORT scale as a postoperative pain instrument in 0 to 3-year-old infants', *Pain*, 84 (2-3): 367–377.

Dubin, A.E. and Patapoutian, A. (2010) 'Nociceptors: the sensors of the pain pathway', *Journal of Clinical Investigation*, 120 (11): 3760–72.

Eidelman, A., Weiss, J.M., Baldwin, C.L., Enu, I.K., McNicol, E.D. and Carr, D.B. (2011) 'Topical anaesthetics for repair of dermal laceration', *Cochrane Database of Systematic Reviews (Online)* (6): CD005364. doi.

Hedström, E.M., Bergström, U. and Michno, P. (2012) 'Injuries in children and adolescents – analysis of 41,330 injury-related visits to an emergency department in northern Sweden', *Injury*, 43 (9): 1403–8.

Hicks, C., von Baeyer, C., Spafford, P.A., van Korlaar, I. and Goodenough, B. (2001) 'The Faces Pain Scale-Revised: toward a common metric in pediatric pain measurement', *Pain*, 93 (2): 173–183.

Hollinworth, H. (2005) 'The management of patients' pain in wound care', *Nursing Standard*, 20 (7): 65.

Hollinworth, H. and Collier, M. (2000) 'Nurses' views about pain and trauma at dressing changes: results of a national survey', *Journal of Wound Care*, 9: 369–78.

Howard, R. and Houghton, C. (2012) 'Improving parental first-aid practices', *Emergency Nurse*, 20 (3): 14–19.

Hudspith, M.J., Siddall, P.J. and Rajesh, M. (2006) 'Physiology of pain', in H.C. Hemmings and P.M. Hopkins (eds), *Foundations of Anesthesia: Basic Sciences for Clinical Practice*, 2nd edn. Philadelphia, PA: Elsevier, pp. 267–85.

Hunt, A., Goldman, A., Seers, K., Crichton, N., Mastroyannopoulu, K., Moffat, V., Oulton, K. and Brady, M. (2004) 'Clinical validation of the paediatric pain profile', *Developmental Medicine and Child Neurology*, 46 (1): 9–18.

Hunt, A., Wisbeach, A., Seers, K., Goldman, A., Crichton, N., Perry, L. and Mastroyannopoulu, K. (2007) 'Development of the paediatric pain profile: role of video analysis and saliva cortisol in validating a tool to assess pain in children with severe neurological disability, *Journal of Pain and Symptom Management*, 33 (3): 276–289.

Jones, C. and Hammig, B. (2012) 'Epidemiology of exercise-related injuries among children', *Health*, 4 (9): 625–8.

Kendrick, D. and Marsh, P. (1999) 'Parents and first aid: I know what to do – but I'm not very confident', *Health Education Journal*, 58 (1): 39–47.

Kipping, B., Rodger, S., Miller, K. and Kimble, R.M. (2012) 'Virtual reality for acute pain reduction in adolescents undergoing burn wound care: a prospective randomized controlled trial', *Burns*, 38: 650–7.

Malloy, K.M. and Milling, L.S. (2010) 'The effectiveness of virtual reality distraction for pain reduction: a systematic review', *Clinical Psychology Review*, 30 (8): 1011–18.

Malviya, S., Voepel-Lewis, T., Burke, C., Merkel, S. and Tait, S.R (2006) 'The revised FLACC observational pain tool: improved reliability and validity for pain assessment in children with cognitive impairment', *Pediatric Anesthesia*, 16 (3): 258–265.

Manworren, R.C.B. and Hynan, L.S. (2003) 'Clinical validation of FLACC: preverbal patient pain scale', *Pediatric Nursing*, 29 (2): 140–146.

McCord, S.S. and Levy, M.L. (2006) 'Practical guide to pediatric wound care', *Seminars in Plastic Surgery*, 20 (3): 192–9.

Merkel, S.I., Voepel-Lewis, T., Shayevitz, J.R. and Malviya, S. (1997) 'The FLACC: a behavioral scale for scoring postoperative pain in young children', *Pediatric Nursing*, 23 (3): 293–297.

Meuleneire, F. (2009) 'A case study evaluation of Safetac® dressings used for paediatric wounds', *Wounds UK*, 5 (2): 12–18.

Miller, K., Rodger, S., Kipping, B. and Kimble, R.M. (2011) 'A novel technology approach to pain management in children with burns: a prospective randomized controlled trial', *Burns*, 37 (3): 395–405.

Moffatt, C.J., Franks, P.J. and Hollinworth, H. (2002) *Understanding Wound Pain and Trauma: An International Perspective*. London: MEP Ltd.

Nilsson, S., Finnströem, B. and Kokinsky, E. (2008) 'The FLACC behavioral scale for procedural pain assessment in children aged 5–16 years', *Pediatric Anesthesia*, 18 (8): 767–774.

Nilsson, S., Hallqvist, C., Sidenvall, B. and Enskär, K. (2011) 'Children's experiences of procedural pain management in conjunction with trauma wound dressings', *Journal of Advanced Nursing*, 67 (7): 1449–57.

Nilsson, S. and Renning, A. (2012) 'Pain management during wound dressing in children', *Nursing Standard*, 26 (32): 50–5.

Pasin, S., Avila, F., de Cavatá, T., Hunt, A. and Heldt, E. (2013) 'Cross-cultural translation and adaptation to Brazilian Portuguese of the paediatric pain profile in children with severe cerebral palsy', *Journal of Pain And Symptom Management*, 45 (1), pp. 120–8.

Price, D.D. (2000) 'Psychological and neural mechanisms of the affective dimension of pain', *Science*, 288 (5472): 1769–72.

Richardson, C. and Upton, D. (2010) 'A discussion of the potential mechanisms for wound dressings' apparent analgesic effects', *Journal of Wound Care*, 19 (10): 424.

Rippon, M., Davies, P. and White, R. (2012) 'Taking the trauma out of wound care: the importance of undisturbed healing', *Journal of Wound Care*, 21 (8): 359–68.

Singer, A.J., Gulla, J., Thode, H.J. and Cronin, K.A. (2004) 'Pediatric first aid knowledge among parents', *Pediatric Emergency Care*, 20 (12): 808–11.

Sundblad, G., Saartok, T., Engström, L. and Renström, P. (2005) 'Injuries during physical activity in school children', *Scandinavian Journal of Medicine & Science in Sports*, 15 (5): 313–23.

Thomas, S. (2003) 'Atraumatic dressings', *World Wide Wounds*, 1: 9.

Thomas, S. (2008) 'The role of dressings in the treatment of moisture-related skin damage', *World Wide Wounds*, 1–8. Available at www.worldwidewounds.com/2008/march/Thomas/Maceration-and-the-role-of-dressings. html (accessed 29 October 2013).

Upton, D. (2009) Stress, pain and wound healing. *The European Wound Management Association Conference*. Mölnlycke Health Care, Holsworthy, UK, 21 May. Available at http://less-pain.com/Documents/EWMA_symposium_proceedings_abstract.pdf (accessed 1 January 2014).

Van Twillert, B., Bremer, M. and Faber, A.W. (2007) 'Computer-generated virtual reality to control pain and anxiety in pediatric and adult burn patients during wound dressing changes', *Journal of Burn Care and Research*, 28 (5): 694–702.

Verhagen, E., Collard, D., Chin, M., Paw, A. and van Mechelen, W. (2009) 'A prospective cohort study on physical activity and sports-related injuries in 10–12-year-old children', *British Journal of Sports Medicine*, 43 (13): 1031–5.

Voepel-Lewis, T., Malviya, S., Merkel, S. and Tait, A.R. (2003) 'Behavioral pain assessment and the face, legs, activity, cry and consolability instrument', *Expert Review of Pharmacoeconomics and Outcomes Research*, 3 (3): 317–325.

Voepel-Lewis, T., Merkel, S., Tait, S.R., Trzcinka, A. and Malviya, S. (2002) 'Reliability and validity of the Faces, Legs, Activity, Cry, Consolability observational tool as a measure of pain in cognitively impaired children', *Anesthesia and Analgesia*, 95(5): 1224–1229.

World Health Organization (2010) *Global Recommendations on Physical Activity for Health*. Geneva: WHO.

Zaman, H.U., Islam, J.M.M., Khan, M.A. and Khan, R.A. (2011) 'Physico-mechanical properties of wound dressing material and its biomedical application', *Journal of the Mechanical Behavior of Biomedical Materials*, 4 (7): 1369–75.

Chapter 13

Non-pharmacological Methods of Pain Relief

Ben's and Maria's Stories

Ben's story

Ben was admitted from the emergency service. His parents had brought him to get relief from terrible pain. His headaches had been previously investigated and nothing serious had been found to explain these. He had had contact with the Child Pain Team. Ben had received prescriptions for medications and also got extra medication at the emergency service. However, nothing had helped this time. When he came to the ward Ben was shouting out, and nothing we did or gave him could ease his pain. He was given a bed in a two-bed room and his mother stayed with him and tried to comfort him. But nothing helped.

It was devastating to hear him and Ben's voice was heard all over the ward, making other children and parents anxious. We asked for the prescription of more effective pharmacological treatment but the paediatrician did not feel it safe to give anything more. I and my colleague suggested trying some non-pharmacological treatment, but the boy was unreachable and unable to come to an agreement. Guided imagery (GI) would have been an option: I have tried this with children suffering from acute pain as a complement to pharmacological treatment, and it used to work well. But when it was not possible to talk with Ben and give proper information, we deemed GI contradictive.

The evening went on and it passed midnight. Ben was still screaming and could not fall asleep, and nearly no one else on the ward could either. Gradually I came to the point where I had to use GI. I just went to Ben and asked him to take some deep breaths, try to blow on his hand (to make him stop hyperventilating) and then started the relaxation exercise, instructed him to focus on one part of the body at a time, from toes to all over the body ending with his fingers.

Then he was a little bit calmer and I asked Ben to think about some pleasant episode. Ben dreamed himself to a beautiful field with flowers. His eyes moved under his closed eyelids and after a while he fell asleep and slept all night. I was not proud about introducing guided imagery like this, and had doubts about what it meant to him to go through the exercise without being able to actively choose the method. Then I was able to meet him the night after. He liked the method and tried it again. We met several times and Ben enjoyed dreaming away.

Preferably children should be involved in decisions about the nursing interventions offered, and especially when using guided imagery the child has to be well informed and then actively chose to try it. However, when a child is panicking it seems appropriate to reach out with the methods you are skilled in and have been proven to help comfort children with the problem the child suffers from. When a child is in pain you are in a panic, you are in need of a lifeline.

Maria's Story

This episode happened on a night shift on a ward caring for children 0–18 years old with different diagnosis, orthopaedic, surgery, medical conditions, infections and so on. This night was a night like any other night. The children I cared for were sleeping and there was a lull in caregiving activities.

My colleague on the other hand was troubled about Maria, a teenage girl, who was in pain. Maria had been involved in a car accident. Maria was seriously injured, with fractures and internal bleeding, pneumothorax and lots of bruises and scrapes all over her body: moreover the driver, her boyfriend, had been killed. The situation was compounded by the fact Maria's boyfriend had been a married man with children. Because of this she risked being rejected by her family, however her sister was on her side and relatives were visiting during the day. Maria's medical condition was taken care of and she had advanced medical treatment for her pain. However, her pain was not relieved. My colleague had tried everything to help Maria but without success. We discussed how to ease her pain, taking everything into consideration: the trauma, her grief, the problematic cultural aspect preventing her mother from sitting by her side, as well as prejudices against her culture even within health care professionals.

Since I am experienced in the use of guided imagery my colleague asked me to go and talk to the girl and ask if she would like to try GI. There was Maria lying in the bed, pale and obviously suffering, not able to fall asleep, though it was past midnight. We had never met before and she was silent and barely answering. I sat down on the chair beside the bed and told her I could see she was in pain and offered some alternatives; contacting the anaesthesiologist, trying GI, listening to music, watching a movie or having massage and so on. Maria still didn't talk and I considered leaving the room, reflecting that the situation was nothing more than could be expected. It is not easy to trust another person and respond to a helping hand when things have turned so bad. But then when I was just about to leave the room Maria told me she would like to have massage on her feet. I am not skilled in massage but I stroked her feet following the instructions from baby massage, and she got relief and could then fall asleep.

Introduction

Ben's story describes a challenging and disturbing situation of a boy in pain, and how it was successfully dealt with through the skill and perseverance of the nurse. There are many issues in the story that may resonate with any nurse who has been faced with a child in distressing pain, and as you read the story the tension on the ward that was created by Ben shouting out in pain is quite palpable, being heard by the whole unit, resulting in other children being distressed. The nurse knew that guided imagery was a potentially successful intervention that she could offer Ben, and she was skilled in its use. However, Ben's lack of acceptance of this offer left the nurse feeling somewhat helpless to intervene to relieve his pain. As time passed Ben's distress did not lessen and the nurse decided to reach out to him in a gentle but skilled way. By approaching him in this way it gave Ben the opening he needed to respond and accept her help. Ben was hyperventilating and needed to relax for any intervention to work. By engaging Ben in focusing on his breathing he became calmer and was more receptive to guided imagery.

Maria was clearly experiencing physical pain from her multiple injuries. This alone would have made managing her pain a challenge. However, compounding her pain were some very distressing issues connected to her accident. Maria was likely to be experiencing grief, anxiety and stress, and perhaps guilt, fear and loneliness, all of which would contribute to exacerbating her pain.

Complex situations such as Maria's can be demanding for health care professionals, requiring an individual approach. It would have been easy for the nurse to have accepted that Maria did not want her offer of pain-relieving intervention and then to leave. However, the nurse's patience in reaching out to this troubled adolescent meant that she could engage effectively in a pain relieving intervention. The nurse recognised that she had not yet developed a therapeutic relationship (Mitchell and Cormack 1998) with Maria, which meant it was more likely that she would not trust her, however, communicating in a skilled way and 'being present' enabled Maria to accept her offer of care.

These two stories have much in common: distressing pain, the rejection of help offered by a nurse, and the skilled communication of nurses in their determination to attempt to reach out and relieve the suffering of the young people in their care.

Guided imagery: its uses and effectiveness

The use of guided imagery for procedural pain has been in place for some time (Lal et al. 2001; MacLaren and Cohen 2005) and has been found to be effective in significantly reducing pain after ambulatory surgery (Huth et al. 2004). Guided imagery has also been used in children with chronic pain who used it alongside muscle relaxation, resulting in increased self-management of their pain (Weydert et al. 2006).

Naparstek (1995), a pioneer of guided imagery, describes it as a process of deliberately using the imagination to help the mind and body heal. It is a directed, deliberate daydream, a purposeful creation of positive sensory images, sights, sounds, smells, tastes, and feelings in the imagination. This state of focused concentration allows a temporary escape and relaxation and produces a sense of physical and emotional well-being. It has a marked impact on pain perception.

Guided imagery is a form of relaxation or meditation that can be used to promote a child's own coping abilities. It has been shown to be extremely useful in a number of situations, for example as demonstrated by Ball et al. (2003) who used guided imagery on a group of ten children who had recurrent abdominal pain. The children were guided to imagine what their pain looked like, using all their senses to make the image more clear, followed by asking the child what could destroy the pain, and were then guided through this second image, making the pain disappear. The children in the study experienced a 67 per cent decrease in their pain during the therapy. Baird et al. (2010) suggest that guided imagery is inexpensive, easy to teach and easy to use, and is effective in pain relief and reducing medication use.

Because of its adaptability guided imagery can be used in many settings: Russell and Smart (2007) report on a number of case studies of children receiving hospice care. The use of guided imagery helped reduce pain and anxiety during medical procedures. Guided imagery has also been tested in relation to children's post-operative pain. Polkki et al. (2008) conducted a randomised controlled trial on 60 children aged 8–12 years following surgery. The experimental group listened to an imagery CD, while those in the control group received standard care. The children in the experimental group were found to have significantly less pain than the children in the control group. However, the study authors suggest that the affect of guided imagery is short-lived. This finding is countered by a study by van Tilberg et al. (2009) who carried out a home-based study with 34 children aged 6–15 years using guided imagery and found that the treatment effects were sustained over a long period of time. An explanation could be that the home-based study involved children expecting to have to repeat the guided imagery process regularly to achieve pain relief, whereas in hospital the approach may have been different.

Guided imagery is simple to undertake and requires little in terms of equipment or preparation: it can be used repeatedly, as well as independently by children and young people. Such an intervention could be seen to be ideal for children experiencing long term or chronic pain, including children with sickle cell disease. Dobson (2006) studied 21 children aged 5–11 years with sickle cell disease for their self-efficacy and use of medication while using guided imagery over time. The findings reported children having less pain, using less opioid medication and increasing their self-efficacy after brief training to use guided imagery.

How does guided imagery work?

Bush (1987) described imagery as a type of distraction that uses many of the main senses, and demands high attention. Attention is a cognitive process in which individuals focus on certain things while ignoring others. How distraction works is explained by Twycross et al. (2009) as a process that works in line with the gate control theory; the use of distraction closes the gate, blocking off the pain pathway and therefore denying the mechanisms that lead to the perception of pain. Pain is put at the periphery of awareness with attention being focused on the distracting device, which in Ben's story involved imagery that guided him to a field of flowers, but other children might focus back to a holiday or a day out, where the child has an image in their mind that evokes the sensations experienced on that day and related to the memory of the image (see Figure 13.1).

Huth et al. (2006) evaluated the effectiveness of a guided imagery compact disc in reducing post-operative pain, increasing relaxation and stimulating imagery in children. Children were asked to use all their senses in the guided imagery; to see,

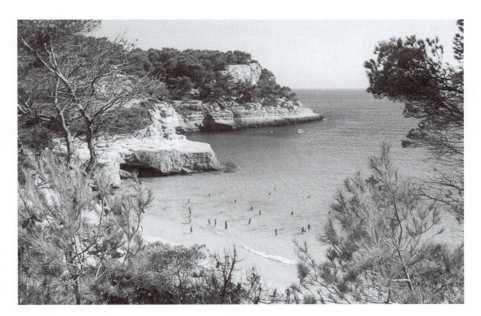

Figure 13.1   An image of a place a child has visited can be used in guided imagery
© Jon Sparks Photography

hear, touch, smell and taste. Pain scores were significantly reduced, demonstrating that school-aged children are capable of using guided imagery to reduce their post-operative pain.

Many studies have been conducted on pain processes and pain pathways, but until recently little was understood about the complex interplay of neurons and messenger modules that leads to an individual perceiving pain. A relatively new area of study is exploring how emotional effects and cognitive functioning actually contribute to the experience of pain (Weich et al. 2008). Ben was in a highly emotional state which is likely to have been exacerbating his pain. The nurse started engaging Ben by focusing on his breathing, and this meant he stopped hyperventilating and began to relax. Relaxation is a necessary precursor to effective guided imagery, because it means the child is in a receptive state to enable them to focus on the imagery. Relaxation causes direct physiologic responses and enhances an individual's ability to physically and psychologically focus on the images used in guided imagery (Selhub 2007).

Huth and Lin (2008) studied the use of imagery with 7–12-year-old children and found that the older children scored higher on imagery when used for post-operative pain, suggesting that older children have an increased ability to cope with stressful situations and focus their attention. This makes them more receptive to the use of guided imagery as a non-pharmacological method of pain relief. Although Ben fits within the age group studied by Huth et al. as likely to be receptive to guided imagery, the skilled actions of the nurse in engaging Ben in guided imagery were pivotal to its success.

The use of massage

In Maria's story there is another example of a challenging situation where a nurse uses a non-pharmacological method to relieve pain, in this case massage. The use of massage as a form of sensory stimulation has been recognised as far back as early civilisations.

Lund (2000) proposed three main mechanisms that occur during massage (see Figure 13.2). In relating these mechanisms to the gate control theory of pain (Melzack and Wall 1965) the effect of massage is to close the gate and therefore block pain perception. The relaxation effect combined with the reduction in pain may explain how Maria's foot massage allowed her to sleep. Grealish et al. (2000) carried out a study on foot massage for pain in patients with cancer and found that it both helped relax patients and promoted sleep.

The use of massage has been studied across many age groups. Jain et al. (2006) studied the use of massage prior to heel stick in infants and showed good effect in reducing pain responses. They suggest that leg massage in infants could close the gate referred to in the gate control theory (Melzack and Wall 1965), or alternately massage works by activating the endogenous opioid pathways to decrease the nociceptic transmission of pain. Further evidence of the benefits of massage was demonstrated in a large randomised controlled trial by Mitchinson et al. (2007) (n = 605) to explore the effect of massage on acute pain. Their findings demonstrated statistically significant reductions in pain intensity and anxiety.

Hand massage has also been found to reduce anxiety, depressed mood and sleep disturbance over a four-week period (Field et al. 2011). Each of these studies may in some way throw light on how Maria, a very anxious and stressed 16–year-old, responded positively to the effects of massage and was able to go to sleep. Massage

| Different types of low threshold mechanoreceptors are most probably activated in the periphery and thus induce activity in the afferent nerve fibres such as Aβ fibres. In a pain experience this activity in the thick myelinated nerve fibres gives rise to a reduced transmission of pain impulses in the dorsal horn of the spinal cord. | Massage also has an anxiolytic effect which has been attributed to the release of the hormone oxytocin from neurons in the supraspinal centres. Oxytocin has anti-stress effects characterised by a decrease in sympatho-adrenergic activity and sedation. |

Figure 13.2   The mechanisms involved in massage

Adapted from Lund (2000)

can reduce stress and anxiety levels as well as interfering with the pain pathways sending messages of pain to the higher centres in the brain. The combination of these three effects was very much suited to Maria's needs as she needed to relax, have less pain, and as a result fall asleep. Wang and Keck (2004) suggest that when medication alone is not sufficient in relieving pain, the use of massage to complement analgesics can provide more effective pain control. Maria had been administered analgesics but needed an adjunct such as massage to reduce her anxiety and allow her medication to work.

Another advantage of massage is that it is easy to use, and does not require any equipment. Maria's nurse had only done massage on babies previously but managed to successfully massage Maria's feet. Wang and Keck (2004) suggest that massage requires little training, is cheap and easy to use and can be taught to patients' families.

The use and effect of non-pharmacological interventions for pain relief

Ben's and Maria's stories exemplify the effective use of two non-pharmacological methods of pain relief. However, there are a range of other methods that can be readily used by nurses in their management of children's pain. Idvall et al. (2005) studied non-pharmacological strategies used with children post tonsillectomy and found that the children's pain was physical and psychological. The physical pain responded to thermal regulation and psychological pain was relieved with emotional support which involved the child not being alone. To relate these findings to Maria, the nurse's presence as well as a choice of intervention may have resulted in Maria being receptive to massage, therefore enhancing its effectiveness. Sutters et al. (2007) suggest that providing children and young people with options for pain relief interventions gives them a feeling of control over their pain, enabling them to cope more effectively.

Lassetter (2006) reviewed 13 articles on the effectiveness of complementary therapies on children's pain, and suggested that analgesics alone may not be sufficient to deal with pain, but a more holistic approach including non-pharmacological methods is likely to be effective. The nurses knew that Maria had received analgesics, but due to her emotional state, something other than medication was required. This finding is supported by Polkki et al. (2008) who suggest that non-pharmacological techniques are needed in conjunction with pain medication for pain relief in children to be adequate.

Complementary therapies represent valuable strategies, particularly for the treatment of acute and chronic pain (Luchetti 2010). Studies are being carried out that demonstrate their place alongside conventional treatments for pain. However, more studies are needed not only to demonstrate their effectiveness, but also to promote their use.

There is very good evidence that non-pharmacological methods of pain relief are effective as demonstrated by the following Cochrane reviews. Uman et al. (2006) conducted a Cochrane review (n = 28) on psychological interventions in children and adolescents. The findings suggest that the most effective method was distraction followed by hypnosis – which is closely related to guided imagery – and then combined cognitive behavioural therapy. Another Cochrane review conducted by Eccleston et al. (2009) focused on the use of psychological therapies for both chronic and recurrent pain. The review included 29 studies and found that psychological treatments are effective in pain control and benefits appear to be maintained for at least three months.

The array of non-pharmacological methods of pain relief and the ease with which they may be deployed are no guarantee of their use. He et al. (2005) studied Chinese nurses' use of non-pharmacological methods of pain relief and found that many factors limited their use, such as being short staffed, a lack of time and a lack of knowledge of non-pharmacological pain-relieving methods. Interventions such as acupuncture have been practised for millennia, without scientific evidence of their effectiveness being required (Luchetti 2010). Acupuncture, due to its association with needles, may reduce its acceptability to many children, but for adolescents such as Maria, it may play a part in pain management.

The need for nurses to instigate pain care

Pain is a complex phenomenon and will be experienced in different ways by different individuals, as well as by the same individual at different times. The complexity is then multiplied by other influencing factors such as the child's emotional state, their past experiences of pain, beliefs about pain and the maturity or personality of the individual in determining their coping skills. Anderson and Weisman (2007) suggest that emotional factors such as anxiety, distress and anger can heighten pain perception. Maria was clearly in a state of emotional turmoil, with the death of her boyfriend, along with, perhaps, conflict or tension with her family, on top of the many physical injuries she sustained in the accident. The nurse had assessed Maria to be in obvious pain, even though she had not asked for help. Nurses have a 24-hour responsibility for pain management and are the only health professional to engage in care in this way. Therefore the onus is on nurses, as front-line carers, to recognise and address pain (APA 2012).

Maria's and Ben's stories exemplify many of the conundrums faced by nurses dealing with children in pain: children do not always express how they are feeling accurately, and they may initially refuse a pain-relieving intervention, only to accept it later. Such contradictions can be frustrating for nurses, and may mean that busy nurses do not have the time to put in the extra effort to ensure an intervention is offered again. Many nurses when asked about the barriers to delivering effective pain relief cite lack of time as the main obstacle (Simons and Macdonald 2004).

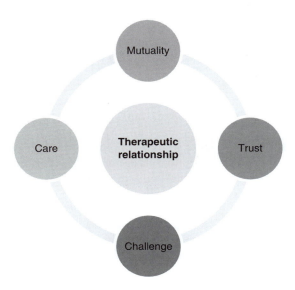

Figure 13.3   The components of a therapeutic relationship
Adapted from Mitchell and Cormack (1998)

It is clear that in these stories the nurse placed the challenge of relieving pain as a high priority and therefore decided to spend time dealing with the challenge of providing relief. In both stories there are clear indications of the development of a therapeutic relationship. Mitchell and Cormack (1998) in their book on the therapeutic relationship suggest that relationships can in and of themselves heal. Based on this belief, they propose a model of treatment as illustrated in Figure 13.3.

Within this framework a patient and practitioner may engage in effective therapy. A successful therapeutic relationship requires the nurse not only to have high-quality communication and interpersonal skills but also to be able to build rapport and trust with the patient (McQueen 2000). Maria's and Ben's nurses recognised the need to spend time offering different options and their persistence managed to engage both Ben and Maria gaining some element of trust and allowing a therapeutic intervention to take place.

The role of parents

Although both guided imagery and massage are beneficial as non-pharmacological pain interventions, nurses rarely incorporate them into their practice (Huth et al. 2006). These findings are similar to a study carried out a decade earlier by Polkki et al. (2001) suggesting there has been little progress in the past ten years in nurses' use of non-pharmacological methods of pain relief. Polkki et al. (2002) suggest that one way forward is for parents to become actively involved in their child's pain management, as this would enhance the likelihood of non-pharmacological methods being utilised. However, it is recognised that parents tend to be passively involved in their child's pain and nurses do not appear to recognise the need to engage them more actively (Simons et al. 2001).

One aspect that is not included in Ben's and Maria's stories is the role of parents. Kankkunen et al. (2002), in a large study with parents on their use of non-pharmacological methods of pain relief, found that parents do use a variety of methods, but these are limited in scope which could imply that there is an opportunity for nurses to engage parents in developing their skills in relation to the use of non-pharmacological methods of pain relief. McCarthy and Kleiber (2006) propose a model focused on the use of parents as distraction coaches when children are undergoing painful procedures. It was found that parents want to help their children, and some are able to successfully coach their children in the use of distraction. McDowell (2005) suggests that massage is the non-pharmacological intervention most frequently used by parents to help relieve their child's pain, and suggests that it should be used with critically ill children.

Implications for practice

Children are often reticent to admit to their pain, for fear of the intervention that might be offered. Nurses need to use skills of knowledge and experience as well as empathy in caring for young people with complex pain. Zagier Roberts (1994), in writing about the unconscious at work and focusing on individual and organisational stresses working in the caring services, suggests that to understand and therefore to help another person requires empathy, and Dihle et al. (2006) suggest the need for empathy and empathic communication in relation to managing pain. Maria's and Ben's nurses clearly showed empathy, but their interventions could be considered unusual in that both cases were somewhat extreme in relation to the pain experienced. In more routine exchanges related to pain it is likely that nurses may not have enough time to reach out to children in a similar way. In fact von Baeyer (2009) suggests that pain management is often ad hoc or based on hunches and assumptions rather than data from children's self-report or observational measures. Arnstein (2010) suggests that pain assessment is the cornerstone of pain management. However, in itself a child's self-report of pain may not be enough to provide the relevant information for a nurse to act upon to relieve that pain. In his groundbreaking book *Thinking Fast and Slow*, Daniel Kahneman (2011) explores our ability to make rational decisions, and what influences our ability to do so. He found that when making judgements even experts in their fields are inferior to algorithms and recommends that to maximise accuracy, decisions should be left to formulas. To relate this to pain management, nurses should not dismiss validated pain assessment tools but instead use them as a cornerstone of their holistic pain management practice. Holistic pain assessment requires us to think slowly to take in all the indicators that are telling you a child is in pain. It requires a nurse to be in the moment with the child, and to not disregard the child's self-report, but to place it in the context of all the other visual cues a child or young person is demonstrating. To build on the information gained from using a validated pain assessment tool there is a need to employ what Covey (2005) states is one of habits of highly effective people: seek first to understand. In other words gain the child's perspective of their pain, namely how they feel, what their pain means to them, and also what part of their body is affected – most pain tools do not include this information. Only once the nurse has gained an understanding of the child's perspective of their pain can they realistically attempt to deal with the pain in a holistic way.

Carter (2004, 2008) outlines some of the core aspects of good nursing practice – reciprocal trust, relational practice, being less distanced, not being passive and listening to children. All of these aspects of practice are demonstrated in Ben's and Maria's stories, where nurses reached out to them and met the very real challenge of dealing with and relieving their pain.

Conclusion

This chapter has focused on two stories of challenging pain where nurses had to adapt their practice to meet the unique needs of a child and young person in their care. By focusing on the needs in each case, balanced with a determination to help them in their pain, both nurses achieved pain relief for the children in their care. The nurses gave the child their undivided attention and by focusing on their very specific needs adapted their approach in attempting to relieve their pain. There was a sense of each nurse being in the moment with Ben and Maria, tuning in to their needs and responding accordingly.

The stories demonstrate just how effective non-pharmacological methods of pain relief can be. The chapter has outlined many examples of studies on non-pharmacological methods of pain relief as well as high-quality evidence that they work. However, it is also clear that much work has to be done in providing nurses with the confidence to use non-pharmacological methods more widely and also to promote their use in parents who are willing to help their child in pain, but need the support to do so.

Key Points

- Guided imagery is a form of relaxation or meditation that can be used to promote a child's own coping. Because of its adaptability it can be used in many settings.
- The use of massage as a form of sensory stimulation has been recognised as far back as early civilisations. The effect of massage is to block pain perception.

- It is recognised that children and young people do not always tell the truth about their pain for fear of the intervention that might be offered.
- Assessment of pain in children and young people requires more than a pain assessment tool. It also demands reciprocal trust, relational practice, being less distanced and passive and listening to children.
- Providing children and young people with options for pain relief interventions gives them a feeling of control over their pain, enabling them to cope effectively.
- There is good evidence that non-pharmacological methods of pain relief are effective.

Additional Resources and Reading

- Two resources you may find useful are:
  - o Twycross, A., Dowden, S.J. and Bruce, E. (2009) *Managing Pain in Children: A Clinical Guide*. Oxford: Wiley Blackwell. In this book there is a chapter on non-drug methods of pain relief which covers a range of non-pharmacological methods of pain relief.
  - o Uman, L.S., Chambers, C.T., McGrath, P.J. and Kisely, S.R. (2010) 'Psychological interventions for needle-related procedural pain and distress in children and adolescents', *The Cochrane Library Reviews*, Issue 11. This review demonstrated that there are a variety of cognitive behavioural interventions that can be used to successfully manage or reduce pain in needle-related procedures. The full review is available at http://onlinelibrary.wiley.com/doi/10.1002/14651858.CD005179.pub2/pdf/standard

References

Association of Paediatric Anaesthetics (APA) (2012) *Good Practice in Postoperative and Procedural Pain Management*, 2nd edn. *Pediatric Anaesthesia*, 22 (S1): 1–81.

Arnstein, P. (2010) *Clinical Coach for Effective Pain Management*. Philadelphia, PA: F.A. Davis Company.

Baird, C.L., Murawski, M.M. and Wu, J. (2010) 'Efficacy of guided imagery with relaxation for osteoarthritis symptoms and medication intake', *Pain Management Nursing*, 11 (1): 56–65.

Ball, T.M., Shapiro, D.E., Monheim, C.J. and Weydert, J.A. (2003) 'A pilot study of the use of guided imagery for the treatment of recurrent abdominal pain in children', *Clinical Pediatrics*, 42: 527–32.

Bush, J.P. (1987) 'Pain in children: a review of the literature from a developmental perspective', *Psychology & Health*, 1: 215–36.

Carter, B. (2004) 'Pain narratives and narrative practitioners: a plea for working "in relation" with children experiencing pain', *Journal of Nursing Management*, 12: 210–16.

Carter, B. (2008) 'What pain assessment guidelines tell us and what they miss', Editorial. *Journal of Child Health Care*, 12 (3): 170–2.

Covey, S. (2005) *The Seven Habits of Highly Effective People*. London: Simon and Schuster.

Cutshall, S.M., Wentworth, L.J., Engen, D., Sundt, T.M., Kelly, R.F. and Bauer, B.A. (2010) 'Effect of massage therapy on pain, anxiety, and tension in cardiac surgical patients: a pilot study', *Complementary Therapies in Clinical Practices*, 16 (2): 92–5.

Dihle, A., Bjolseth, G. and Helseth, S. (2006) 'The gap between saying and doing in postoperative pain management', *Journal of Clinical Nursing*, 15 (4): 469–79.

Dobson, C. (2006) *Guided imagery for pain management by children with sickle cell disease ages 6–11 years*. Doctoral Dissertation, Columbia University.

Eccleston, C., Palermo, T.M., Williams, A.C.D.C., Lewandowski, A. and Morley, S. (2009) 'Psychological therapies for the management of chronic and recurrent pain in children and adolescents. Intervention review', *Cochrane Database of Systematic Reviews*, Issue 2.

Field, T., Diego, M., Delgado, J., Garcia, D. and Funk C.G. (2011) 'Hand pain is reduced by massage therapy', *Complementary Therapies in Clinical Practice*, 17: 226–9.

Grealish, L., Lomasney, A. and Whiteman, B. (2000) 'Foot massage: a nursing intervention to modify the distressing symptoms of pain and nausea in patients hospitalised with cancer', *Cancer Nursing*, 23 (3): 237–43.

He, H.G., Jahja, R., Lee, T.L., Neo Kim Ang, E., Sinnappan, R., Vhevilainen-Julkunen, K. and Fai Chan, M. (2010) 'Nurses' use of non-pharmacological methods in children's postoperative pain management: educational intervention study', *Journal of Advanced Nursing*, 66 (1): 2398–2409.

Huth, M.M., Broome, M.E. and Good, M. (2004) 'Imagery reduces children's post-operative pain', *Pain*, 110: 439–48.

Huth, M.M. and Lin, L. (2008) 'Relationships among postoperative pain, imagery, and child characteristics', *Journal of Pediatric Nursing*, 23 (2): e17.

Huth, M.M., Van Kukken, D.M. and Broome, M.E. (2006) 'Playing in the park: what school-age children tell us about imagery', *Journal of Pediatric Nursing*, 21 (2): 115–25.

Idvall, E., Holm, C. and Runeson, I. (2005) 'Pain experiences and non-pharmacological strategies for pain management after tonsillectomy', *Journal of Child Health Care*, 9 (3): 196–207.

Jain, S., Kumar, P. and McMillan, D.D. (2006) 'Prior leg massage decreases pain responses to heel stick in preterm babies', *Journal of Pediatrics and Child Health*, 42: 505–8.

Kahnemann, D. (2011) *Thinking Fast and Slow*. Harmondsworth: Penguin Books.

Kankkunen, P., Vehvilainen-Julkunen, K., Pietila A.M. and Halonen, P. (2002) 'Parents use of nonpharmacological methods to alleviate postoperative pain at home', *Journal of Advanced Nursing*, 41 (4): 367–75.

Khan, K.A and Weisman, S.J. (2007) 'Nonpharmacologic pain management strategies in the pediatric emergency department', *Pediatric Emergency Medicine*, 8: 240–7.

Lal, M.K., McClelland, J., Phillips, J., Taub, N.A. and Beattie, R.M. (2001) 'Comparison of EMLA cream versus placebo in children receiving distraction therapy for venipuncture', *Acta Paediatrica*, 90: 54–9.

Lassetter, J.H. (2006) 'The effectiveness of complementary therapies on the pain experience of hospitalized children', *Journal of Holistic Nursing*, 24 (3): 196–208.

Luchetti, M. (2010) 'Complimentary medicine and pain treatment: one size does not fit all', Editorial. *The Open Pain Journal*, 3: 37.

Lund, I. (2000) 'Massage as a pain relieving method', *Physiotherapy*, 86 (12): 638–54.

MacLaren, J.E. and Cohen, L.L. (2005) 'A comparison of distraction strategies for venipuncture distress in children', *Journal of Pediatric Psychology*, 30: 387–96.

McCarthy, A.M. and Kleiber, C. (2006) 'A conceptual model of factors influencing children's responses to a painful procedure when parents are distraction coaches', *Journal of Pediatric Nursing*, 21 (2): 88–98.

McDowell, B.M. (2005) 'Nontraditonal therapies for the PICU – Part 2', *Journal of Specialists in Pediatric Nursing*, 10 (2): 81–5.

McQueen, A. (2000) 'Nurse–patient relationships and partnerships in hospital care', *Journal of Clinical Nursing*, 9 (5): 723–31.

Melzack, R. and Wall, P. (1965) 'Pain mechanisms: a new theory', *Science*, 150: 971–9.

Mitchell, A. and Cormack, M. (1998) *The Therapeutic Relationship in Complementary Health Care*. Edinburgh: Churchill Livingstone.

Mitchinson, A.R., Kim, H.M., Rosenberg, J.M., Geisser, M., Kirsh, M., Cikrit, D.B. and Hinshaw, D.B. (2007) 'Acute postoperative pain management using massage as an adjuvant therapy: a randomized trial', *Archives of Surgery*, 142 (12): 1158–67.

Naparstek, B. (1995) *Staying Well with Guided Imagery*. New York: Grand Central Publishing.

Polkki, T., Pietila, A.M., Vehvilainen-Julkunen, K., Laukkala, H. and Kivivluoma, K. (2008) 'Imagery-induced relaxation in children's postoperative pain relief: a randomized pilot study', *Journal of Pediatric Nursing*, 23 (3): 217–24.

Polkki, T., Vehvilainen-Julkunen, K. and Pietila, A.-M. (2001) 'Nonpharmacological methods in relieving children's postoperative pain: a survey on hospital nurses in Finland', *Journal of Advanced Nursing*, 34: 483–92.

Pollki, T., Vehvilainen-Julkunen, K. and Pietila, A.M. (2002) 'Parents' roles in using non-pharmacological methods in their child's postoperative pain alleviation', *Journal of Clinical Nursing*, 11: 526–36.

Russell, C. and Smart, S. (2007) 'Guided imagery and distraction therapy in paediatric hospice care', *Paediatric Nursing*, 19 (2): 24–5.

Selhub, E. (2007) 'Mind–body medicine for treating depression: using the mind to alter the body's response to stress', *Alternative & Complementary Therapies*, 13 (1): 4–9.

Simons, J., Franck, L.S. and Roberson, E. (2001) 'Parent involvement in children's pain care: views of parents and nurses', *Journal of Advanced Nursing*, 36 (4): 591–9.

Simons, J. and Macdonald, L.M. (2004) 'Pain assessment tools: children's nurses' views', *Journal of Child Health Care*, 8 (4): 264–78.

Sutters, K.A., Savedra, M.C., Misakowski, C., Holdridge-Zeuner, D., Waite, S., Paul, S.M. and Lanier, B. (2007) 'Children's expectations of pain, perceptions of analgesic efficacy, and experiences with nonpharmacologic pain management strategies at home following tonsillectomy', *Journal of Specialists in Pediatric Nursing*, 12 (3): 139–47.

Twycross, A., Dowden, S.J. and Bruce, E. (2009) *Managing Pain in Children: A Clinical Guide*. Oxford: Wiley Blackwell.

Uman, L.S., Chambers, C.T., McGrath, P.J. and Kisely, S.R. (2006) 'Psychological interventions for needle-related procedural pain and distress in children and adolescents. (Review)', *The Cochrane Library*, Issue 11.

van Tilberg, M.A.L., Chitkara, D.K., Palsson, O.S., Turner, M., Blois-Martin, N., Ulshen, M. and Whitehead, W.E. (2009) 'Audio-recorded guided imagery treatment reduces functional abdominal pain in children: a pilot study', *Pediatrics*, 124: e890–e897.

von Baeyer, C. (2009) 'Children's self-report of pain intensity: what we know, where we are headed', *Pain Research & Management*, 14 (1): 39–45.

Wang, H.L. and Keck, J.F. (2004) 'Foot and hand massage as an intervention for postoperative pain', *Pain Nursing Management*, 5 (2): 59–65.

Weich, K., Ploner, M. and Tracey, I. (2008) 'Neurocognitive aspects of pain perception', *Trends in Cognitive Science*, 12 (8): 306–13.

Weydert, J.A., Shapiro, D.E., Acra, S.A., Monheim, C.J., Chambers, A.S. and Ball, T.M. (2006) 'Evaluation of guided imagery as treatment for recurrent abdominal pain in children: a randomized controlled trial', *BMC Pediatrics*, 6: 29. Available at www.biomed central.com/1471-2431/6/29 (accessed 16 January 2013).

Zagier Roberts, V. (1994) 'The self assigned impossible task', in A. Obholzer and V. Zagier Roberts (eds), *The Unconscious at Work*. London: Routledge, pp. 110–20.

Chapter 14

Neuropathic Pain

Sam's Story

Dave's and Sam's Story

My son Samuel (now 23) developed chronic neuropathic pain in his right leg at the age of 11: this was secondary to a congenital vascular abnormality that compressed the main sciatic nerve. Until that time Sam had been a fit and healthy child, but as he grew into puberty, the compression developed. Sam described his pain as like 'someone poured burning petrol on his leg'. He was seen by experts (many experts!!) from all over the country and it was decided that nothing could be done to help him – surgery would have only left him worse off. And so it began … Sam lost his ability to walk, he could not go to school, he could not sleep or eat normally. Occasionally he would go into remission, walk and be pain free for brief periods of time, only to relapse again. High doses of opiates barely touched his pain, and he grew to manhood with constant disabling pain. There was disbelief from some – was he faking it? was it all 'just in his head'? did he have a 'low pain threshold'? after all there was nothing externally to see. But there was also support from many – not that this seemed to change anything. The stories we could tell are endless and I kept a detailed diary. At 13, Sam had an opiate-induced hallucinatory episode – and the impact of that on his younger brother was to put him into counselling. The impact on my elder son cannot be underestimated either, and on my wife and I. At 21 years Sam was suicidal, depressed and defeated. As a family we were at our wits' end. One night in 2008 he was 'blue lighted' into hospital screaming in pain – only to be told that he was being manipulative, and that he had a substance abuse problem because he was asking for morphine.

Introduction

This story outlines the dramatic and devastating consequences untreated pain can have on a teenager and his family. The length of time the pain persisted compounded by the inefficacy of the treatment clearly had serious repercussions for Samuel. This chapter will explore the nature of neuropathic pain, examining studies on what treatments have been attempted as well as studies outlining the complexity of neuropathic pain. It is recognised that not enough is known about this type of pain and its unpredictable nature. Studies on the impact of chronic pain on parents and on adolescents will also be reviewed in an attempt to understand how Samuel and his family were affected by his ongoing suffering.

Implications for practice will be drawn out, in particular the issue of not believing someone who is pain.

Neuropathic pain

Acute neuropathic pain is a condition that is under-recognised, difficult to treat and one that may over time progress to persistent pain (Gray 2008). Pain sensations can be broadly categorised into two main groups – protective and non-protective pain. Protective pain sensations are also known as nociceptive pain and non-protective pain sensations are known as abnormal or neuropathic pain (Twycross et al. 2009). Characteristic symptoms include a heightened response to noxious stimuli (hyperalgesia) and innocuous stimuli (allodynia) as well as spontaneous, shooting electric shock-like pain (Rahman and Dickinson 2011). The Australian and New Zealand College of Anaesthetists (2010) suggests that acute and chronic pain are part of the same continuum. For example, acute pain following surgery, which becomes persistent, can lead to chronic pain. Similarly neuropathic pain may be a component of acute pain due to trauma or surgery.

The International Association for the Study of Pain (IASP) define neuropathic pain as pain arising as a direct consequence of a lesion or disease affecting the somatosensory system (Dickenson 2011). Jensen (2002) suggests the key clinical features of neuropathic pain are:

- Ongoing spontaneous pain
- Pain located in an area where sensation is disrupted due to a nervous system lesion
- Abnormal evoked pain
- A build-up of pain following repetitive stimulation
- Referred pain and after sensations
- Sympathetic involvement.

Another perspective is offered by Gilron et al. (2006) who suggest slightly different features as the key components of neuropathic pain:

- Continuous or paroxysmal pain that increases rather than improves over time
- Burning or electric shock-like, stabbing or aching, throbbing or cramping pain
- Pain that it disproportionate to the injury or disease process.
- Hyperalgesia: increased response to a stimulus that is normally painful
- Allodynia: pain that can be evoked by a non-painful stimulus
- Dysaesthesia: unpleasant abnormal sensations, either spontaneous or evoked.

These two sets of features provide a picture of pain that is unpredictable, disproportionate and complex. This goes some way to providing an explanation as to the challenges of diagnosing and managing such pain. Samuel's story graphically illustrates the nature of his pain when he described this as like 'someone poured burning petrol on his leg'. Anghelescu et al. (2012) suggest that neuropathic pain is more difficult to treat than non-neuropathic pain, requiring a longer follow-up, more hospital visits, complex pharmacological management and the frequent addition of non-pharmacological interventions. One obvious area to start to gain an understanding of neuropathic pain is its physiology.

Physiology of neuropathic pain

There is a lack of understanding regarding the physiology of neuropathic pain, which leads to some of the challenges in dealing with this type of pain. Gilron et al. (2006) suggest that neuropathic pain is likely to occur as a result of a combination of nociceptic pain and abnormal sensory processing of sensory inputs by the nervous system. The effect of repeated nociceptic activity is sensitisation of the nervous system and this can, if it continues, lower the threshold for pain transmission (known as wind up), which may lead to central sensitisation, which may have an integral role in chronic pain. Schwartzman et al. (2001) proposes that the result of central sensitisation is a hypersensitivity to all incoming nerve impulses, resulting in non-painful stimuli being perceived as pain. The long-term consequences of this sensitisation can lead to physiological changes occurring in the peripheral nervous system as well as at the dorsal horn of the spinal cord.

Effects of neuropathic pain

Meyer-Rosberg et al. (2001) found that neuropathic pain is thought to be a particularly distressing pain condition and is associated with a high degree of suffering, not only because of the intensity of the pain but also because of the long duration of the condition, as the pain does not generally decline over time (Dickenson 2011). In many cases no effective treatments exist and no oral drugs are licensed for the treatment of neuropathic pain. The intensity of pain, other troublesome symptoms, limited efficacy and tolerability of available treatments, together with impaired work status, amount to a substantial burden for patients with neuropathic pain. In the case of a young person suffering neuropathic pain, the consequences affect not only the young person, but also their entire family. Samuel's father describes how his son was in constant disabling pain, that high doses of opiates barely touched his pain and how distressing this was for the family.

Diagnosing neuropathic pain

An abiding area of complexity in relation to neuropathic pain is the area of diagnostics. Much work has been done in attempting to design diagnostic tools, with only limited success. Two pain scoring systems have been developed for use in diagnosing neuropathic pain: the Neuropathic Pain Scale (NPS) (Galer and Jensen 1997); and the Neuropathic Pain Questionnaire (NPQ) (Krause and Backonja 2003). Behrman et al. (2007) conducted a study to assess the diagnostic accuracy of the two pain-scoring systems, using logistical regression and artificial neural networks as methods of data analysis. The result of the study was that the accuracy of the NPS was 55.5 per cent and the NPQ was 68.4 per cent. With such low diagnostic accuracy, Hanson and Haanpää (2007) suggest that tools such as these must not replace the diagnostic work-up procedure in children where neuropathic pain is suspected.

Rowbotham (2002) suggests neuropathic pain is complex and therefore requires a sophisticated assessment tool to enable an appropriate evaluation of the patients' pain to take place. A simple numerical pain rating tool is too reductionist for chronic or neuropathic pain. Measuring the quality and nature of pain provides only one-dimensional information. A short and simple screening tool for neuropathic pain, the Douleur Neuropathique 4(DN4) has been developed by Bouhassira et al. (2005).

The first seven items of the DN4 tool focus on pain characteristics and sensations, and the last three items relate to examination of the painful area. For each item a score of 'yes' is given 1, and a score of 'no' is given 0. The patient is defined as having neuropathic pain if the total score is 4 or more.

Table 14.1   Questionnaire Douleur Neuropathique 4 (DN4)

Questionnaire DN4 (Douleur Neuropathique 4)				
Please complete this questionnaire by ticking one answer for each item in the four questions below:				
Interview of the patient				
Question 1.				
Does the pain have one or more of the following characteristics?			**Yes**	**No**
	1	Burning		
	2	Painful cold		
	3	Electric shocks		
Question 2.				
Is the pain associated with one or more of the following symptoms in the same area?	4	Tingling		
	5	Pins and needles		
	6	Numbness		
	7	Itching		
Examination of the patient				
Question 3.				
Is the pain located in an area where the physical examination may reveal one or more of the following characteristics?	8	Touch hypoesthesia		
	9	Pricking hypoesthesia		
Question 4.				
In the painful area, can the pain be caused or increased by:	10	Brushing		
Patient score: out of 10				

Bouhassira et al. (2005)

Neuropathic pain sufferers often experience depression, anxiety and sleep distur-bances alongside their pain, leading to a significantly reduced quality of life (Rahman and Dickinson 2011). There is a need therefore to assess patients' quality of life in relation to the impact of their pain. Becker et al. (1997) suggest that quality of life measures have become standard practice in many pain clinics. Rowbotham (2002) acknowledges that it is generally recognised that neuropathic pain is associ-ated with reduced quality of life, but there is a dearth of literature on the area. Poole et al. (2009) developed a measure specifically focused on patients with neuropathic pain; the Neuropathic Pain Impact on Quality of Life (NePIQoL) questionnaire is a valid patient-derived neuropathic pain specific measure. Otto et al. (2007) found a link between neuropathy patients' responses to analgesics and their quality of life. It is recognised that there is a need to assess the multiple components of quality of life as an integral part of the evaluation of a patient's neuropathic pain. There are a number of quality of life scales designed to measure the impact of chronic pain but there is a need for a specific tool focused on neuropathic pain such as that devised by Poole et al. (2009). The tool assesses six different areas of relevance (see Figure 14.1) to the quality of life of those suffering from neuropathic pain.

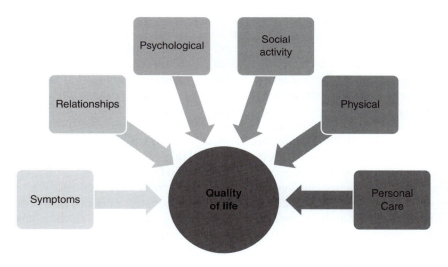

Figure 14.1   Areas of relevance to quality of life in those suffering from neuropathic pain

Treatment and pharmacological management of neuropathic pain

Jensen (2002) suggests that part of the difficulty in finding effective methods of treatment of neuropathic pain is due to the traditional approach to the classification of pain, where pain is categorised based on aetiology and location. There is a need to understand the underlying mechanisms in neuropathic pain. However, there is no simple relationship between symptoms and signs, aetiology and location, mechanisms and response to treatment. The challenge is to determine the interrelationships between these categories in order to gain insight into methods of effective relief of neuropathic pain.

The complexity of neuropathic pain has given rise to considerable challenges to health professionals in its treatment, resulting in many novel approaches. Attal et al. (2004) reported a study on the use of oral cannabinoids in a small sample of eight patients with refractory neuropathic pain. No overall benefit was found.

For many years the clinical consensus has been that opioids were ineffective in the treatment of neuropathic pain, but recent studies are suggesting they have a place in its management. Watson (2007) carried out a long-term study of 145 patients with neuropathic pain on the efficacy of opioids for their pain. The findings were that both long- and short-term opioids were effective and had a positive effect on quality of life. In a study by Dickenson and Suzuki (2005) it was found that opioids could work, but the sensory deficits such as numbness occurring in neuropathic pain pose challenges. It was also found that negative influences could be overcome by titration of the doses used.

Gormsen et al. (2007) suggest pain is often associated with anxiety and depression, which could be a result of disturbances in common neurotransmitter systems, e.g. monoamines in the brain and spinal cord. Samuel is described by his father as being defeated and depressed after suffering with neuropathic pain for 10 years. This was as a result of many different unsuccessful attempts at treatment.

The Australian and New Zealand College of Anaesthetists (2010) suggests that the treatment of acute neuropathic pain is based largely on evidence from trials for the treatment of a variety of chronic neuropathic pain disorders. A number of studies, both large randomised clinical trials as well as systematic reviews (Attala et al. 2006; Dworkin et al. 2007), have been conducted on the pharmacological treatment of neurological pain. However, despite the available evidence many patients still do not get sufficient relief from their pain. Hanson et al. (2009) suggest that it is customary to consider patients who respond to treatment to be those patients who report pain relief of up to 30–50 per cent. However, in neuropathic pain this goal is difficult to achieve as only one-third report relief from their pain despite all the pharmacological strategies that have been tried (Finnerup et al. 2005). Friedrichsdorf (2010) propose a twofold approach to deal with children suffering from neuropathic pain receiving palliative care (see Figure 14.2).

The use of gabapentin, an anticonvulsant, has been widely recognised in the treatment of neuropathic pain. Butkovic et al. (2006) conducted a small study of adolescents with intractable neuropathic pain who were administered gabapentin, and found a rapid improvement in their pain scores. They suggest that gabapentin should be included earlier in the treatment of neuropathic pain in adolescents.

The challenge of alleviating neuropathic pain has driven a number of studies to search for solutions. Bessiere et al. (2010) found that in animal studies the use of 50 per cent nitrous oxide over a prolonged period of time delivered a delayed and sustained reduction of pain hypersensitivity, which lasted a month. Such findings

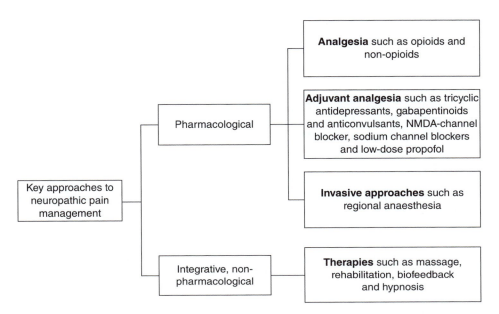

Figure 14.2   Twofold approach to neuropathic pain in children receiving palliative care

Developed from Friedrichsdorff (2010)

need to be translated into human studies and expanded upon in an attempt to find a reliable treatment for neuropathic pain.

Despite many studies on interventions to relieve neuropathic pain, the IASP (Jensen et al. 2011) suggests that only 30 per cent of patients respond to drug treatments: clearly alternative approaches should also be explored. A non-pharmacological approach that has been explored in the use of neuropathic pain is music therapy (Akin Korhan et al. forthcoming). Thirty patients received one hour of music therapy, resulting in their mean pain intensity scores reducing after 30 minutes and reduced further after 60 minutes. Non-pharmacological approaches such as this are easy to deliver and could be a strategy that nurses employ with all patients who have neuropathic pain. The effect of music is likely to relax patients and reduce their fears. Simons et al. (2012) found that the impact of fear on neuropathic pain was significantly related to disability and depression. The unpredictable nature of neuropathic pain means that adolescents are likely to have very real fear in relation to pain. A non-pharmacological approach such as music therapy could be taught to adolescents for use at home to promote relaxation and reduce fear and anxiety.

Neuropathic pain in adolescence

Adolescence is a period characterised by rapid and extensive social, psychological and physical maturation. The goal of successful adolescence is the emergence of independent behaviour, reduction in dependence on parents, with an increase in peer dependence, experimentation with identity and the development of emotional skills (Eccleston et al. 2008).

Peers and social networks are a crucial part of identity exploration; challenges to this process hinder the development of emotional skills. Eccleston et al. (2008) explored three issues of cognitive development with 110 adolescents focusing on self-perception, the importance of social development while living with chronic pain, and how it is affected by disability, anxiety, depression, family and peer functioning, in addition to pain severity. Over half of the sample felt they were less developed than their peers. It was found that peer support acted as a protective mechanism against the negative consequences of pain in relation to their development. One aspect in which the sample scored high was in the area of problem solving – their experience of having to develop coping mechanisms to deal with their pain meant they had developed problem-solving skills ahead of their peers.

Huguet et al. (2009a) studied 561 healthy school attending children aged 8–16 years of age, to examine the role of cognitive appraisal in the relationship between chronic pain and the level of functioning. They found that positive expectations about ability, the responsibility to exert control over the pain, and the belief that medication and doctors will help to control the pain, were found to be protective of normal functioning in chronic pain. Compared to younger children in the sample, older children perceived themselves to be less able to control their pain, agreed more strongly that pain means something is being hurt in the body, trusted less that the medical profession could cure their pain and trusted less in medication for pain relief.

Samuel experienced disbelief from health care professionals and such responses to complex, unpredictable pain are not uncommon. Newton et al. (2010) conducted a narrative review of the wider social contexts in which individuals with chronic pain may experience disbelief towards their pain. Three main themes emerged from the review: stigma, the experience of isolation, and the experience of emotional distress. Stigma can result in a challenge to one's integrity and subsequent effect on one's identity. The loss of relationships associated with being disbelieved can lead to the experience of isolation, and disbelief can lead to emotional distress which can take the form of guilt, depression or anger. The resulting consequences of experiencing stress, isolation and stigma can lead to mental health issues. Over time, due to the impact of unrelenting pain and not being believed, Samuel developed mental health issues. This is evident where his father described him as being suicidal at one point. Gormsen et al. (2010) found that chronic pain patients with neuropathic pain had significantly more mental distress including depression and anxiety than healthy controls both by self-rating and professional rating.

Effect on parents

Parents such as Samuel's, who are unable to achieve the relief of their adolescent's chronic pain and suffering, report significant personal distress that is exemplified by the repetitive search for legitimacy of their child's pain via a 'diagnosis'. In the absence of a diagnosis, parents reported an unwelcome suspension of normal parenting which is replaced with an unusual pattern of parenting, resembling the infant phase of parenting (Jordan et al. 2007).

Although parents feel responsible in some way for alleviating their adolescent's pain, the area of assessing and understanding the severity and consequences of their pain can be challenging. Cohen et al. (2010) suggest that an accurate assessment of adolescent chronic pain is critical in guiding treatment decisions. Their study explored the correlations between adolescents' and their parents' reports of pain. Although there were high correlations between the raters, there was also significant discordance: mothers rated their adolescents as having greater disability in social functioning, depression and pain specific anxiety than the adolescents rated themselves. Analysis suggested that high pain and being older predicted greater concordance in ratings.

The effect of having a child with chronic neuropathic pain can be devastating not only on the child or young person, but as evidenced in Samuel's story it can also have a profoundly negative effect on the whole family. Samuel's parents are described as being at their 'wits' end' at one point and Samuel's brother suffered long-lasting stress as a result of Samuel having an opiate-induced hallucinatory episode resulting in the need for counselling.

Parents of a child with undiagnosed pain have been found to embark on all-consuming attempts to find a diagnosis and cure for their child's pain. Gaughan et al. (2012) interviewed parents of children and young people aged 8–18 years who had chronic neuropathic pain. Parents described an exhausting and difficult journey in search of pain relief for their child. In their search for answers they encountered both a lack of understanding and conflict. Their parenting skills were undermined and they were left with a feeling of a lack of control and disempowerment. It is clear that some parents need help to modify their parenting style in response to their child having neuropathic pain. Health professionals need to be aware of the needs of parents in providing support to their children in pain, and the coping strategies that can help, such as adapting a rehabilitative focus.

Coping with pain

Coping with pain is a process that may affect children's adjustment to pain (Eccleston et al. 2004). Information-seeking, problem-solving, seeking social support and the use of positive self statements, were found to be related to pain controllability. Females reported a greater use of problem-solving, information-seeking, seeking social support and positive self statements than their male counterparts and girls only reported a greater use of seeking social support. The difference may be partly due to socialisation patterns. This is to say, females are educated to be more comfortable talking about their feelings than males.

With regard to using pain coping strategies, children with the most severe headaches seek more social support, they internalise and externalise more, they use less behavioural and cognitive distraction techniques, and seek information less (Bandell-Hoekstra et al. 2002).

One study that suggests the potential for positive outcomes was undertaken by McCracken et al. (2010). Their research has identified that when adolescents can positively adapt to the consequences of a health condition, rather than attempt to change the condition itself, they also function better and experience less distress. Three approaches to coping are suggested: assimilative; accommodative; and passive coping (see Figure 14.3).

Adolescents such as Samuel would require support in the form of professional advice to develop techniques that are effective in positively adapting to coping with neuropathic pain. However, it is necessary to acknowledge the challenges such complex and unpredictable pain poses for health professionals, many of whom have not had the education or support in dealing with complex cases like Samuel's. As a result it is not uncommon for health professionals to be unsure of how to deal with complex pain, and they may even disbelieve a patient who says they are suffering apparently inexplicable pain such as neuropathic pain. Samuel was confronted with disbelief, being told he was manipulative and had a substance abuse problem when he asked for morphine because he was in severe pain. Such a response from a health professional can lead to a negative relationship between them and their patient. Clarke and Iphofen (2008) suggest that such reactions can mean that patients begin to feel alienated from those they expect to help them and this can cause them to seek alternative help from other sources, compounding the fruitless search for a cure.

There is a clear need for health professionals to have a greater understanding of the vagaries of neuropathic pain, and to be less ready to disbelieve a child or young

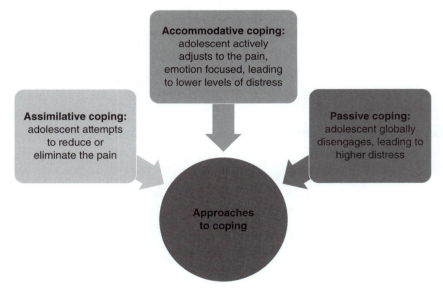

Figure 14.3   Approaches to coping

Developed from McCracken et al. (2010)

person in pain. In fact believing that a child or young person is in pain is likely to have a therapeutic effect in itself, and the effort put into trying to gain credibility can be used to manage pain more effectively. Huguet et al. (2009b) found that positive expectations about ability, the responsibility to exert control over the pain, and the belief that medication and doctors will help to control the pain, were protective of normal functioning in chronic pain.

Conclusion

This chapter has explored Dave's story of being a father and experiencing years of Sam's unrelieved neuropathic pain, a condition that is under-recognised, difficult to treat and in Sam's case over time progressed to persistent pain. There is a growing body of literature on this type of complex pain, although there appears to have been limited impact on clinical practice. Our understanding of the mechanisms of neuro-pathic pain is becoming clearer, but treatment with an array of drugs has, to date, been successful in the treatment of only a minority of neuropathic pain sufferers.

The management of such a complex type of pain requires a sophisticated approach, with nurses and doctors becoming better informed about the indications of neuro-pathic pain. The use of diagnostic tools such as the DN4, which is specifically designed to screen for pain characteristics and pain sensations in neuropathic pain, may help health care professionals to identify neuropathic pain early and therefore help patients avoid protracted periods of undiagnosed pain, as well as disbelief on the part of health professionals.

It is likely that a combination of pharmacological treatments could be comple-mented by a non-pharmacological approach that could provide children and fami-lies with coping strategies to deal with persistent pain.

Key Points

- Neuropathic pain is pain arising as a direct consequence of a lesion or disease affecting the somatosensory system.
- Neuropathic pain is a particularly distressing pain condition associated with a high degree of suffering, not only because of the intensity of the pain but also because of the long duration of the condition.
- Young people suffering from neuropathic pain often experience depression, anxi-ety and sleep disturbances alongside their pain, leading to a significantly reduced quality of life.
- Experiencing neuropathic pain in adolescence can hinder a young person's devel-opment cognitively, emotionally and socially.
- Parents who are unable to achieve the relief of their adolescent's chronic pain and suffering report significant personal distress.
- Young people experiencing neuropathic pain require support to develop tech-niques that are effective in positively adapting to coping with neuropathic pain.

Additional Resources and Reading

- If you would like to read further on the subject of neuropathic pain you may find the following two articles and WHO guideline of interest:
  - Gaughan, V., Logan, D. and Sethna, N. (2012) 'Parents' perspective of their journey caring for a child with chronic neuropathic pain', *Pain Managment Nursing*. doi: 10.1016/j.pmn.2012.09.002.
  - Korhan, E.A. Uyar, M., Eyigor, C., Hakverdioglu Yont, G., Celik, S. and Khorshid, L. (2013) 'The effect of music therapy on pain in patients with neuropathic pain', *Pain Managment Nursing*, e-pub doi: 10.1016.j.pmn.2012.10.006.
- This WHO (2012) document is 178 pages long and provides useful information on neuropathic pain and pharmacological approaches.
  - WHO (2012) Guidelines on the *Pharmacological Treatment of Persisting Pain in Children with Medical Illness* can be downloaded from the following site. www.who.int/medicines/areas/quality_safety/guide_on_pain/en/index.html.

References

Anghelescu, D.L., Faughnan, L.G., Popenhagen, M.P., Oakes, L.L., Pei, D. and Burgoyne, L.L. (2012) 'Neuropathic pain referrals to multidisciplinary pediatric cancer pain service', *Pain Managment Nursing*. Available online 25 August 2012. In press, corrected proof.

Attal, N., Brasseur, L., Guirimand, D., Clermond-Gnamien, S., Atlami, S. and Bouchassira, D. (2004) 'Are oral cannabinoids safe and effective in refractory neuropathic pain?', *European Journal of Pain*, 8: 173 –7.

Attal, N., Cruccu, G., Haanpää, M., Hansson, P., Jensen, T.S., Nurmikko, T., Sampaio, C., Sindrup, S. and Wiffen, P. (2006) 'EFNS guidelines on pharmacological treatment of neuropathic pain', *European Journal of Neurology*, 13: 1153–69.

Australian and New Zealand College of Anaesthetists (2010) *Acute Pain Management: Scientific Evidence*, 3rd edn. Melbourne: Australian and New Zealand College of Anaesthetists and Faculty of Pain Medicine.

Bandell-Hoekstra, I.E.N.G, Abu-Saad, H.H., Passchier, J., Frederiks, C.M.A., Feron, F.J.M. and Knipschild, P. (2002) 'Coping and qualilty of life in relation to headache in Dutch school children', *European Journal of Pain*, 6: 315–21.

Becker, N., Thomsen Bondegaard, A., Olsen Kornelius, A., Sjorgen, P., Bech, P. and Erikson, J. (1997) 'Pain epidemiology and health related quality of life in chronic non malignant pain patients referred to a Danish multidisciplinary pain center', *Pain*, 73: 393–400.

Behrman, M., Linder, R., Assadi, A.H., Stacey, B.R. and Backonja, M. (2007) 'Classification of patients with pain based on neuropathic pain symptoms: comparison of an artificial neural network against an established scoring system', *European Journal of Pain*, 11 (4): 370–6.

Bessiere, B., Laboureyras, E., Chateauraynaud, J., Laulin, J.P. and Simonet, G. (2010) 'A single nitrous oxide (N$_2$O) exposure leads to persistent alleviation of neuropathic pain in rats', *The Journal of Pain*, 11 (1): 13–23.

Bouhassira, D., Attal, N., Alchaar, H., Boureau, F., Brochet, B., Bruxelle, J., Cunin, G., Fermanian, J., Ginies, P., Grun-Overdyking, A., Jafari-Schluep, H., Lanteri-Minet, M., Laurent, B., Mick, G., Serrie, A., Valade, D. and Vicaut, E. (2005) 'Comparison of pain syndromes associated with nervous or somatic lesions and development of a new neuropathic pain diagnostic questionnaire (DN4)', *Pain*, 114: 29–36.

Butkovic, D., Toljan, S. and Mihovilovic-Novak, B. (2006) 'Experience with gabapentin for neuropathic pain in adolescents: report of five cases', *Pediatric Anesthesia*, 16: 325–9.

Clarke, K.A. and Iphofen, R. (2008) 'Effects of failing to believe patients' experiences of pain', *Nursing Times*, 104 (8): 30–1.

Cohen, L.L., Vowles, K.E. and Eccleston, C. (2010) 'Adolescent chronic pain-related functioning: Concordance and discordance of mother-proxy and self-report ratings', *European Journal of Pain*, 14: 882–6.

Dickenson, A.H. (2011) 'Neuropathic pain', Editorial. *Reviews in Pain*, 5 (11): 1–2.

Dickenson, A.H. and Suzuki, R. (2005) 'Opioids in neuropathic pain: clues from animal studies', *European Journal of Pain*, 9: 113–16.

Dworkin, R.H., O'Connor, A.B., Backonja, M., Farrar, J.T., Finnerup, N.B., Jensen, T.S., Kalso, E.A., Loesser, J.D., Miaskowski, C., Nurmikko, T.J., Portenoy, R.K., Rice, A.S., Stacey, B.R. and Treede, R.D. (2007) 'Pharmacologic management of neuropathic pain: evidence based recommendations', *Pain*, 132: 237–51.

Eccleston, C., Crombez, G., Scotford, A., Clinch, J. and Connell, H. (2004) 'Adolescent chronic pain: patterns and predictors of emotional distress in adolescents with chronic pain and their parents', *Pain*, 108: 221–9.

Eccleston, C., Wastell, S. and Jordan, A. (2008) 'Adolescent social development and chronic pain', *European Journal of Pain*, 12: 263–70.

Finnerup, N.B., Sindrup, S.H. and Jensen, TS. (2005) 'Chronic neuropathic pain: mechanisms, drug targets and measurement', *Fundamental Clinical Pharmacology*, 21: 129–36.

Friedrichsdorf, S. (2010) 'Managing neuropathic pain in pediatric palliative care', *Journal of Pain and Symptom Management*, 39 (2): 365.

Galer, B.S. and Jensen, M.P. (1997) 'Development and preliminary validation of a pain measure specific to neuropathic pain. The Neuropathic Pain Scale', *Neurology*, 48: 332–8.

Gaughan, V., Logan, D. and Sethna, N. (2012) 'Parents' perspective of their journey caring for a child with chronic neuropathic pain', *Pain Management Nursing*, doi: 10.1016/j.pmn.2012.09.002.

Gilron, I.,Watson, P. and Cahill, C. (2006) 'Neuropathic pain: a guide for the clinician', *Canadian Medical Association Journal*, 175 (3): 265–75.

Gormsen, L., Rosenberg, R., Bach, F.W. and Jensen, T.S. (2007) 'Pain, anxiety and depression in neuropathic and non neuropathic pain patients compared with healthy controls: a quantitative study', *European Journal of Pain*, 11 (S1): S59–S207.

Gormsen, L., Rosenberg, R., Bach, F.W. and Jensen, T.S. (2010) 'Depression, anxiety, health-related quality of life and pain in patients with fibromyalgia and neuropathic pain', *European Journal of Pain*, 14 (127): e1–e8.

Gray, P. (2008) 'Acute neuropathic pain: diagnosis and treatment', *Current Opinion in Anaesthesiology*, 21 (5): 590–5.

Hanson, P. and Haanpää, M. (2007) 'Diagnostic work of neuropathic pain: computing, using questionnaires or examining the patient?', Editorial. *European Journal of Pain*, 11: 367–9.

Hanson, P.T., Attal, N. and Baron, R. (2009) 'Towards a definition of pharmacoresistant neuropathic pain', *European Journal of Pain*, 13: 439–40.

Huguet, A., Gauntlett-Gilbert, J., Miro, J. and Eccleston, C. (2009a) 'Young people making sense of pain: cognitive appraisal, function and pain in 8–16-year-old children', *European Journal of Pain*, 13: 751–8.

Huguet, A., Miro, J. and Nieto, R. (2009b) 'The factor structure and factorial invariance of the Pain-Coping Questionnaire across age: evidence from community-based samples of children and adults', *European Journal of Pain*, 13: 879–89.

Jensen, T.S. (2002) 'An improved understanding of neuropathic pain', *European Journal of Pain*, 6 (Supplement B): 3–11.

Jensen T.S., Baron R., Haanpää M., Kalso E., Loeser J.D., Rice A.S.C. and Treede R.D. (2011) 'A new definition of neuropathic pain', *Pain: Journal of the International Association for the Study of Pain*, 152(10): 2204–5.

Jordan, A.L., Eccleston, C. and Osborn, M. (2007) 'Being a parent of the adolescent with complex chronic pain: an interpretive phenomenological analysis', *European Journal of Pain*, 11: 49–56.

Korhan, E.A., Uyar, M., Eyigor, C., Hakverdioglu Yont, G., Celik, S. and Khorshid, L. (2013) 'The effect of music therapy on pain in patients with neuropathic pain', *Pain Managment Nursing*, e-pub doi: 10.1016.j.pmn.2012.10.006.

Krause, S.J. and Backonja, M.M. (2003) 'Development of a neuropathic pain questionnaire', *Clinical Journal of Pain*, 19: 306–14.

McCracken, L.M., Gauntlett-Gilbert, J. and Eccleston, C. (2010) 'Acceptance of pain in adolescents with chronic pain: validation of an adapted assessment instrument and preliminary correlation analysis', *European Journal of Pain*, 14: 316–20.

Meyer-Rosberg, K., Kvarnstrom, A., Kinman, E., Gordh, T., Nordfors, L. and Kristofferson, A. (2001) 'Peripheral neuropathic pain – a multidimensional burden for patients', *European Journal of Pain*, 5: 379–89.

Newton, B.J., Southall, J.L., Raphael, J.H., Ashford, R.L. and Lermarchand, K. (2010) 'A narrative review of the impact of disbelief in chronic pain', *Pain Management Nursing*, 14 (3): 161–71.

Poole, H.M., Murphy, P. and Nurmikko, T.J. (2009) 'Development and preliminary validation of the NePIQoL: a quality-of-life measure for neuropathic pain', *Journal of Pain and Symptom Management*, 37 (2): 233–45.

Rahman, W. and Dickinson, A.H. (2011) 'Recent developments in neuropathic pain mechanisms: implications for treatment', *Reviews in Pain*, 5 (2): 21–31.

Rowbotham, D.J. (2002) 'Neuropathic pain and quality of life', *European Journal of Pain*, 6 (Supplement B): 19–24.

Schwartzman, R., Grothusen, J. and Kiefer, T. (2001) 'Neuropathic central pain: epidemiology, etiology and treatment options', *Archives of Neurology*, 58 (10): 1547–50.

Simons, L.E., Kaczynski, K.J., Conroy, C. and Logan, D.E. (2012) 'Fear of pain in the context of intensive pain rehabilitation among children and adolescents with neuropathic pain: associations with treatment response', *The Journal of Pain*, 13 (12): 1151–61.

Twycross, A., Dowden, S.J. and Bruce, E. (2009) *Managing Pain in Children*. Oxford: Wiley Blackwell.

Watson, C.P.N (2007) 'Chronic non-cancer pain predominantly neuropathic pain and the long term safety and efficacy of opioids', *European Journal of Pain*, 11 (S1): S1–S57.

Chapter 15

Organisational Imperatives and Individual Responsibility to Avoid Poor Pain Management

Tom's Story

Ruth's and Tom's Story

I have given a great deal of thought to this and following a discussion with my husband, Adrian, we wonder if you would be interested in our story as parents.

I am not sure whether you know Bernie, but our son Tom, aged nineteen, died four years ago following six months of chemo and radiotherapy from a rare malignant brain tumour. Tom's end of life care was poor in hospital particularly in relation to pain control. He had spinal and brain secondaries and was paralysed for the last few weeks of his life. On the children's ward in the teaching hospital where he was cared for he had several breakdowns in pain which were distressing for him as well as his family and friends. Adrian and I were very distressed for him not only because of the pain Tom suffered but what we thought were humiliating circumstances for him; these episodes, as you can imagine, haunt us still.

In fact, we totally lost confidence in the nursing and medical team and it was only when he returned home that his pain came under control because of input from our dedicated GP who visited us daily and daily phone calls from a wonderful adult consultant at the local Marie Curie Hospice.

After Tom died we complained in writing to the hospital about his poor care and pain control, giving instances (I kept a diary), but in their response we did not even get an apology or acknowledgement that there was any poor practice. This, on top of our grieving, was hard to bear but we persisted and in the end got some changes put in place by going to see the Professor (of Palliative Care) who contacted the Chief Executive of the hospital. The Chief Executive ordered an audit to take place; the findings showed that: (1) there were no standards in place, and (2) there were poor working practices. As a result of this, all teenagers in pain are now being referred to the Adult Pain Team for hospital-based management rather than being 'managed' by the staff on the children's ward. There is now a dedicated Teenage Cancer Unit which may also help other young people like Tom.

However, I remain sceptical about pain control in general on children's wards and young people's units. I hope you are brave enough in your book to highlight the many bad practices that can happen and basically be a 'warts and all' book.

Adrian's and Tom's Story

Bernie, I have just read the chapter. What Ruth may not have told you is that Tom's pain stemmed mainly from the spinal mets, so it was neurological and manifested itself as a severe 'burning' in his legs. They tried many pain relief options – including methadone! The staff did not seem to have a clue about cancer pain management – did not know about fentanyl patches or lollypops. They were clueless about patient tolerance to morphine-based drugs and the cancer-related doubling protocols.

They had no knowledge of the side effects of radiotherapy – Tom had 8 Grays to his spinal column and this, as you would expect, gave him severe diarrhoea. They also had no knowledge of the short-term and long-term effects of cytotoxic Cx drugs! After I brought this to their attention it took them 36 hours to prescribe imodium – I purchased it from Boots and gave it to him myself.

However, when I checked his drug charts I saw that he was still being given a laxative, as he had been constipated prior to the Rx. When I brought this to the ward sister's attention she said I was a grieving parent and over-reacting.

Tom was 19 years old, 5'6' tall and about 14 stone; paralysed from the waist down. It took them five days to get a portable hoist onto the ward and when it arrived there were only two people who knew how to make the transfer using the slings – myself and a third year student nurse.

To put these comments in perspective, at the time of Tom's illness I was a third year student on the Radiotherapy and Oncology course at [name of hospital] and can say that the treatment Tom received at [name] Centre was far more caring and professional that he received on [name of hospital ward].

The only good thing I can say about the ward is that they had a day room and operated a relaxed visiting regime so Tom had his friends with him, coming and going, from 11a.m. until 11p.m.

Introduction

Ruth's, Adrian's and Tom's story are infinitely painful to read. Ruth and Adrian had to face Tom's death while having to deal with the distress and humiliation that resulted from the inadequate management of his pain. Watching your child experience persistent and severe pain is a terrifying experience for parents. It reduces their capacity to be 'proper' parents. Despite a desperate desire to protect, help and make things better for their child, they are often helpless, emotionally drained and reliant on professionals to act on their behalf. The experiences that Ruth and Adrian describe frame their memories of Tom and these continue to hurt them and 'haunt them'. The loss of confidence in nursing staff and the poor practice they witnessed reflect a setting in which care was inadequate and staff had insufficient expertise to instigate appropriate pain management. Many things seem to have gone wrong in the hospital setting and it is with a sense of relief that we read how Tom's pain 'came under control' once he was home and when he and his family became enfolded within a compassionate, caring and expert team of people.

Tom certainly deserved better pain management than he received when he was in hospital and Tom and his parents should have been better supported. He deserved to have 'access to specialised treatment and services' and 'access to suitably qualified multi-disciplinary medical specialists' (Cancer Charter Org 2013).

Tom's parents are perhaps unusual in that at the time of Tom's illness Adrian was a 'third year student on the Radiotherapy and Oncology course' and his mother, Ruth, is a children's nurse whose research and writing address chronic illness and end of life care.[1] However, first and foremost they were Tom's parents and they found it difficult to influence his care in hospital. In Ruth's chapter in a textbook on palliative care for children and their families, she writes that a failure to manage children's pain at end of life is 'unpardonable, precisely because modern medicine does have the technical means to reduce nearly all pain' (Davies 2009: 178). Ruth and Adrian intimately know how unpardonable it is for professionals to fail to provide good pain management and compassionate care. We take the failure that is the centre of Ruth's and Adrian's stories[2] as the focal point for this chapter and we explore some of the key issues related to pain management and palliative care. We also consider how good pain management for end of life care is an individual, organisational, societal and – ultimately a moral – responsibility.

Prevalence of persisting pain at end of life

Inadequate treatment of pain is a global problem. The World Health Organization (WHO) (2012: 1) estimates that 'around 5.7 billion people live in countries where moderate and severe pain is not adequately treated' and 'over 80% of the world population will have insufficient analgesia'. This figure provides a clear and stark context for the significantly different issues facing professionals managing end of life pain in countries such as the UK compared with those working in developing countries. The WHO (2012: 1) state that 'more than 90 percent of the global consumption of strong opioids occurred in Australia, Canada, New Zealand, the United States of America, the United Kingdom and several other European countries'.

It might be expected that societies would, as a matter of moral course, provide good services for children suffering pain and distress. Yet despite the availability of opioids, other medications and additional fundamental resources, many children in apparently resource-rich countries do experience unrelieved pain at the end of life. Houlahan et al. (2006) note that most children in the USA do not receive high-quality end of life care, and only 1 per cent of children who need end of life care have hospice care (Stephenson 2000). Most children's hospitals in the USA do not have trained paediatric palliative

---

[1]Ruth emailed me a copy of her chapter not long after she had sent me her story. In the email she 'wondered if I would be interested in the chapter'. I was interested because it acts as a kind of academic companion text to her 'personal' story.

[2]Adrian and Ruth were kind and brave enough to read a close to final draft of this chapter. I cannot begin to imagine how much courage that takes but I am thankful that they did this. In response to the chapter, Adrian emailed me 'his story' which provides additional context and he was happy for this to be used in the book.

care specialists and in 2007, very few had designated paediatric palliative care services (Friedrichsdorf et al. 2007b). In contrast, Ellis et al.'s (2003: 26) survey in Canada found that mostly children with cancer have 'access to the components of best practice pain management'. Compared to the provision for adult patients, provision of services for end of life and palliative care for children in the UK is not as good (Friedrichsdorf et al. 2007b). As a result of this deficit in service provision, access to specialist services is often patchy and inequitable (National Institute for Health and Clinical Excellence 2005a) and depends as much on geographical good or bad luck as on genuinely coherent planning and commissioning. The report *When Children Die* (Field et al. 2002) asserts that even though better care is possible, organisational and financial issues mean that some families have to 'choose between curative or life-prolonging care and palliative services, in particular, hospice care'.

However, although the numbers of children requiring paediatric palliative care are low compared to the adult population, prevalence studies suggest that in the UK 1.5–1.9/10,000 of children aged 0–19 years die each year from a life-limiting condition. In the USA figures vary between >11,000 children and young adults (Wiener et al. 2012) and >13,000 children (Houlahan et al. 2006) dying per year from life-limiting illness. From a purely statistical perspective, these numbers may be small and the health economics of providing services may not financially 'add up' but the costs and consequences to those families who have to manage without specialist pain support are immense.

Suffering and distress at the end of life

Many children experience a range of distressing symptoms at the end of life (Houlahan et al. 2006) and many children are highly symptomatic (Friedrichsdorf et al. 2007b). During the last week of life children with life-limiting illness and/ or cancer suffer from a mean of more than 10 different symptoms (Drake et al. 2003; Schiessl et al. 2008). The more severe the symptoms, the greater the potential delay in instigating effective treatment (Miller et al. 2011). Pain and nausea were the symptoms that parents most commonly associated with their child's suffering (von Lützau et al. 2012). Pain and fear are often co-associated and pain is regularly identified as a fear-inducing symptom for hospitalised children with cancer (Enskär et al. 2007) and children with life-limiting illness (Friedrichsdorf et al. 2007b).

The 'absolute number of children who die in pain is not known' (Friebert 2009) although Schiessl et al. (2008) state that between 75–92 per cent of dying children do experience pain as a leading symptom. Despite the fact that better and more consistent care could result in radical improvements in the management of a child's pain and the associated anticipatory distress, all too often fear is added to the already toxic mix of a child's suffering. Wolfe et al. (2000: 332) report that 'substantial suffering' in the last month of life was not uncommon.

A more recent study conducted in Australia found that 84 per cent of parents reported that their child had suffered 'a lot' or 'a great deal' from at least one symptom, most commonly pain (46 per cent) in their last month of life – although 'treatment was successful in 47% of those with pain' (Heath et al. 2010). Pain was also shown to add to the load of suffering experienced by children in Tomlinson et al.'s (2011) Canadian study. Clearly if the findings of these studies from the USA, Canada and Australia are indicative of children's experiences elsewhere there is certainly room for substantial improvement in pain management services and practices. All too often children's physical, emotional, and spiritual needs fail to be met (Field et al. 2002).

These studies focus on management of pain and suffering in the developed world where there is generally ready access to core resources such as analgesia. The situation faced by children and families in less well-resourced settings is worse. Even within 'rich' countries there are inequities of provision, for example, children receiving Medicaid are shown to be prescribed disproportionately less opioid analgesia than 'non-Medicaid' children.

Woodgate and Degner's (2003) grounded theory study found that children and their families equated cancer with suffering and expressed the feeling that suffering is perceived to be necessary to fight cancer. This partial and somewhat uneasy acceptance of 'short term pain for long term gain' (Woodgate and Degner 2003: 29) makes some sense in the light of cancer survival being perceived as more important than the pain that accompanies cancer and its treatment. However, when hope for survival is lost, then pain and other distressing symptoms cannot easily be associated with any gains.

Managing cancer pain: an overview of issues

Raphael et al.'s (2010) thought-provoking discussion paper about the management of cancer pain emphasises the need for a more comprehensive, multi-modal, mechanism-based model of managing cancer pain. Interestingly and paradoxically Raphael et al. (2010: 745) note that the:

> [the] trend over the past two decades to exclude pain specialists from mainstream cancer pain management means that they tend to be called in at a very late stage as 'last resort.' Patients may be missing out on benefits of combined multidisciplinary care from palliative care as well as pain medicine.

Cancer pain is complex. It can involve multiple sites and can arise from inflammatory, ischaemic, neuropathic and compression mechanisms resulting from disease, procedural or metastatic processes. It can be acute as well as chronic and, for children who survive, then persisting pain may be an ongoing feature of their survivorship. Adrian describes Tom's pain as 'stemming mainly from the spinal mets [metastases], so it was neurological and manifested itself as a severe "burning" in his legs' and he goes on later to explain that Tom 'was paralysed from the waist down'. The combination suggests an imaginably awful experience which required – but did not get – immediate, ongoing and undivided professional attention.

The complexity of pain arising from different causes and requiring different approaches to treatment clearly creates challenges and can be overwhelming for less experienced practitioners trying to provide care for the young person and their family. This may have been what occurred in Tom's situation. However, even if this did occur, an assessment of Tom's pain should have indicated that the situation was out of control, and this in turn should have triggered a request for additional support. Lack of experience does not excuse inaction. A multidisciplinary approach should be used drawing on a range of different management strategies (Bennett and Givens 2011).

Traditionally the WHO ladder has provided a three-stepped pharmacological approach to pain management, with the middle of the three steps focusing on the use of mild to moderate opioids. However, for children with persisting pain due to medical illness, the recommendation is now for a two-stepped approach for pharmacological intervention which misses out the 'middle step' (see Figure 15.1).

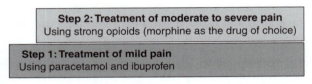

Figure 15.1   The WHO two-step ladder

Medical illness is defined by the WHO (2012: 4) in their guidance on persisting pain as being 'specific situations of on-going tissue damage where there is a clear role for pharmacological treatment'.

If used effectively, the four key concepts (World Health Organization 2012) are expected to be able to relieve pain for most children experiencing pain as a result of medical illness:

1. *A two-stepped strategy* (as in Figure 15.1) for the use of analgesic medicines:
   Step 1: Treatment of mild pain with paracetamol and ibuprofen; and
   Step 2: Treatment of moderate pain with morphine as the drug of choice
2. *Dosing at regular intervals* rather than on an 'as-needed' basis
3. *Using the appropriate route of administration* which, wherever possible and appropriate, should be oral. The subcutaneous can also be considered when the oral route is not available. The intramuscular route should be avoided.
4. *Adapting treatment to the individual child* and adjusting the dose to the child's changing needs, providing rescue doses when there is breakthrough pain and acknowledging that there is no fixed maximum dose for a child with persisting pain.

Each of these concepts provides a clear basis for analgesic treatment and also a starting point for evaluation of the effectiveness of the intervention. Although Ruth does not give details of Tom's medication, it appears that his breakthrough pain was poorly managed and rescue doses were either inadequate or not provided. Breakthrough pain is a challenge but in most circumstances it can be managed reasonably effectively (Friedrichsdorf et al. 2007a).

However, as good as the WHO's (2012) clear pharmacological-based approach is, it concentrates solely on analgesia and does not acknowledge the equally important contribution of a biopsychosocial approach to pain management. Supportive, holistic care considers three strands of therapeutic intent – disease, patient and family – across the whole of the patient trajectory (Figure 15.2). Had Ruth and Adrian felt that they and Tom were receiving adequate levels of supportive care and pain management, then it is likely that their overall experience would have been less stressful.

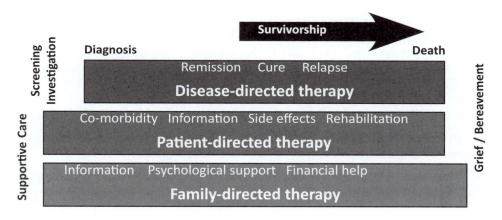

Figure 15.2   Models of cancer pain therapies
Developed from Raphael et al. (2010)

The need to closely link disease-directed, patient-directed and family-directed pain therapies is clearly a sounder approach than solely focusing on the administration of medication as the panacea for suffering and treatment of pain. This is particularly important because psychological distress increases with the intensity of cancer. Had the staff caring for Tom used Raphael et al.'s (2010) model to frame his management then maybe some of the small but vital elements would not have been overlooked. Adrian's despair about the lack of knowledge of adverse effects of cytotoxic drugs is evident. Having asked for Tom to be prescribed medication to manage diarrhoea, he takes things into his own hands by going out and buying it from the local chemist and then 'gave it to him myself'. He then notes that Tom was still being given a laxative. Even if staff were not familiar with the side effects of cytotoxics they should have been to alert to stopping the administration of laxatives when Tom was having diarrhoea. When we are caring for young people like Tom, we need to be able to think holistically about what we are doing and look at the big picture (cancer) as well as the small picture (such as diarrhoea) and act appropriately

Palliative care and early integration

Hui et al. (2012) discuss the lack of definitional clarity for many of the terms used within the supportive and palliative care literature and the consequences of this in terms of generating a clear and consistent understanding of this area of practice. However, the WHO definition states:

> Palliative care for children represents a special, albeit closely related, field to adult palliative care. WHO's definition of palliative care appropriate for children and their families is as follows; the principles apply to other paediatric chronic disorders;

> - Palliative care for children is the active total care of the child's body, mind and spirit, and also involves giving support to the family.

> - It begins when illness is diagnosed, and continues regardless of whether or not a child receives treatment directed at the disease.

> - Health providers must evaluate and alleviate a child's physical, psychological, and social distress.

> - Effective palliative care requires a broad multidisciplinary approach that includes the family and makes use of available community resources; it can be successfully implemented even if resources are limited.

> - It can be provided in tertiary care facilities, in community health centres and even in children's homes.

Early integration of palliative care into curative care is proposed as being an important means of managing symptoms (National Institute for Health and Clinical Excellence 2005b), improving care and helping families (Field et al. 2002). Research shows that there are often delays in early integration (Bruera and Hui 2010, 2012), that paediatricians do not easily adopt early referral for palliative care (Thompson et al. 2013) and early integration was not always triggered sufficiently early to make the best use of the skills and expertise of the palliative care team (Gaertner et al. 2012).

Organisational and individual imperatives

Managing end of life pain well requires a commitment from the individuals who provide care as well as from the organisations in which those individuals work. Where care breaks down it is often as a result of failures at different organisational levels. The barriers that impede good care and the factors which promote good care need to be understood in order to prevent situations such as Ruth and Adrian describe occurred during Tom's hospitalisation.

Barriers to effective pain management

Beyond the usual barriers to effective pain management (Kost-Byerly and Chalkiadis 2012), there are considerable and diverse barriers to optimal pain management in paediatric palliative care. These include medical, psychosocial, cultural, financial (Sourkes et al. 2005) and geographical problems (World Health Organization 2012). Cultural issues relate both to the ethnic and cultural background of the children and families but also to organizational and professional cultures in which palliative care occurs. In some settings, palliative care is seen as 'giving-up' on the child (Sourkes et al. 2005) rather than providing a richer, enhanced and more comprehensive care pathway. There are a number of different ways of overcoming these barriers. Some barriers are societal (e.g., lack of policy drivers that prioritise pain, lack of funding and other resources). Other barriers are at the level of the individual (e.g., lack of knowledge and/or fear of opioid use, perceptions that curative and palliative care are mutually exclusive). Some barriers can be overcome through changes of attitude and a shift in established but outmoded practices.

Imperatives to improve pain management

The fact that many children still experience unrelieved pain at end of life is, as Solomon and Browning (2005: 9055) state, a 'symptom of insufficient commitment'. There are many different elements that contribute to an effective organisational approach including a commitment at an individual and organisational level to getting things right for children and their families. Organisational planning is essential if pain management is to be effective. Based on their own experience of enhancing care, Friedrichsdorf et al. (2007a: 541–2) propose that a plan includes: 'assessment and goal definition'; 'workgroup formation'; 'assessment of opportunities, allies and stakeholders'; 'assessment of barriers'; 'development of action plan'; and 'reassessment'. Other factors include the use of guidelines, the implementation of best practice, auditing pain management practice, undertaking quality improvement of services, education of staff, and planning and commissioning services

Individual responsibility, leadership and self-awareness

Everyone involved in a child's care has a responsibility to ensure that that child receives the best possible pain management and they also have a responsibility for ensuring that barriers are broken down and factors that support success are in place. This would seem to be an obvious statement to make. However, Thompson et al.'s (2010, 2013) research showed that only 32.3 per cent of paediatricians, generalists and specialists in their study perceived themselves as having primary and individual responsibility for managing severe, chronic pain; most saw this responsibility as lying with pain specialists. Although onward referral to a specialist or an acute care centre might be the most appropriate action, this does not in and of itself absolve the referrer from continuing responsibility.

Not every health care professional will have expertise in palliative pain management. Stayer (2012) notes that nurses caring for children who require palliative care may not always be sufficiently well prepared to undertake this complex role. Friebert (2009: 749) acknowledges that sometimes health professionals overestimate their own skills. However, every professional should be able to assess a child's pain and suffering and seek advice on best management and/or refer for specialist support whilst continuing to be active in their efforts to effectively, actively and compassionately manage the child's pain and suffering.

Looking in from the outside it would appear that one of the failures in Tom's care was a lack of leadership. Without leadership, even strong and committed people can fail to do their best. Understandings of, and approaches to, leadership have evolved from the notion of individual leadership to more recent approaches that include transformational leadership (Burns 1978) through action-centred leadership (Adair 2002), to various forms of distributed leadership (e.g., Diamond and Spillane 2007). In distributed leadership, 'leadership agency' is undertaken by many members of the organisation (Currie and Lockett 2011; Mackian and Simons 2013). If there had been an action-oriented leader or more distributed leadership on Tom's ward, it is likely that Tom's pain management would have been of a higher standard because pain management, maintaining standards and improving performance would have been prioritised. All pain management requires good leadership, and this is especially so when the pain is complex and outside of the ordinary parameters of a practice setting.

Guidelines, policies and the importance of audit

As Ellis et al. (2003: 26) note, the 'prevention and relief of pain and distress should be part of an institutional commitment to comfort for children with cancer'. Many policies, guidelines and best practice documents identify appropriate standards of pain management and care and are readily available on the Internet. For example, detailed advice on the care and management of teenagers with cancer, that acknowledges their particular needs, is now readily available (National Institute for Health and Clinical Excellence 2005b; Smith and Case 2012). In brief, the core recommendations state that 'multidisciplinary protocols should be in place to support the safe and effective use of analgesia', 'daily access to play specialists or, for older children and young people, activity coordinators to assist in preparation for painful procedures' and 'adequate provision of general anaesthesia for patients undergoing regular painful procedures' (National Institute for Health and Clinical Excellence 2005b: 60).

However, although clinical practice guidelines exist, they are not consistently used within practice and clinical settings may not have local pain protocols to guide practice (Tyc et al. 1998); this has consequences for determining standards for clinical practice. Implementation of pain protocols can be challenging (Megens et al. 2008; Ang and Chow 2010) and it is disappointing that in many cases pain practice does not improve consistently or to the level hoped for. However, the use of protocols and audit does highlight where practice needs improvement so that measures can be implemented. Without a rigorous commitment to evidence-based practice guided by protocols, poor practice is invisible (National Institute for Health and Clinical Excellence 2005b). The findings of the audit instigated as a result of Ruth's complaint were 'there were no standards in place ... poor working practices'. Ruth describes a setting which failed her son and which probably had no idea that it was failing. The results of the audit are shocking and probably were shocking to the professionals working in the setting.

However, significant quality improvements in pain practice can occur as a result of comprehensive approaches to the implementation of local guidelines and protocols (Simons and MacDonald 2006; Oakes et al. 2008). One excellent example of this is the detailed model of care developed by Houlahan et al. (2006) to improve the end of life care for children suffering from escalating and intractable symptoms. Zernikow et al.'s (2008) impressive nationwide quality improvement plan for the management of children's cancer pain in Germany was successful in terms of improving the structure, process and outcome quality in the settings which were actively engaged. Audit and feedback strategies can be effective in helping to promote the implementation of clinical practice guidelines (Dulko 2007; Dulko et al. 2010).

Scrupulous documentation is key to good pain management. However, pain management documentation is not always consistently completed and there are often omissions in recording: this has consequences for the quality of pain management and benchmarking (Samuels and Fetzer 2009; Samuels 2012; Simons 2012).

Education

Education is an important element in promoting good pain management in end of life care as it can address deficits in core issues such as knowledge, skills and attitudes. Education also provides an opportunity for 'cultivating the moral imagination' which helps to promote the concept that pain management is a personal and professional moral duty (Browning et al. 2005). Many different approaches to education about pain management and palliative care have been developed with varying degrees of success. Adriaansen and van Achterberg (2008) conclude that the most successful courses were those that were integrated, focused on several themes and were underpinned by a diversity of didactical methods.

The outcomes of effective education are clear: for example: Enskär et al. (2007) show that staff who had increased knowledge of symptom management demonstrated better attitudes and that increased education of health professionals results in better symptom management.

Conclusion

Near the end of Ruth's story she talks of being 'sceptical about pain control in general on children's wards and young people's units'. Based on her experience with Tom's lack of care, this is hardly surprising. In fact, looking at the broader picture both within the UK and globally, Tom's experience is not unusual. Although it is clear that the pain associated with end of life can be well managed and we know what the barriers and success factors are, it is also clear that too many children suffer persistent and breakthrough pain. Ruth, writing in 2009 as both a nurse and a mother, is emphatic that this situation is 'unpardonable'.

What is clear is that the situation can be changed, providing health professionals have the will and commitment to make the change and to accept that they can either be part of the problem or the solution. When Adrian brought the fact that Tom was still being prescribed a laxative even though he had diarrhoea and had just been prescribed imodium to deal with the diarrhoea to her attention, the ward sister could have accepted responsibility and dealt with the situation. Instead, Adrian explains that 'she said I was a grieving parent and over-reacting'. Parents watching their child suffer are under unimaginable pressure and their responses are not over-reactions – they are reactions to what is happening. As health care professionals we need to accept that we are responsible for our actions and improve our practice and act as leaders.

Accepting individual responsibility for making changes and improving practice is essential. The National Council for Palliative Care (2010: 2) talk about how everyone involved in end of life care can 'change care here and now in the small and thoughtful things that they do'. Every act of kindness and compassion that we show to a child and their family is important. Every time we reflect on our care and determine to learn more, do better, check protocols, read the evidence underpinning practice, and lobby for change and improvement, this is helping to advance the care and management of children suffering pain.

Suffering at the end of life should not be seen as inevitable. Our humanity should help guide our practice and if it does so this should mean that Tom's story, which is set in the mid-2000s, becomes a story from our past rather than from our present.

Key Points

- Inadequate treatment of persisting pain at the end of life is a global problem even in resource-rich countries.
- Many children experience a range of distressing symptoms at the end of life.
- Persisting plan is complex as it arises from different causes and required different treatment approaches.
- The WHO recommends a two stepped approach for pharmacological intervention for children with persisting pain due to medical illness.
- A bio-psychological approach to pain management is vital.
- Early management of persisting pain requires both good leadership and individuals accepting responsibility.
- Clinical practice guidelines exist but they are not consistently used and not all clinical settings not have local pain protocols to guide practice.
- Effective pain managment is a personal and professional moral duty.

Additional Resources and Reading

- Recommendations for pain management from *Improving Outcomes with Children and Young People with Cancer*:
  - www.nice.org.uk/nicemedia/live/10899/28876/28876.pdf
- Lucy Grealy's book is an evocative read about some of the challenges that a child faces dealing with cancer treatment, surgery and becoming an adult:
  - Grealy, L. (2003) *Autobiography of a Face*. Boston, MA: Harper Perennial.
- Stupidcancer addresses the particular needs of young adults with cancer:
  - stupidcancer.org/index.shtml
- Information written for young people with cancer can be found at:
  - www.macmillan.org.uk/Cancerinformation/teensandyoungadults/Infoforteensandyoungadults.aspx
- Elliot Krane's video 'The mystery of chronic pain' can be viewed by linking to:
  - www.ted.com/talks/elliot_krane_the_mystery_of_chronic_pain.html
- Anne Grinyer's books provide a good starting point for reading about palliative care, e.g.
  - Grinyer, A. (2012) *Palliative and End of Life Care for Children and Young People*: *Home, Hospice and Hospital*. Oxford: Wiley Blackwell.
- An interesting talk on leadership can be viewed at:
  - www.ted.com/talks/drew_dudley_everyday_leadership.html
- There are some great materials at the NHS Leadership Academy website:
  - www.leadershipacademy.nhs.uk/discover/leadership-framework-self-assessment-tool/

References

Adair, J. (2002) *Effective Strategic Leadership*. London: Macmillan.

Adriaansen, M. and van Achterberg, T. (2008) 'The content and effects of palliative care courses for nurses: a literature review', *International Journal of Nursing Studies*, 45 (3): 471–85.

Ang, E. and Chow, Y.L. (2010) 'General pain assessment among patients with cancer in an acute care setting: a best practice implementation project', *International Journal of Evidence-based Healthcare*, 8 (2): 90–6.

Bennett, R. and Givens, D. (2011) 'Easing suffering for a child with intractable pain at the end of life', *Journal of Pediatric Health Care*, 25 (3): 180–5.

Browning, D.M., Solomon, M.Z. and Initiative for Pediatric Palliative Care (IPPC) Investigator Team (2005) 'The initiative for pediatric palliative care: an interdisciplinary educational approach for healthcare professionals', *Journal of Pediatric Nursing*, 20 (5): 326–34.

Bruera, E. and Hui, D. (2010) 'Integrating supportive and palliative care in the trajectory of cancer: establishing goals and models of care', *Journal of Clinical Oncology*, 28 (25): 4013–17.

Bruera, E. and Hui, D. (2012) 'Conceptual models for integrating palliative care at cancer centers', *Journal of Palliative Medicine*, 15 (11): 1261–9.

Burns, J.M. (1978) *Leadership*. London: Harper and Row.

Cancer Charter Org (2013) *International Charter of Rights for Young People with Cancer*. Available at www.cancercharter.org/issues.html (accessed 30 May 2013).

Currie, G. and Lockett, A. (2011) 'Distributing leadership in health and social care: concertive, conjoint or collective?', *International Journal of Management Reviews*, 13 (3): 286–300.

Davies, R. (2009) 'Caring for the child at end of life', in J. Price and P. McNeilly (eds), *Palliative Care for Children and Families: An Interdisciplinary Approach*. Basingstoke: Palgrave Macmillan, pp. 172–91.

Diamond, J.B. and Spillane, J.P. (2007) *Distributed Leadership in Practice*. Columbia University, New York: Teachers College.

Drake, R., Frost, J. and Collins, J.J. (2003) 'The symptoms of dying children', *Journal of Pain and Symptom Management*, 26 (1): 594–603.

Dulko, D. (2007) 'Audit and feedback as a clinical practice guideline implementation strategy: a model for acute care nurse practitioners', *Worldviews on Evidence-based Nursing*, 4 (4): 200–9.

Dulko, D., Hertz, E., Julien, J., Beck, S. and Mooney, K. (2010) 'Implementation of cancer pain guidelines by acute care nurse practitioners using an audit and feedback strategy', *Journal of the American Academy of Nurse Practitioners*, 22 (1): 45–55.

Ellis, J.A., McCarthy, P., Hershon, L., Horlin, R., Rattray, M. and Tierney, S. (2003) 'Pain practices: a cross-Canada survey of pediatric oncology centers', *Journal of Pediatric Oncology Nursing*, 20 (1): 26–35.

Enskär, K., Ljusegren, G., Berglund, G., Eaton, N., Harding, R., Mokoena, J., Chauke, M. and Moleki, M. (2007) 'Attitudes to and knowledge about pain and pain management, of nurses working with children with cancer: a comparative study between UK, South Africa and Sweden', *Journal of Research in Nursing*, 12 (5): 501–15.

Field, M.J., Behrman, R.E. and Committee on Palliative and End-of-Life Care for Children and Their Families (2002) *When Children Die: Improving Palliative and End-of-Life Care for Children and Their Families*. Washington, DC: The National Academies Press.

Friebert, S. (2009) 'Pain management for children with cancer at the end of life: beginning steps toward a standard of care', *Pediatric Blood and Cancer*, 52 (7): 749–50.

Friedrichsdorf, S.J., Finney, D., Bergin, M., Stevens, M. and Collins, J.J. (2007a) 'Breakthrough pain in children with cancer', *Journal of Pain and Symptom Management*, 34 (2): 209–16.

Friedrichsdorf, S.J., Remke, S., Symalla, B., Gibbon, C. and Chrastek, J. (2007b) 'Developing a pain and palliative care programme at a US children's hospital', *International Journal of Palliative Nursing*, 13 (11): 534–42.

Gaertner, J., Wolf, J., Frechen, S., Klein, U., Scheicht, D., Hellmich, M., Toepelt, K., Glossmann, J., Ostgathe, C., Hallek, M. and Voltz, R. (2012) 'Recommending early integration of palliative care – does it work?', *Supportive Care in Cancer*, 20 (3): 507–13.

Heath, J.A., Clarke, N.E., Donath, S.M., McCarthy, M., Anderson, V.A. and Wolfe, J. (2010) 'Symptoms and suffering at the end of life in children with cancer: an Australian perspective', *Medical Journal of Australia*, 192 (2): 71–5.

Houlahan, K.E., Branowicki, P.A., Mack, J.W., Dinning, C. and McCabe, M. (2006) 'Can end of life care for the pediatric patient suffering with escalating and intractable symptoms be improved?', *Journal of Pediatric Oncology Nursing*, 23 (1): 45–51.

Hui, D., Mori, M., Parsons, H.A., Kim, S.H., Li, Z., Damani, S. and Bruera, E. (2012) 'The lack of standard definitions in the supportive and palliative oncology literature', *Journal of Pain and Symptom Management*, 43 (3): 582–92.

Kost-Byerly, S. and Chalkiadis, G. (2012) 'Developing a pediatric pain service', *Paediatric Anaesthesia*, 22 (10): 1016–24.

Mackian, S. and Simons, J. (2013) *Leading, Managing, Caring: Understanding Leadership and Management in Health and Social Care*. London: Routledge in association with The Open University.

Megens, J.H.A.M., Van der Werff, D. and Knape, J.T.A. (2008) 'Quality improvement: implementation of a pain management policy in a university pediatric hospital', *Pediatric Anesthesia*, 18 (7): 620–7.

Miller, E., Jacob, E. and Hockenberry, M.J. (2011) 'Nausea, pain, fatigue, and multiple symptoms in hospitalized children with cancer', *Oncology Nursing Forum*, 38 (5): E382–E393.

National Council for Palliative Care (2010) *Small is Beautiful*. London: National Council for Palliative Care.

National Institute for Health and Clinical Excellence (2005a) *Improving Outcomes in Children and Young People with Cancer*. London: National Institute for Health and Clinical Excellence.

National Institute for Health and Clinical Excellence (2005b) *Improving Outcomes with Children and Young People with Cancer*. London: Department of Health.

Oakes, L.L., Anghelescu, D.L., Windsor, K.B. and Barnhill, P.D. (2008) 'An institutional quality improvement initiative for pain management for pediatric cancer inpatients', *Journal of Pain and Symptom Management*, 35 (6): 656–69.

Raphael, J., Ahmedzai, S., Hester, J., Urch, C., Barrie, J., Williams, J., Farquhar-Smith, P., Fallon, M., Hoskin, P., Robb, K., Bennett, M.I., Haines, R., Johnson, M., Bhaskar, A., Chong, S., Duarte, R. and Sparkes, E. (2010) 'Cancer pain: part 1: pathophysiology; oncological, pharmacological, and psychological treatments: a perspective from the British Pain Society endorsed by the UK Association of Palliative Medicine and the Royal College of General Practitioners', *Pain Medicine*, 11 (5): 742–64.

Samuels, J.G. and Fetzer, S. (2009) 'Pain management documentation quality as a reflection of nurses' clinical judgment', *Journal of Nursing Care Quality*, 24 (3): 223–31.

Samuels, J.G. (2012) 'Abstracting pain management documentation from the electronic medical record: comparison of three hospitals', *Applied Nursing Research*, 25 (2): 89–94.

Schiessl, C., Gravou, C., Zernikow, B., Sittl, R. and Griessinger, N. (2008) 'Use of patient-controlled analgesia for pain control in dying children', *Supportive Care in Cancer*, 16 (5): 531–6.

Simons, J. (2012) 'Nurses do assess pain, they just don't write it down!', *Journal of Child Health Care*, 16 (1): 3–4.

Simons, J. and MacDonald, L.M. (2006) 'Changing practice: implementing validated paediatric pain assessment tools', *Journal of Child Health Care*, 10 (2): 160–76.

Smith, S. and Case, L. (2012) *Blueprint of Care for Teenagers and Young Adults with Cancer*. London: Teenage Cancer Trust & Teenagers and Young Adults with Cancer.

Solomon, M.Z. and Browning, D. (2005) 'Pediatric palliative care: relationships matter and so does pain control', *Journal of Clinical Oncology*, 23 (36): 9055–7.

Sourkes, B., Frankel, L., Brown, M., Contro, N., Benitz, W., Case, C., Good, J., Jones, L., Komejan, J., Modderman-Marshall, J., Reichard, W., Sentivany-Collins, S. and Sunde, C. (2005) 'Food, toys, and love: pediatric palliative care', *Current Problems in Pediatric and Adolescent Health Care*, 35 (9): 350–86.

Stayer, D. (2012) 'Pediatric palliative care: a conceptual analysis for pediatric nursing practice', *Journal of Pediatric Nursing*, 27 (4): 350–6.

Stephenson, J. (2000) 'Palliative and hospice care needed for children with life-threatening conditions', *Journal of the American Medical Association*, 284 (19): 2437–8.

Thompson, L.A., Knapp, C.A., Feeg, V., Madden, V.L. and Shenkman, E.A. (2010) 'Pediatricians' management practices for chronic pain', *Journal of Palliative Medicine*, 13 (2): 171–8.

Thompson, L.A., Meinert, E., Baker, K. and Knapp, C. (2013) 'Chronic pain management as a barrier to pediatric palliative care', *The American Journal of Hospice & Palliative Care*, doi: 10.1177/1049909112473632.

Tomlinson, D., Hinds, P.S., Bartels, U., Hendershot, E. and Sung, L.L. (2011) 'Parent reports of quality of life for pediatric patients with cancer with no realistic chance of Cure', *Journal of Clinical Oncology*, 29 (6): 639–45.

Tyc, V.L., Bieberich, A.A., Hinds, P. and Sifford, L. (1998) 'A survey of pain services for pediatric oncology patients: their composition and function', *Journal of Pediatric Oncology Nursing*, 15 (4): 207–15.

von Lützau, P., Otto, M., Hechler, T., Metzing, S., Wolfe, J. and Zernikow, B. (2012) 'Children dying from cancer: parents' perspectives on symptoms, quality of life, characteristics of death, and end-of-life decisions', *Journal of Palliative Care*, 28 (4): 274–81.

Wiener, L., Zadeh, S., Battles, H., Baird, K., Ballard, E., Osherow, J. and Pao, M. (2012) 'Allowing adolescents and young adults to plan their end-of-life care', *Pediatrics*, 130 (5): 897–905.

Wolfe, J., Grier, H.E., Klar, N., Levin, S.B., Ellenbogen, J.M., Salem-Schatz, S., Emanuel, E.J. and Weeks, J.C. (2000) 'Symptoms and suffering at the end of life in children with cancer', *The New England Journal of Medicine*, 342 (5): 326–33.

Woodgate, R.L. and Degner, L.F. (2003) 'Expectations and beliefs about children's cancer symptoms: perspectives of children with cancer and their families', *Oncology Nursing Forum*, 30 (3): 479–91.

World Health Organization (2012) *Persisting Pain in Children. Highlights for Policymakers Extracted from the WHO Guidelines on the Pharmacological Treatment of Persisting Pain in Children with Medical Illnesses*. Geneva: World Health Organization.

World Health Organization. Definition of Palliative Care for Children. Available at www. who.int/cancer/palliative/definition/en/ (accessed January 2014).

Zernikow, B., Hasan, C., Hechler, T., Huebner, B., Gordon, D. and Michel, E. (2008) 'Stop the pain! A nation-wide quality improvement programme in paediatric oncology pain control', *European Journal of Pain*, 12: 819–33.

Conclusion

An Ending as Well as Potential New Beginnings

In this book on pain stories we have gained a very privileged insight into the sensory, affective and evaluative aspects of children's and their families' pain alongside the reactions of health care professionals as they engage and respond to children's pain.

Time and again as you read the stories you are drawn into the first-hand experiences of pain, which create very moving accounts. They range from Erik's story of existential pain (Chapter 6), focusing on how the nurse used all her skills and judgement in stepping forward and stepping back to facilitate a family being together at the end of life, to the anger and sheer powerlessness of Dave (Chapter 9) where he describes his son Sam as 'crushed by pain', and wanting to scream and the pain to go away.

A common thread running through all the stories and fundamental to the management of children's pain is the issue of engagement. In the stories where there is ineffective management of pain the consequence is usually unnecessary suffering on the part of the child or young person. Samuel (Chapter 14), for example, experienced denial of this pain when attending accident and emergency, and Tom (Chapter 15) experienced severe cancer-related pain due to the unit he was on having no protocols for pain and perhaps nurses feeling overwhelmed by this pain. On the other hand where nurses reach out to a child or young person we hear inspiring stories of engagement. In Maria's story (Chapter 13), for example, her nurse's offer of pain-relieving interventions are initially refused but, through gentle persistence and reaching out to Maria, the nurse gains Maria's trust which results in her pain being relieved.

The stories also evoke the stress and emotional burden for those caring for children and young people in pain. In Lily's and Lucas's story (Chapter 1) we hear from an ANNP using her skill and judgement to prevent or limit neonatal pain, hoping that the pharmacological and non-pharmacological methods of pain relief had been effective but being unsure due to Lily's level of prematurity. Tilli's mother (Chapter 3) talks of her despair over her small daughter's suffering from the repeated attempts at cannulation, and asks 'What about compassion, empathy and basic human kindness?' Rosie's mother (Chapter 8) expresses her frustration when those caring for her have not recognised her pain: 'Surely you can see the pain in her eyes, and her face and her body?'

Reading the stories can also throw surprising insights into children's perceptions of pain, for example Luci (Chapter 12) warns other children 'Don't let mums put things on your legs only if the doctor gave it to you!!' Luci's pain story focused not on her cuts and bruises from cartwheeling across the handle bars of her scooter, but on the pain of having her wounds dressed. In other stories children have used insightful descriptions to convey the power of their pain. Tanya Tia (Chapter 11) says 'pain is like a poison moving through my veins', and Hattie (Chapter 11) describes pain as 'like a monster I couldn't hide from'. These eloquent descriptions, which are poetic in nature, leave the reader in no doubt as to the overwhelming nature of these young persons' pain bringing into stark focus the limitations of a question that just asks for a 0–10 intensity score. The depth of feelings of anxiety and fear due to severe pain is very likely to be daunting for health care professionals to deal with, and may in some cases make them feel powerless to relieve such pain.

The concept of power is highlighted in the stories where helath care professionals are frustrated either with colleagues, as in Jennie's story (Chapter 2) where unhelpful advice is given to a mother as she takes her child home following surgery. Parents' stories have also suggested feelings of powerlessness where inequality is alluded to between parents and health care professionals, such as in Georgina's story (Chapter 3) or Rosie's story (Chapter 8) told by her mother, where she can clearly and unquestioningly recognise her daughter's pain but none of the health care professionals understand her perspective. In such situations those caring for Rosie appear to be in a position of authority. However, formal authority is only one source of power in an organisation; other sources include personal characteristics, expertise, and opportunity (Gaventa 2003). Furthermore, influential French philosopher Michael Foucault (1994) suggests that the power of interactions does not belong to an individual or a group of individuals but rather is a force in itself. This stance is developed by Wong's (2003) web of power (discussed in Chapter 2), which conveys clearly the relational aspects of power.

An understanding of power creates the possibility of forming more equitable relationships which recognise and acknowledge the complex operation of power between people. For example Wong's 'power-with' and-'power-from-within' can both be seen at work in many of the positive examples of effective management of children's pain, such as Becky's story (Chapter 7), where the two PICU nurses used their power to influence her analgesic prescriptions until Becky gained relief of her complex pain. Power is evident in Ahmet's story (Chapter 10) where his nurse decides to review his care and introduce a comprehensive pain assessment tool in order to facilitate Ahmet communicating his pain, followed by an effective pain management plan that resulted in his six months of pain coming to an end.

From Wong's web of power the expression of 'power-with', which focuses on finding common ground among practitioners' different interests and building collective strengths, is the form of power most likely to be beneficial in dealing with the everyday challenges of managing children's pain. The three positive aspects of Wong's model of power – power from within, power to and power with – provide sources of power that have considerable potential for positive action by health care professionals. Such a stance provides opportunities for both the prevention and reduction of pain, as well as the promotion of a culture of managing pain proactively, rather than reactively.

However, nurses are unlikely to engage in effective management of children's pain if they feel overwhelmed or burdened by the challenge of children's pain. Menzies' (1960) seminal work outlined how nurses who feel anxious develop a defence against anxiety, which acts to protect them emotionally, thereby distancing them from engaging in the very emotions portrayed so evocatively in the stories in this book. Perhaps nurses' defence against anxiety can be overcome by providing them with the confidence, skills and self-belief that they have the power to deal effectively with children's pain and the satisfaction of doing so successfully. To achieve such an empowering situation there is a need for a cultural change in relation to the management of children's pain. There is a need for institutions to recognise that children have a right to pain management and that as health care providers they have a duty of care not only to do no harm but also to do good (Simons 2011) when dealing with children in pain and their families.

For Max Landsberg (2002), the essence of leadership is the ability to create vision, inspiration and momentum in a group of people. Vision is a component of leadership that motivates people to higher levels of effort and performance. However, to achieve a vision within an organisation it needs to be communicated to all levels of the work-force in order to gain their support. Reflecting on the stories we have collected for this book, there is real energy and commitment conveyed in many of them. It is entirely possible that if such energy were to be harnessed and used synergistically, aligned to a vision of effective pain management through leadership, health care providers would feel both emancipated and empowered to step forward and engage in effective pain management practice every day. The real challenge for institutions providing health care to children, who experience pain, is to provide the support at all levels to realise such a vision.

References

Foucault, M. (1994) *Power: Essential Works of Foucault 1954–1984*, edited by J.D. Faubion. London: Penguin Books.

Gaventa, J. (2003) *Power After Lukes: A Review of the Literature*. Brighton: Institute of Development Studies.

Landsberg, M. (2002) *The Tools of Leadership: Vision, Inspiration, Momentum*. London: Profile Books.

Menzies, I.E.P. (1960) 'A case study in the functioning of social systems as a defence against anxiety', *Human Relations*, 13: 95–121.

Simons, J. (2011) 'Above all else do no harm: an ethical evaluation of paediatric nurses' management of children's pain', in G.M. Brykczynska and J. Simons (eds), *Ethical and Philosophical Aspects of Nursing Children and Young People*. Oxford: Wiley-Blackwell, pp. 155–63.

Wong, K.F. (2003) 'Empowerment as a panacea for poverty – old wine in new bottles? Reflections on the World Bank's conception of power', *Progress in Development Studies*, 3 (4): 307–22.

Index

Bold entries indicate tables, *italic* entries indicate figures